Abnormal Psychology: An Integrative Approach

Abnormal Psychology: An Integrative Approach

Editor: Julian Hodges

AMERICAN
MEDICAL PUBLISHERS
www.americanmedicalpublishers.com

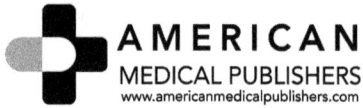

AMERICAN
MEDICAL PUBLISHERS
www.americanmedicalpublishers.com

Cataloging-in-Publication Data

Abnormal psychology : an integrative approach / edited by Julian Hodges.
   p. cm.
Includes bibliographical references and index.
ISBN 978-1-63927-433-8
1. Psychology, Pathological. 2. Mental health. 3. Psychiatry. I. Hodges, Julian.
RC435 .A26 2022
616.89--dc23

American Medical Publishers,
41 Flatbush Avenue,
1st Floor, New York,
NY 11217, USA

ISBN 978-1-63927-433-8 (Hardback)

Contents

Permissions

List of Contributors

Index

Preface

Abnormal psychology is a branch of psychology that deals with the study of unusual behavior, emotion and thought. The study of adaptive behavior and maladaptive behavior falls under this domain. Abnormal psychology also deals with behavior in a clinical context and identifies several causes for different conditions. It involves diverse theories from the general field of psychology and focuses on what exactly is meant by abnormal. It has three different categories to classify mental disorders that are subnormal, supernormal and paranormal. Abnormal psychology revolves around two major paradigms for explaining mental disorders i.e. the psychological paradigm and the biological paradigm. The psychological paradigm deals with humanistic, cognitive and behavioral causes and effects of psychopathology. The biological paradigm involves theories that focus more on physical factors. This book unravels the recent studies in the field of abnormal psychology. It analyzes and upholds the pillars of this field and its utmost significance in modern times. This book is appropriate for students seeking detailed information in this area as well as for experts.

Various studies have approached the subject by analyzing it with a single perspective, but the present book provides diverse methodologies and techniques to address this field. This book contains theories and applications needed for understanding the subject from different perspectives. The aim is to keep the readers informed about the progresses in the field; therefore, the contributions were carefully examined to compile novel researches by specialists from across the globe.

Indeed, the job of the editor is the most crucial and challenging in compiling all chapters into a single book. In the end, I would extend my sincere thanks to the chapter authors for their profound work. I am also thankful for the support provided by my family and colleagues during the compilation of this book.

Editor

Hyperprolactinemia and insulin resistance in drug naive patients with early onset first episode psychosis

Maria Giuseppina Petruzzelli[1]*[iD], Mariella Margari[1], Antonia Peschechera[1], Concetta de Giambattista[1], Andrea De Giacomo[1], Emilia Matera[1] and Francesco Margari[2]

Abstract

Background: Hyperprolactinemia and glucose and lipid metabolism abnormalities are often found in patients with schizophrenia and are generally considered secondary to the use of antipsychotic drugs. More recent studies have shown these same neuroendocrine and metabolic abnormalities in antipsychotic naïve patients with first episode psychosis (FEP), rising the hypothesis that schizophrenia itself may be related to an abnormal regulation of prolactin secretion and to impaired glucose tolerance. The aim of this study was to compare prolactin levels, glycometabolism parameters and lipid profile between a sample of 31 drug-naive adolescents in the acute phase of FEP and a control group of 23 subjects at clinical high risk (CHR) of developing psychosis.

Methods: The assessment involved anthropometric data (weight, height, BMI index, pubertal stage) and blood tests (levels of glucose, glycated hemoglobin, serum insulin, triglycerides, total and fractionated cholesterol, prolactin). Insulin resistance (IR) was calculated through the homeostatic model of assessment (HOMA-IR), assuming a cut-off point of 3.16 for adolescent population. FEP patients and CHR controls were compared by using Student's t-distribution (t-test) for parametric data. $P < 0.05$ was considered significant.

Results: Significant higher level of prolactin was found in FEP group than in CHR group (mean = 28.93 ± 27.16 vs 14.29 ± 7.86, $P = 0.009$), suggesting a condition of hyperprolactinemia (HPRL). Patients with FEP were more insulin resistant compared to patients at CHR, as assessed by HOMA-IR (mean = 3.07 ± 1.76 vs 2.11 ± 1.11, $P = 0.043$). Differences of fasting glucose (FEP = 4.82 ± 0.71, CHR = 4.35 ± 0.62, $P = 0.016$) and HbA1c (FEP = 25.86 ± 13.31, CHR = 33.00 ± 2.95, $P = 0.013$), were not clinically significant as the mean values were within normal range for both groups. No significant differences were found for lipid profile. A BMI value within the range of normal weight was found for both groups, with no significant differences.

Conclusion: We suggested that HPRL, increase in HOMA-IR, and psychotic symptoms may be considered different manifestations of the acute onset of schizophrenia spectrum psychosis, with a common neurobiological vulnerability emerging since adolescence. The influence of age and gender on clinical manifestations of psychotic onset should be considered for early prevention and treatment of both schizophrenia spectrum psychosis and neuroendocrine-metabolic dysfunctions.

Keywords: Prolactin regulation, Glucose tolerance, Neuroendocrine dysfunctions, Schizophrenia spectrum psychosis, Clinical high risk of psychosis, Adolescence, Stress,

* Correspondence: maria.petruzzelli@uniba.it
[1]Child Neuropsychiatry Unit, Department of Basic Medical Sciences, Neuroscience and Sense Organs, University of Bari "Aldo Moro", Azienda Ospedaliero-Universitaria Policlinico di Bari, Piazza Giulio Cesare 11, 70124 Bari, Italy
Full list of author information is available at the end of the article

Background

Hyperprolactinemia (HPRL) and glucose and lipid metabolism abnormalities are often found in patients with schizophrenia and are usually considered secondary to the use of antipsychotic drugs [1–4]. The production of prolactin (PRL) is inhibited by dopamine release in the hypothalamo-pituitary circuit and can be increased by blocking type 2 (D2) dopamine receptors [5]; therefore HPRL in patients with psychosis seems to be related mainly to the D2-receptors affinity of antipsychotic drugs [6]. Moreover, second generation antipsychotics (SGAs) have a marked propensity to induce increased levels of blood glucose, glycosylated hemoglobin and insulin, higher IR, alterations of blood lipid profiles, weight gain and sometimes frank diabetes mellitus (T2DM) [7–9]. The focus of these metabolic abnormalities is on the phenomena of hyperglycemia and IR, but the mechanism through which SGAs induce glucose metabolism disorders is not clearly understood and is likely multifactorial [3].

In more recent years it's been purposed that HPRL and impaired glucose tolerance may be independent of antipsychotic treatment, at least in a subgroup of patients with psychotic disorders. Some authors have identified variations in PRL secretion in drug-free patients, suggesting that schizophrenia itself may be characterized by an abnormal regulation of PRL levels [5, 10–13]. Likewise some studies showed that antipsychotic naive patients with first episode psychosis (FEP) had increased prevalence of impaired glucose tolerance and were more insulin resistant than their healthy comparison subjects [14–16]. These findings lead to the hypothesis that schizophrenia spectrum psychosis is implicated in the pathophysiology of diabetes [15] although conflicting data on the risk of T2DM in patients with schizophrenia prior to antipsychotic treatment has been published [17, 18].

In this study we moved from the hypothesis that at least a subgroup of patients with schizophrenia spectrum psychosis may have a specific vulnerability for abnormalities of regulation of PRL secretion and impaired glucose tolerance, independent of antipsychotic treatment. We purposed that HPRL and abnormalities of glucose and lipid metabolism parameters may be related to the acute phase of psychosis. To verify this hypothesis we compared PRL levels, glycometabolism parameters and lipid profile between a sample of drug-naive adolescents in the acute phase of FEP and a control group of subjects at clinical high risk (CHR) of developing psychosis, age and sex matched.

Method

Subjects

The study sample included 31 patients of both sexes, aged between 8 and 18, consecutively referred over a three-years period, from 2014 to 2017, among the inpatients of the Child Neuropsychiatry Unit, Department of Basic Medical Sciences, Neurosciences and Sense Organs, University "Aldo Moro" of Bari, Italy. They were in the acute phase of their FEP, defined as the manifestation of delusion, hallucination and/or disorganization symptoms of less than 6 months'duration at the time of the assessment. Diagnoses of early onset first-episode schizophrenia spectrum psychosis (schizophrenia, schizophreniphorm disorder, schizoaffective disorder, psychosis not otherwise specified) were made in accordance to Diagnostic and Statistical Manual for Mental Disorders-fifth edition (DSM-5) criteria, on the basis of clinical evaluations and supported by using of the Italian version of the Kiddie-Schedule for Affective Disorders and Schizophrenia-Present and Lifetime Version, (K-SADS-PL), a semi-structured diagnostic interview [19]. All patients were clinically assessed within the first 72 h after their admission to the Child Neuropsychiatry Unit, by the validated Italian version of the Positive and Negative Syndrome Scale (PANSS), a standardized instrument including 30 items on a seven point scale to assess positive, negative and general symptoms [20]. The assessment was performed following a semi-structured interview to ensure that all content domains were covered during the evaluation session; the scores were assigned according to PANSS rating criteria. The control sample consisted of 23 patients, referred to the same Child Neuropsychiatry Unit, age and sex matched, defined as at CHR state of psychosis on the basis of the ultra-high risk (UHR) and the basic symptoms criteria, as indicated by the European Psychiatric Association (EPA) guidance on the early detection of clinical high risk states of psychosis [21]. The UHR criteria, defined as the presence of al least one of attenuated psychotic symptoms (APS), brief limited intermittent psychotic symptoms (BLIPS) or genetic risk and functional decline (GRFD), were assessed with the Italian version of Comprehensive Assessment of At Risk Mental State (CAARMS), a semi-structured interview developed to measure a range of sub-threshold symptoms associated with the prodromal phase of psychotic disorders [22]. The basic symptoms criteria were assessed with the Italian version of Schizophrenia Proness Instrument - Child & Youth version (SPI-CY), a semi-structured interview developed to assess basic symptoms in 8 to 18 year olds [23]. Two experienced child and adolescent psychiatrists from the research group, trained in the use of the above mentioned instruments, interviewed parents and patients; all the evaluations were discussed in regular reliability meetings, supervised by the senior researcher. Body weight (Kg) and height (m) of each study participant were measured and their body mass index (BMI, kg/m^2) was calculated. The pubertal stage was evaluated using visual inspection and palpation, according to Tanner classification for breast development in girls and for genitalia in boys. Exclusion criteria were age < 8 years or > 18 years, antipsychotics intake before the enrolment, evidence form medical history, physical examination, laboratory and instrumental findings that psychotic symptoms were substance induced or due to another medical condition, clinical and instrumental evidences of medical causes of HPRL, no history of diabetes or other serious medical condition associated with glucose intolerance or IR. After providing complete description about the study, we obtained written informed consent from the parents of all subjects. The study was approved by the Ethical Committee of the Hospital Consortium Policlinico of Bari, Italy.

Biochemical analyses

Peripheral blood samples from all partecipants were collected between 7 and 8 AM, following an overnight fast. Serum PRL levels were measured by Advia Centaur XP Immunoassay System (Siemens, Erlangen, Germany). HPRL was defined as a PRL level more than 20 ng/ml in males and more than 25 ng/ml in females. Serum glucose was estimated by enzymatic method; levels between 4 and 5,5 mmol/L were considered normal for both sexes. Glycated hemoglobin (HbA1c) was determined by High Performance Liquid Chromatography; levels between 20 and 42 mmol/L were considered normal for both sexes. Serum insulin was determined by chemioluminescence. Hyperinsulinemia was defined as a value more than 16 microUI/mL, for both male and female patients. HOMA-IR was calculated through the homeostatic model of assessment as the product of the fasting plasma insulin level (μU/mL) and the fasting plasma glucose level (mmol/L), divided by 22.5; a HOMA value > 3.16 was considered indicative of IR [24, 25]. Total cholesterol (mg/dl) levels were determined by a traceable IFCC standardized method. Levels of $156 \pm 4,9$ (mg/dl) for male and $173 \pm 4,5$ (mg/dl) for female were considered normal. High-density lipoprotein cholesterol (HDLc) was measured by clearance assay. Levels between $39 \pm 1,4$ mg/dl for male and $45 \pm 1,2$ for female were considered normal. Fasting plasma levels of low-density lipoprotein cholesterol (LDLc) were calculated by using of Friedewald et al. (1972). LDLc levels of $101 \pm 4,6$ mg/dl for male and $108 \pm 3,9$ mg/dl were considered normal.

Triglycerides levels were determined by a traceable IFCC standardized method. Levels within the range 22–138 mg/dl were considered normal for both sexes.

Statistical analyses

Data analysis was performed by using SPSS 13.0 software. Data were expressed as mean ± standard deviation (S.D.) for continuous variables; qualitative variables were expressed as percentage. Demographic and clinical characteristics were compared using χ^2 test or Mann-Withney U test as appropriate. Clinical observed variables between groups were compared by using Student's t-distribution (t-test) for parametric data. $P < 0.05$ was considered significant.

Results

The demographic and clinical features of the two samples of study were resumed in Table 1. Patients with FEP did not differ from patients at CRH with respect to age, gender and Tanner stage. Table 2 described data on PRL levels, glycometabolism parameters, lipid profile and BMI. The FEP group showed a significant higher level of PRL than the CRH group ($P = 0.009$), with a mean value corresponding to a condition of HPRL (28.93 ± 27.16). When we compared glucose metabolism parameters we found significant differences of fasting glucose ($P = 0.016$) and HbA1c ($P = 0.013$) between FEP and CRH. These data were not clinically significant as the mean values for both groups were within normal range. We found a significant difference of mean value of HOMA-IR between FEP and CRH ($P = 0.043$), with a value of 3.07 ± 1.76 close to the reported cut off of IR. No significant differences were found for parameters of lipid metabolism, with values within normal range. A BMI value within normal range was found in both groups, with no significant statistical difference between FEP and CRH.

Discussion

The main findings of this study were significantly higher values of PRL and HOMA-IR in the sample of early onset drug-naive FEP when compared with subjects at CHR of developing psychosis. These data suggested that dysfunctions of regulation of PRL serum levels and abnormalities of glucose metabolism parameters could be related to acute phase of FEP more than to a clinical risk of psychotic illness, excluding the iatrogenic effects of antipsychotic drugs.

Some previous studies on patients with adult onset FEP showed that HPRL may be a condition pre-existing the introduction of antipsychotic drugs, at least in a subgroup of cases [10–13]. In addition genetic studies suggested that some patients with schizophrenia may have a predisposition to HPRL consisting in functional – 1449 g/t polymorphism of the PRL gene [26, 27]. In a review on the literature of the relationship between PRL and schizophrenia Rajkumar R.P. recommended a reappraisal of the role of prolactin in the various stage of schizophrenia, particularly with regard to its onset [5]. At this purpose an important concern involves the relationship between stress, psychosis onset and increased release of PRL. As is known acute stress leads to an increased serum level of PRL [28] and, in addition to it,

Table 1 Sociodemographic and clinical characteristics in FEP and CHR group

	FEP (n = 31)	CHR (n = 23)	P value
Age in years [a](mean ± S.D.)	15.8(±1.30)	14(±1.41)	0.064
Gender [b]			0.56
Male n(%)	10(32.26%)	8 (34.78%)	
Female n(%)	21 (67.74%)	15 (65.22%)	
Tanner stage[b] n(%)*			0.68
I	–	1 (4.35%)	
II	–	3 (13.04%)	
III	6 (19.35%)	8 (34.78%)	
IV	13 (41.93%)	6 (26.08%)	
V	12 (38.72%)	5 (21.75%)	
PANSS total score(mean ± S.D.)	92(± 8.54)	–	
At risk criterion			
UHR n(%)	–	16 (69.57%)	
Coper/COGDIS n(%)	–	7 (30.43%)	

[a] Mann-Whitney U test
[b] χ^2 test

patients with FEP report more stressful life events and perceived stress when compared to healthy subjects [29]. An increased level of PRL triggers dopamine release by a feedback mechanism, therefore it is reasonable to infer that patients with schizophrenia may have an exaggerated PRL response to stress mediated by a dysfunction in dopaminergic transmission [5]. Moreover, it has been hypothesized that in early psychosis a stress related hormonal dysregulation leads to a greater activation of the hypothalamic-pituitary-adrenal axis (HPA) with an increase in the number and size of corticotroph cells [30, 31]. The pituitary gland is a dynamic structure changing in response to different conditions. Nordholm et al.

Table 2 Comparison between FEP and CHR of prolactin values, glucose metabolic parameters, lipid profile and BMI

	FEP (n = 31)	CHR (n = 23)	P values
Prolactin (ng/ml)	28.93 (27.16)	14.29 (7.86)	**0.009**
Glucose metabolic parameters			
Fasting glucose (mmol/l)	4.82 (0.71)	4.35 (0.62)	**0.016**
HbA1c (mmol/mol)	25.86 (13.31)	33.00 (2.95)	**0.013**
Fasting insulin (µUI/ml)	14.01 (6.88)	11.08(4.67)	0.098
HOMA-IR	3.07 (1.76)	2.11 (1.11)	**0.043**
Lipid profile			
Total cholesterol (mg/dl)	137.23 (22.30)	150.56 (25.27)	0.051
HDL-cholesterol (mg/dl)	54.96 (12.96)	53.18 (12.68)	0.628
LDL-cholesterol (mg/dl)	71.6 0(18.89)	79.54 (19.59)	0.156
Tryglicerides (mg/dl)	58.83 (19.14)	91.95 (19.44)	0.156
BMI (kg/m²)	21.13(2.80)	21.50 (4.07)	0.731

Values are shown as mean (SD). Bold font is indicative of P < 0.05

published a systematic review and meta-analysis on pituitary gland volume showing that the onset of psychosis, more than the high-risk state, is associated with an enlargement of the pituitary gland and that this is independent of antipsychotics [30]. On the other hand, pituitary size may be influenced by age and gender [32], so that subjects in juvenile age (puberal and post-puberal stage) and female in gender may be more easy to have an increase of pituitary gland volume and activation during the early stage of psychosis [32, 33]. All these evidences give more consistency to our finding of HPRL in acute phase of FEP more than in CHR subjects, so we suggest that neurobiological abnormalities related to the acute phase of full emergence of psychotic symptoms in adolescent patients may be involved in dysregulation of PRL secretion. Considering the development and sexual dimorphism of the pituitary gland, further studies could be useful to examine the relevance of age and gender differences on early onset psychiatric disorders in which pituitary dysfunctions has been implicated. In addition, the early identification of HPRL in drug naïve adolescents with FEP may be useful in clinical setting to guide treatment decisions and to manage antipsychotic drugs over the time.

A complex and multifactorial relationship it's been purposed also to explain the risk of diabetes in psychotic disorders [2]. In a recent meta analysis examining data of glucose tolerance, insulin and insulin resistance from drug naïve adult patients with non affective psychosis (mean age of 28.7) Greenhalgh et al. purposed that an increased risk of diabetes may be apparent in acute phase of psychosis prior to antipsychotic use. The authors found that at the time of first clinical contact for psychosis, patients have a slight increase in fasting glucose, which most of them maintain in the normal range, despite a small increase in IR, by secreting additional insulin [34]. According to these evidences, we found a higher fasting glucose in the FEP group then in the CHR group, with no clinical significance, as the mean values for both groups were within normal range. The mean value of HbA1c, reflecting the average plasma glucose, was within normal range for both groups too, so we can assume that the statistical difference (HbA1c was higher in the CHR group than in the FEP group) was not of clinical significance. Actually, some previous studies showed that determination of fasting plasma glucose or HbA1c is not very useful in the screening of impaired glucose tolerance [35, 36]. Conversly Garcia-Rizo et al. have recently suggested that at the onset of psychosis HOMA-IR may be considered a more useful predictor of cardiometabolic risk than other metabolic syndrome criteria [37]. The HOMA-IR is a proxy estimate of IR, based upon the relationship between fasting glucose and insulin levels, with higher value of HOMA-IR representing more severe IR [38]. Several authors have recently purposed a definition of HOMA-IR values across the age continuum from childhood to adolescence, identifying IR with more specificity and sensibility [39, 40]. Actually, there is no consensus regarding the reference value of HOMA-IR for the diagnosis of IR in the pediatric age group and several cut off points have been reported in the literature according to age, gender, pubertal status and BMI [38, 41, 42]. The most used cut off value is 3.16 for obese children, considering that in obese young individuals IR may exceed physiological values especially at the time of puberty [24, 25, 41]. Different population-based studies in the world on normal weight healthy children and adolescents found that a HOMA-IR ≥ 2.6 was associated with a greater cardiovascular and metabolic risk [38, 43, 44]. According to these data we can assume that the mean value of HOMA-IR of 3.07 we found in the FEP group was indicative of IR, since the BMI of these patients was in the range of normal weight. So we suggest that since adolescence, as up to now purposed for adulthood [34], a higher risk of impaired glucose homeostasis, assessed by an increase in HOMA-IR, may be evident in the acute phase of FEP, also in absence of other risk factors as overweight and independently by antipsychotic intake. This is of substantial clinical importance to identify adolescent patients with FEP at increase cardiovascular risk, in order to implement preventive strategies and optimize therapies to reduce the burden of weight gain relate to antipsychotic drugs.

We reserved one last comment to the hypothesis of a deep relationship between HPRL and IR in schizophrenia spectrum psychosis. In a 2016 review Gragnoli et al. suggested that in schizophrenic patients neuroendocrine dysfunctions involving dopamine-prolactin pathway might contribute to both diabetes and schizophrenia [45]. This hypothesis recalls the multifunctional role of PRL that, beside the lactogenic activity, has different functions broadly classified as reproductive, metabolic, osmoregulatory and immunoregulatory [46]. As "metabolic hormon" increasing evidence showed that PRL has different effects on glucose metabolism and may be involved in the manifestation of IR [47, 48]. On the other hand we know that IR is not an endocrine disorder per se but more a disorder of several systems that appears in many inflammatory conditions with an activated immune/repair system and/or in different conditions with increased mental activation via stress axes [49, 50]. So Gragnoli et al. purposed that PRL and/or PRLreceptor gene may carry risk variants associated with schizophrenia, T2DM and/or their clinical association [45]. This hypothesis is in line with a contemporary conceptual model of schizophrenia as a complex disorder with several manifestations outside the brain, so that some "non-psychiatric" abnormalities, traditionally considered as "comorbid" conditions, actually appear as integral parts of the illness, sharing etiopathophisiological factors [51] (Brian Kirkpatrick 2015). In this framework we can suggest that our finding of co-occurring HPRL, increase in HOMA-IR and psychotic symptoms may be considered different manifestations of the acute phase of psychotic onset with a common neurobiological vulnerability.

Some limitations need to be considered. Certainly the small sample size of this study limited the statistical power of the results and made difficult to evaluate the effect of age, sex, pubertal stage, phase of disease on neuroendocrine and metabolic parameters. We must consider, in addition, that this is a cross-sectional study. Further replications trough longitudinal studies including larger samples would be needed to a better understanding of the relationship between schizophrenia spectrum psychosis, regulation of prolactin secretion and IR, according to different age of onset and different stage of disease.

Conclusion

In conclusion this study showed HPRL and an increase in HOMA-IR in the acute phase of early onset FEP but not in CHR of developing psychosis, rising the needs to look at schizophrenia spectrum psychosis as a complex and multifactorial clinical condition in which neuroendocrine and metabolic abnormalities may be considered integral parts of a wide spectrum of neurobiological dysfunctions. Genetic predisposition, immune system activation, stress related factors are most likely the common mediators explaining the co-occurrence of neuroendocrine and metabolic dysfunctions in acute phases of psychosis and will become important directions for further research. A better understanding of the influence of age and gender on clinical manifestations of psychotic onset may be useful for early prevention and treatment of both schizophrenia spectrum psychosis and neuroendocrine-metabolic dysfunctions.

Abbreviations

APS: Attenuated Psychotic Symptom; BLIPS: Brief Limited Intermittent Psychotic Symptom; BMI: Body Mass Index; CAARMS: Comprehensive Assessment of At Risk Mental States; CHR: Clinical High Risk; D2: Dopamine 2; DSM-5: Diagnostic and Statistical Manual for Mental Disorders-fifth edition; EPA: European Psychiatric Association; FEP: First Episode Psychosis; GRFD: Genetik Risk and Functional Decline; HbA1c: Glycated Hemoglobin; HDLc: High-density Lipoprotein cholesterol; HOMA-IR: Homeostatic Model of Assessment-Insuline Resistance; HPA: Hypothalamic-Pituitary-Adrenal axis; HPRL: Hyperprolactinemia; IR: Insuline Resistance; LDLc: Low Density Lipoprotein cholesterol; PANSS: Positive and Negative Syndrome Scale; PRL: prolactine; SD: Standard Deviation; SGAs: second generation antipsychotics; SPI-CY: Schizophrenia Proness Instrument, Child & Youth Version; T2DM: Type 2 Diabetes Mellitus; UHR: Ultra-High Risk

Availability of data and materials

The datasets generated and/or analysed during the current study are not pubblically available due to ongoing analyses for further publications but are available from the corresponding author on reasonable request.

Authors' contributions

MGP, designed the study and drafted the manuscript; MM contributed in the enrollment and assessment of the patients; AP contributed in the enrollment and assessment of the patients; DGC performed the statistical analysis; DGA contribute in the literature searches and analyses and in the enrollment of the patients; EM contributed in the literature searches and in revising critically of the manuscript; MF coordinated the study group and has been involved in revising critically of the manuscript. All the authors read and approved the final manuscript.

Consent for publication

All parents of the participants gave written consent to publish all data reported in this and other publications arising from study.

Competing interests

The authors declare that they have no competing interests.

Author details

[1]Child Neuropsychiatry Unit, Department of Basic Medical Sciences, Neuroscience and Sense Organs, University of Bari "Aldo Moro", Azienda Ospedaliero-Universitaria Policlinico di Bari, Piazza Giulio Cesare 11, 70124 Bari, Italy. [2]Psychiatry Unit , Department of Basic Medical Sciences, Neuroscience and Sense Organ, University of Bari "Aldo Moro", Azienda Ospedaliero-Universitaria Policlinico di Bari, Piazza Giulio Cesare 11, 70124 Bari, Italy.

References

1.   Werner FM, Covenas R. Safety of antipsychotic drugs: focus on therapeutic and adverse effects. Expert Opin Drug Saf. 2014;13(8):1031–42.
2.   Ward M, Druss B. The epidemiology of diabetes in psychotic disorders. Lancet Psychiatry. 2015;2(5):431–51.
3.   Girgis RR, Javitch JA, Lieberman JA. Antipsychotic drug mechanisms: links between therapeutic effects, metabolic side effects and the insulin signaling pathway. Mol Psychiatry. 2008;13(10):918–29.
4.   Margari L, Matera E, Petruzzelli MG, Simone M, Lamanna AL, Pastore A, Palmieri VO, Margari F. Prolactin variations during risperidone therapy in a sample of drug-naive children and adolescents. Int Clin Psychopharmacol. 2015;30(2):103–8.
5.   Rajkumar RP. Prolactin and psychopathology in schizophrenia: a literature review and reappraisal. Schizophr Res Treatment. 2014;2014:175360.
6.   Montejo AL. Prolactin awareness: an essential consideration for physical health in schizophrenia. Eur Neuropsychopharmacol. 2008;18(Suppl 2):S108–14.
7.   Paredes RM, Quinones M, Marballi K, Gao X, Valdez C, Ahuja SS, Velligan D, Walss-Bass C. Metabolomic profiling of schizophrenia patients at risk for metabolic syndrome. Int J Neuropsychopharmacol. 2014;17(8):1139–48.
8.   Scaini G, Quevedo J, Velligan D, Roberts DL, Raventos H, Walss-Bass C. Second generation antipsychotic-induced mitochondrial alterations: implications for increased risk of metabolic syndrome in patients with schizophrenia. Eur Neuropsychopharmacol. 2018;28(3):369–80.
9.   Margari L, Matera E, Craig F, Petruzzelli MG, Palmieri VO, Pastore A, Margari F. Tolerability and safety profile of risperidone in a sample of children and adolescents. Int Clin Psychopharmacol. 2013;28(4):177–83.
10. Riecher-Rossler A, Rybakowski JK, Pflueger MO, Beyrau R, Kahn RS, Malik P, Fleischhacker WW, Group ES. Hyperprolactinemia in antipsychotic-naive patients with first-episode psychosis. Psychol Med. 2013;43(12):2571–82.
11. Garcia-Rizo C, Fernandez-Egea E, Oliveira C, Justicia A, Parellada E, Bernardo M, Kirkpatrick B. Prolactin concentrations in newly diagnosed, antipsychotic-naive patients with nonaffective psychosis. Schizophr Res. 2012;134(1):16–9.
12. Aston J, Rechsteiner E, Bull N, Borgwardt S, Gschwandtner U, Riecher-Rossler A. Hyperprolactinaemia in early psychosis-not only due to antipsychotics. Prog Neuro-Psychopharmacol Biol Psychiatry. 2010;34(7):1342–4.
13. Segal M, Avital A, Berstein S, Derevenski A, Sandbank S, Weizman A. Prolactin and estradiol serum levels in unmedicated male paranoid schizophrenia patients. Prog Neuro-Psychopharmacol Biol Psychiatry. 2007; 31(2):378–82.
14. Petrikis P, Tigas S, Tzallas AT, Papadopoulos I, Skapinakis P, Mavreas V. Parameters of glucose and lipid metabolism at the fasted state in drug-naive first-episode patients with psychosis: evidence for insulin resistance. Psychiatry Res. 2015;229(3):901–4.
15. Chen S, Broqueres-You D, Yang G, Wang Z, Li Y, Wang N, Zhang X, Yang F, Tan Y. Relationship between insulin resistance, dyslipidaemia and positive symptom in Chinese antipsychotic-naive first-episode patients with schizophrenia. Psychiatry Res. 2013;210(3):825–9.
16. Wu X, Huang Z, Wu R, Zhong Z, Wei Q, Wang H, Diao F, Wang J, Zheng L, Zhao J, et al. The comparison of glycometabolism parameters and lipid profiles between drug-naive, first-episode schizophrenia patients and healthy controls. Schizophr Res. 2013;150(1):157–62.
17. Fernandez-Egea E, Garcia-Rizo C, Zimbron J, Kirkpatrick B. Diabetes or prediabetes in newly diagnosed patients with nonaffective psychosis? A historical and contemporary view. Schizophr Bull. 2013;39(2):266–7.
18. Sengupta S, Parrilla-Escobar MA, Klink R, Fathalli F, Ying Kin N, Stip E, Baptista T, Malla A, Joober R. Are metabolic indices different between drug-naive first-episode psychosis patients and healthy controls? Schizophr Res. 2008;102(1–3):329–36.
19. Kaufman J, Birmaher B, Rao U, Ryan N: Test K-SADS-PL - Intervista diagnostica per la valutazione dei disturbi psicopatologici in bambini e adolescenti Erickson edn; 2004.
20. Pancheri P, Brugnoli R, Carilli L, Delle Chiaie R, Marconi PL, Petrucci RM. Valutazione dimensionale della sintomatologia schizofrenica. Validazione della versione italiana della Scala per la valutazione dei Sintomi Positivi e Negativi (PANSS). Giorn Ital Psicopat. 1995;1:60–75.
21. Schultze-Lutter F, Michel C, Schmidt SJ, Schimmelmann BG, Maric NP, Salokangas RK, Riecher-Rossler A, van der Gaag M, Nordentoft M, Raballo A, et al. EPA guidance on the early detection of clinical high risk states of psychoses. Eur Psychiatry. 2015;30(3):405–16.
22. Pelizza L, Paterlini F, Azzali S, Garlassi S, Scazza I, Pupo S, Simmons M, Nelson B, Raballo A. The approved Italian version of the comprehensive assessment of at-risk mental states (CAARMS-ITA): field test and psychometric features. Early Interv Psychiatry. 2018.
23. Schultze-Lutter F. In: Fioriti G, editor. STRUMENTO DI VALUTAZIONE PER LA PROPENSIONE ALLA SCHIZOFRENIA, Versione per bambini e adolescenti; 2010.
24. Shikha D, Singla M, Walia R, Potter N, Mercado A, Winer N. Vascular compliance in lean, obese, and diabetic children and adolescents: a cross-sectional study in a minority population. Cardiorenal Med. 2014;4(3–4):161–7.
25. Keskin M, Kurtoglu S, Kendirci M, Atabek ME, Yazici C. Homeostasis model assessment is more reliable than the fasting glucose/insulin ratio and quantitative insulin sensitivity check index for assessing insulin resistance among obese children and adolescents. Pediatrics. 2005; 115(4):e500–3.
26. Rybakowski JK, Dmitrzak-Weglarz M, Kapelski P, Hauser J. Functional −1149 g/t polymorphism of the prolactin gene in schizophrenia. Neuropsychobiology. 2012;65(1):41–4.
27. Ivanova SA, Osmanova DZ, Boiko AS, Pozhidaev IV, Freidin MB, Fedorenko OY, Semke AV, Bokhan NA, Kornetova EG, Rakhmazova LD, et al. Prolactin gene polymorphism (−1149 G/T) is associated with hyperprolactinemia in patients with schizophrenia treated with antipsychotics. Schizophr Res. 2017;182:110–4.
28. Jaroenporn S, Nagaoka K, Kasahara C, Ohta R, Watanabe G, Taya K. Physiological roles of prolactin in the adrenocortical response to acute restraint stress. Endocr J. 2007;54(5):703–11.
29. Labad J, Stojanovic-Perez A, Montalvo I, Sole M, Cabezas A, Ortega L, Moreno I, Vilella E, Martorell L, Reynolds RM, et al. Stress biomarkers as predictors of transition to psychosis in at-risk mental states: roles for cortisol, prolactin and albumin. J Psychiatr Res. 2015;60:163–9.
30. Nordholm D, Krogh J, Mondelli V, Dazzan P, Pariante C, Nordentoft M. Pituitary gland volume in patients with schizophrenia, subjects at ultra high-risk of developing psychosis and healthy controls: a systematic review and meta-analysis. Psychoneuroendocrinology. 2013;38(11):2394–404.
31. Pariante CM. Pituitary volume in psychosis: the first review of the evidence. J Psychopharmacol. 2008;22(2 Suppl):76–81.
32. MacMaster FP, Keshavan M, Mirza Y, Carrey N, Upadhyaya AR, El-Sheikh R, Buhagiar CJ, Taormina SP, Boyd C, Lynch M, et al. Development and sexual dimorphism of the pituitary gland. Life Sci. 2007;80(10):940–4.
33. Soni BK, Joish UK, Sahni H, George RA, Sivasankar R, Aggarwal R. A comparative study of pituitary volume variations in MRI in acute onset of psychiatric conditions. J Clin Diagn Res. 2017;11(2):TC01–4.
34. Greenhalgh AM, Gonzalez-Blanco L, Garcia-Rizo C, Fernandez-Egea E, Miller B, Arroyo MB, Kirkpatrick B. Meta-analysis of glucose tolerance, insulin, and insulin resistance in antipsychotic-naive patients with nonaffective psychosis. Schizophr Res. 2017;179:57–63.

35. Carnevale Schianca GP, Rossi A, Sainaghi PP, Maduli E, Bartoli E. The significance of impaired fasting glucose versus impaired glucose tolerance: importance of insulin secretion and resistance. Diabetes Care. 2003;26(5):1333–7.

36. Hu Y, Liu W, Chen Y, Zhang M, Wang L, Zhou H, Wu P, Teng X, Dong Y, Zhou J, et al. Combined use of fasting plasma glucose and glycated hemoglobin A1c in the screening of diabetes and impaired glucose tolerance. Acta Diabetol. 2010;47(3):231–6.

37. Garcia-Rizo C, Fernandez-Egea E, Oliveira C, Meseguer A, Cabrera B, Mezquida G, Bioque M, Penades R, Parellada E, Bernardo M, et al. Metabolic syndrome or glucose challenge in first episode of psychosis? Eur Psychiatry. 2017;41:42–6.

38. Shashaj B, Luciano R, Contoli B, Morino GS, Spreghini MR, Rustico C, Sforza RW, Dallapiccola B, Manco M. Reference ranges of HOMA-IR in normal-weight and obese young Caucasians. Acta Diabetol. 2016;53(2):251–60.

39. Singh Y, Garg MK, Tandon N, Marwaha RK. A study of insulin resistance by HOMA-IR and its cut-off value to identify metabolic syndrome in urban Indian adolescents. J Clin Res Pediatr Endocrinol. 2013;5(4):245–51.

40. Bussler S, Penke M, Flemming G, Elhassan YS, Kratzsch J, Sergeyev E, Lipek T, Vogel M, Spielau U, Korner A, et al. Novel insights in the metabolic syndrome in childhood and adolescence. Horm Res Paediatr. 2017;88(3–4):181–93.

41. Nogueira-de-Almeida CA, de Mello ED. Different criteria for the definition of insulin resistance and its relation with dyslipidemia in overweight and obese children and adolescents. Pediatr Gastroenterol Hepatol Nutr. 2018;21(1):59–67.

42. Tang Q, Li X, Song P, Xu L. Optimal cut-off values for the homeostasis model assessment of insulin resistance (HOMA-IR) and pre-diabetes screening: developments in research and prospects for the future. Drug Discov Ther. 2015;9(6):380–5.

43. Yin J, Li M, Xu L, Wang Y, Cheng H, Zhao X, Mi J. Insulin resistance determined by homeostasis model assessment (HOMA) and associations with metabolic syndrome among Chinese children and teenagers. Diabetol Metab Syndr. 2013;5(1):71.

44. Burrows R, Correa-Burrows P, Reyes M, Blanco E, Albala C, Gahagan S. Healthy Chilean Adolescents with HOMA-IR >/= 2.6 Have Increased Cardiometabolic Risk: Association with Genetic, Biological, and Environmental Factors. J Diabetes Res. 2015;2015:783296.

45. Gragnoli C, Reeves GM, Reazer J, Postolache TT. Dopamine-prolactin pathway potentially contributes to the schizophrenia and type 2 diabetes comorbidity. Transl Psychiatry. 2016;6:e785.

46. Bernabeu I, Casanueva FF. Metabolic syndrome associated with hyperprolactinemia: a new indication for dopamine agonist treatment? Endocrine. 2013;44(2):273–4.

47. Ben-Jonathan N, Hugo E. Prolactin (PRL) in adipose tissue: regulation and functions. Adv Exp Med Biol. 2015;846:1–35.

48. Daimon M, Kamba A, Murakami H, Mizushiri S, Osonoi S, Yamaichi M, Matsuki K, Sato E, Tanabe J, Takayasu S, et al. Association between serum prolactin levels and insulin resistance in non-diabetic men. PLoS One. 2017; 12(4):e0175204.

49. Straub RH. Insulin resistance, selfish brain, and selfish immune system: an evolutionarily positively selected program used in chronic inflammatory diseases. Arthritis Res Ther. 2014;16(Suppl 2):S4.

50. Blaslov K, Kruljac I, Mirosevic G, Kirigin Bilos LS, Vrkljan M. The possible role of stress induced hormonal disbalance in the patophysiology of insulin resistane in lean individuals. Med Hypotheses. 2018;114:8–10.

51. Kirkpatrick B, Miller B, Garcia-Rizo C, Fernandez-Egea E. Schizophrenia: a systemic disorder. Clin Schizophr Relat Psychoses. 2014;8(2):73–9.

2

To die or not to die: a qualitative study of men's suicidality in Norway

Birthe Loa Knizek[*] (iD) and Heidi Hjelmeland

Abstract

Background: Previous research has shown that men who adhere to traditional beliefs about masculinity have increased health risks compared to those who do not. Single marital status, unemployment, retirement, and physical illness are commonly known risk factors for male suicidal behavior. Most men struggling with these risk factors are, however, not suicidal. To find out more about what makes some men vulnerable to suicidal behavior, risk factors must be analyzed in light of men's life history as well as the social context where they live their masculinity.

Method: We conducted semi-structured qualitative in-depth interviews with 15 men (20–76 years old) who were admitted to hospital after a suicidal act. We analyzed the data by means of qualitative content analysis with a directed approach. The analysis was directed by the participants' reports on whether they had wanted to die or not at the time of the suicidal act. On this basis, they were divided into two groups: a "to die" and a "not to die" group. We then analyzed each group separately before comparing them.

Results: In both groups, the main reason or trigger for the suicidal act were problems in intimate relationships. These problems were complex and connected to the men's lived masculinity, ranging from shame, or tainted masculine honor, to taking responsibility as a man for the wife. Some men pointed to pain and ennui as reasons or triggers for their suicidal act. Only one in the "not to die" group took full responsibility for the suicidal act, whereas all but one did the same in the "to die" group. The men not taking responsibility described the suicidal act as involuntary because of either alcohol or a kind of "black-out". Not taking responsibility for the act may be a way of preserving masculine identity.

Conclusion: Relationship problems are the main reason or trigger of the suicidal act for most participants, but in very different ways, mirroring lived masculinity. The most striking finding is the uniqueness of each story, questioning the utility of standardized suicide prevention efforts.

Keywords: Suicidal acts, Men, Masculinity, Relationship problems, Attributed responsibility

Background

In 1998, Canetto and Sakinovsky [1] described the gender paradox of suicidal behavior: "In most Western countries, females have higher rates of suicidal ideation and behavior than males, yet mortality from suicide is typically lower for females than for males". This paradox has puzzled suicide researchers for decades. Thus, gender has increasingly been emphasized as crucial for understanding suicidal behavior [2]. This is, for instance, reflected in the following comprehensive publications: In 2012, Canetto and Cleary [2] edited a part special issue of *Social Science & Medicine* on *Men, Masculinities and*

Suicidal Behavior. In the same year, the Samaritans [3] in the UK published the research report *Men, Suicide and Society: Why Disadvantaged Men in Mid-Life Die by Suicide.* This report provided an extensive overview of factors leading to men's suicide. In 2014, Lester, Gunn III and Quinnett [4] published the anthology *Suicide in Men: How Men Differ from Women in Expressing Their Distress,* with chapters from many different socio-cultural contexts. The editors' aim with this book was to start a discussion on men's vulnerability.

It is, however, necessary to be cautious since gender is one of the most frequently used sociodemographic variables as well as one of the most oversimplified and misused concepts in epidemiological and risk factor suicide studies [5–7]. Consequently, Krysinska et al. [5] underlined

* Correspondence: Birthe.l.knizek@ntnu.no
Department of Mental Health, Norwegian University of Science and
Technology, NO-7491 Trondheim, Norway

that "… it remains a serious challenge for both researchers and clinicians to identify risk and protective factors which make "some men" vulnerable to suicide, while others remain resilient when faced with life adversity or psychopathology".

From research conducted to date, we know some of the circumstances that may make some men vulnerable to suicidal behavior. Evans et al. [8] and Scourfield & Evans [9] have, for instance, pointed out that men are challenged more by changing gender roles than are women. They also maintain that marriage may be a more positive experience for men than for women, that the care of children has become culturally more important and expected for men, and that men do not employ their social network for support when experiencing emotional difficulties. Hence, marriage breakdown may have worse consequences for men than for women.

Cleary [6] interviewed young Irish men after a suicide attempt and found that they had high levels of emotional pain. In addition, they had fewer coping skills as they had problems recognizing their symptoms as well as disclosing their pain to others because of dominating masculine norms of being in control. Also others have found men to be less likely than women to express emotions [10], which again has been assumed to account for the report of higher psychological distress among women, but higher suicide rates in men [6, 11]. A consequence of the inability to disclose emotional distress is that relationship problems and breakups might carry different weight for men than for women. However, the financial and ideological context of severe relationship problems must be considered as mediating factors [8, 12, 13] as cultural condemnation of divorce or women's financial dependency influence the effect of relationship breakup. In addition, one has to consider when in the life course the breakup happens as it carries different weight during different age groups. According to a systematic review by Evans et al. [14] middle-aged men appear to be more affected than women and younger men by a breakdown in their marital/romantic relationships since these relationships may be their main source of intimacy and their only possibility for sharing their vulnerable sides. In another review study Evans et al. [8] find "… no definitive evidence of a gender differential in suicidal behaviors following the breakdown of a relationship" as they do not find any clear trend that goes across age. Nor do they find consistent patterns across countries or regions.

Previous research has shown that men who adhere to traditional beliefs about masculinity seem to have increased health risks compared to those who do not aspire to traditional forms of masculinity [15]. This must be seen in relation to the fact that traditional masculine behavior underplays the role of emotion as the man is expected to be in total control of himself and the

situation, and thus reluctant to report distress [16]. This, in turn, then allows stress to build up and a vulnerability to suicidal behavior may develop. However, the development of masculinity occurs in interplay with the actual and constantly changing context. The life of an 80-year old man has developed in a considerably different context than what is the case for a 20-year old man. From the existing research, some male risk factors like single marital status, unemployment, retirement and physical illness are identified [17], but they all must be seen in light of the actual social and normative context, the specific life history and age and what they mean for each man.

Historically, masculinity norms in Norway were influenced by harsh physical environment and being a fishing nation [18]. Dangerous and hard work was fundamental for being able to provide for the family and necessary periods of absence built the fundament for the women to take responsibility. According to Lease et al. [18] this created cultural values of self-sufficiency, independence, and courage of men, but lay also the foundation for egalitarianism between the genders. Men supported changes at home and working-place but they may have received incongruent messages about appropriate masculine behavior. The news featured Norwegian men who felt a devaluation of traditional masculine roles [19]. In addition, the Norwegian society is changing rapidly through immigration and masculine norms from other cultures are blended into society.

In a changing society like Norway, context sensitive research is needed and qualitative research comes to the fore. Such research is able to take more of the context and actual life situation of individuals into consideration in the analysis, compared to what quantitative risk factor research is able to [8, 20]. Qualitative research also allows us to focus on the individual and to highlight contextualized individual differences in circumstances related to suicidality. This is important in order to develop our understanding of what suicidality might mean to people who are suicidal, in their context, and beyond the common simplistic risk factor categories. Franklin et al.'s [21] recent meta-analysis of 50 years of risk factor research demonstrated the limited value of risk factors in terms of understanding suicidality and hence for suicide prevention. For example, "relationship problems" is a commonly found risk factor for suicidal behavior. In her comprehensive review study on Muslim women and suicide, Canetto [22], however, found that relationship problems can cover many, and very different issues for these women. There is no reason to believe that this would be any different for women in general, as well as for men. This will in turn have consequences for suicide prevention. The purpose of the present qualitative interview study was thus to investigate what men who have engaged in a suicidal act perceived as crucial for their decision to harm themselves or attempt to take their life. We analyze this in the context of their actual life situation, and hence look deeper into aspects that might be overlooked or not described in traditional quantitative risk factor research.

Method

We conducted semi-structured qualitative in-depth interviews with men admitted to hospital following a suicidal act. Before the interview, we knew nothing about the participants other than the fact that they had harmed themselves sufficiently to require hospitalization. We chose this approach deliberately in order to be as open as possible to the men's own descriptions of the circumstances around their suicidal act.

Participants

We interviewed 15 men (20–76 years old), recruited through the hospital. Six of the men were in a stable relationship, five were currently going through, or had just been through a divorce, whereas the rest were single. Five had a job, six were unemployed, two were retired, and two were on sick leave and/or underwent re-education. Two of the men had higher education. Four lived alone, whereas the others lived with a wife, a male/female lover, a child, or a friend. Only one of the men mentioned that he had some mental disorder diagnoses, namely anxiety and depression, and that he was on psychopharmacological medication. Some others said they had been offered antidepressants after incidents/accidents, after which they had felt depressed. Two of the men revealed having been sexually abused from childhood. As regards methods used in their suicidal acts, 13 had taken an overdose of medication, one had swallowed a diluent, and one had tried to hang himself. Alcohol was involved in five of the suicidal acts, whereas only two claimed to have problems with alcohol in general, and two others admitted taking drugs. Almost two thirds ($n = 9$) reported sleeping problems.

Procedure

The second author interviewed the participants one to four weeks after their suicidal acts. The semi-structured interview guide was composed of a narrative part and a problem-focused part. In the narrative part, the men were requested to describe the circumstances leading to their suicidal act, the suicidal act itself, as well as what reactions they had been met with after the act. In the problem-focused part, the interviewer asked questions related to their health if this was not sufficiently covered in the narrative part. The interviews lasted between 19 and 160 min, with most of them lasting about one hour. The interviews were recorded and transcribed verbatim.

Data analysis

We analyzed the data by means of qualitative content analysis [23] following a directed approach [24]. Berelson, 1952, developed content analysis originally as an exclusively quantitative approach. Since then it has undergone comprehensive changes and has moved into the qualitative realm and interpretative perspective [25]. In contrast to context analysis in the positivistic paradigm, here the assumption is that data and interpretation are co-creations of interviewer and participant. In the analysis the co-creation is between the researchers and the text. In our approach we have combined an inductive and a deductive approach. In the initial inductive analysis, the entire material was read by the two authors and the observation of a difference between the men who wanted to die and those who did not want to, triggered a more deductive approach looking at differences between those two groups in the further analysis. Our analysis became more directed [24], which implies coding of the text directed by theory or research findings. In our case, the analysis was directed by the participants' reports on whether they had wanted to die or not at the time of the suicidal act. Two thirds ($n = 10$) explicitly stated that they had wanted to die, whereas one third ($n = 5$) said they had not wanted to die. Consequently, we divided the sample into two groups: a "to die" group and a "not to die" group. In the further process, we stayed close to the text and coded it in line with phenomenological guidelines and developed categories, which were further developed into themes. We then compared the two groups of men in relationship to these themes. This flexible analytical approach has been described as the researcher taking various scientific positions depending on the aim of the study [25]. The aim of this study was thus to investigate what men who had engaged in a suicidal act perceived as crucial for their decision to harm themselves or attempt to take their life and analyze this in the context of their actual life situation.

Ethical considerations

The Regional Committee for Medical and Health Research Ethics approved the study. All the participants had given informed consent before the interview. All interviews took place in an office at the outpatient clinic that was responsible for the participants' follow-up after their suicidal act. The participants were offered a follow-up by the staff at the outpatient clinic after the interview. None of the participants needed such follow-up.

A main purpose of the present paper was to highlight some contextualized individual differences regarding what the men perceived as crucial for their decision to harm themselves or attempt to take their life. This has the potential to challenge the principle of anonymity, which we have handled in the following ways. With the quotations, we report age groups rather than exact age: young adults, middle-aged, and elderly, here defined as 20–35 years, 36–60 years, and 60–76 years, respectively. We have also changed some potentially identifying features of the participants of whom we present rather detailed descriptions and quotations (features presumed to be unimportant for understanding the suicidality).

Results

Two themes were developed through the analysis: *Reasons or triggers for the suicidal act* and *Attributed responsibility for the suicidal act.* They are described and substantiated by quotations in the following.

Perceived reasons or triggers of the suicidal act

All the men in the "not to die" group reported problems with or loss of partner/wife as main triggering factor for their suicidal act. Even though they admitted that problems had accumulated for some time, they pointed to the relational problem as the last straw that broke the camel's back: "It was her that triggered it. And I mean it, that it was her that triggered that this happened. The way that she made me look like a fool in that situation" (middle-aged man). The situation that triggered his suicidal act was that his partner in the presence of friends tried to change some plans they had made as a couple, and instead wanted to plan things that included the friends. His narrative pointed at the situation rather than the partner as the trigger, even though his way of expression was equivocal. He even repeatedly expressed sympathy with his partner's situation after his suicidal act. In the situation he felt let down, excluded, and ridiculed, and then harmed himself. He felt he had lost face in the situation and could not bear the shame. This man was the only one in the "not to die" group who still lived together with his partner (at the time of the interview).

All the other men in the "not to die" group were separated or divorced, and reported feeling lonely or let down. One found it problematic to describe a reason or trigger for his self-harm, but finally ended up saying: "But I went through a separation, which was pretty hard and was much unexpected" (middle-aged man). Before the separation, his parents-in-law had promised to support his business financially on the condition that his wife divorced him. He refused to separate, but his wife divorced him anyway and he did not receive any financial support. He consequently ended up alone with financial problems, felt deceived by his in-laws, and abandoned by his wife. Another middle-aged man had led a life dominated by alcohol and illness that ended up with impotence and a separation from his wife. One young man met a previous girlfriend, who had dumped him earlier, as a pregnant woman in a new relationship. Although the circumstances of these two latter men

were quite different, both struggled with loneliness and the loss of relationship and were unable to accept the separation.

As the men illustrated above, a breakdown in relationships involved many different issues, such as impotence, loneliness, betrayal, abandonment, and shame.

Half of the larger "to-die" group also reported relationship problems as main reason or trigger for their suicidal act, and again this covered very different issues. Of the 10 men, four lived alone and three of these four were currently undergoing separation/divorce. One of the other five still lived with his parents, whereas the rest lived in stable relationships. Two of the men still living with their partner mentioned infidelity or suspicion of infidelity as a triggering factor. One man reported having been institutionalized and helpless when his wife took all their valuables and went away with another man. His helplessness deepened the feeling of being betrayed by his wife. He describes himself as wanting to be independent and able to manage his problems by himself, but admits that there is a limit to what one can take. Another participant was the victim of rumors regarding his wife's infidelity; rumors that eventually turned out to be false. Both reported perceived infidelity as the factor that triggered their suicide attempt, although the circumstances were very different.

Three men mentioned illness/pain and, not surprisingly, the two oldest participants were among them. The third was a young man with serious health problems. All three experienced no quality of life and were without hope for improvement of their condition. The two elderly men expressed explicitly that they did not want to be a burden. They seem to adhere to the traditional masculine values of independence and autonomy, and for one of them death became almost a practical solution in order to take care of the wife: "And have talked about it [with wife] that maybe it is easier for you if I was gone. You could just have sold everything and then bought a flat, easy" (elderly man). He was worried that his wife was overwhelmed by the workload since he could not contribute the way he wanted anymore, and she had to take care of him in addition. At the same time, he insisted that he was *not* depressed, because he did not see himself as the "depressive type". Another elderly participant also suffered from severe illness, which would increasingly disable him and make him dependent on others. He described himself as a modest person, who did not like to ask for continuous assistance and as a consequence he could not bear the thought of the future based on dependency.

The younger man who mentioned pain as a trigger for his suicide attempt had completely lost hope in the health care system, whose lack of ability to understand and help he found scandalous:

"I just get more and more sick and become a larger and larger problem for the health care system (...) and I feel totally ignored and overlooked. Everything that has been found out I have found out myself." (...) You know, I know a lot about bodily processes and then, then the doctors get grumpy (...) Then you get pushed like a thing, well, like a hot potato, which nobody wants to hold in his hands (young man).

The pain and the treatment from the health care system seemed too much and he attempted suicide twice. He felt that there was no hope left and that life was nothing but pain.

The last two men reported being tired of life as the reason for their suicide attempt. Their life situation and history were, however, very different. One was a young man living with his parents, with whom he felt he had nothing in common. He claimed to have no friends, no interests and no energy and insisted that he would not change. In his opinion, he did not fit into his family or into the world as such. Without a prospect of change, he had no hope for the future:

"I tell you that I will take my life regardless what happens in the future and I will do it as soon as ... .well, as soon as possible. And that is nothing people can do anything about. (...) The way I see it is that if you are going to live, you must have something to live for or at least something to look forward to, and that I have never had and will never get. So I see no reason why I should stay here then" (young man).

He lived in a social vacuum and without interests or energy to make a change, he felt tired of life. He was the only participant reporting having been diagnosed with any mental disorders (depression and anxiety).

The other participant being tired of life was middle-aged and had lived an active life with a lot of interests and engagements. Despite a turbulent upbringing, he managed to get an education and a family. He had been politically engaged and had strong ideals for how the world should be. Now his children had grown up, he and his wife had divorced amicably, and he was not happy with the changes in the world. He felt that the world had become cold and cynical: "I don't like the world we live in today (...) I don't feel at home in the world, we live in" (middle-aged man). For the last 10 years, he had not wanted to live anymore and felt burned out. He had attempted suicide before, but in the last moments of consciousness, "a spark of life" emerged and then he got ambivalent. He underlined that it is not necessary to be depressed for not wanting to live in the world as it looks now. He saw his decision as a conscious choice.

In summing up the reasons or triggers, the men mentioned for their suicide attempts, it is evident that their stories are *very* different. Even when it is possible to categorize them as, for instance, having relationship problems or physical pain, the differences in these categories seem larger than the similarities.

Attributed responsibility for the suicidal act

Most of the men explicitly allocated responsibility for their suicidality. In the "not-to-die" group, only one man felt entirely responsible for the suicidal act himself. He was, however, ambivalent as he found the telephone number for the emergency services before harming himself. The others in this group insisted on not having been in possession of their faculties, for instance, because of alcohol:

"I have sleeping problems during night or rather always. Thus, I got sleeping pills from my doctor ... and .... I took all of them at once. Ninety pills. And that was after a large consumption of alcohol, so ... I don't think I knew that I took them" (middle-aged man).

One of the other participants in this group only drinks occasionally, while another one admitted having problems with "King Alcohol", which makes him crazy. Another man mentioned that the brain had "clicked" in the moment of the suicidal act:

It did not hurt. Because I was gone. I was - it was not me who did this. It was not I, who took the rope in the staircase and put it up. It was not me. It was a different side of me, it was a "click" up in my brain, which made it happen. As simple and easy as that (middle-aged man).

He distanced himself entirely from the act. This made it possible for him to sympathize with the reactions of his partner and even to admit that the purpose of the act probably had been to scare his partner, without displaying any guilt. He emphasized that his case shows that suicidality can happen to "completely normal people": "It was not I who was that person obviously, because I remember nothing."

The picture in the "not-to-die" group differed significantly from the one in the "to-die" group; only one in the latter group was not ready to take responsibility for the suicidal act, whereas the rest took full responsibility. The youngest one of the participants, who was tired of life, distanced himself completely from the act and underlined that he did not do it of his own free will:

"I would never have a serious suicide attempt, because an attempt is not what I stand for. I mean that if you have to do it, you do it. And therefore I think it is a bit embarrassing what happened, because that, that was a thing that goes against everything I stand for. But as I said, I would never have done it if I had been conscious of what I was doing. So, I don't know what happened or why it happened, but it is probably some blackout, as they have called it. But I shall not discuss that" (young man).

He felt his honor tainted, because if he had been in possession of his full faculties, he would have been dead. The suicidal act was for him an embarrassing failure and he was ashamed because of it. He ascribed the failure to a blackout.

Some of the other men in the "to-die" group reported having thought about it a long time in advance, while others spent some time contemplating about it in the course of the suicidal act, for example: "... .and then it was, it was totally calm, it was precisely as it should be when I had done it. It was entirely appropriate" (middle-aged man). This participant lost hope when he lost both partner and job and as a result felt worthless and unwanted. He did not regret the attempt at that moment and seemed content with his fate and he emphasized that a theme in his life was to think that he probably did not deserve anything better.

For all men in the "to-die" group, suicide seemed to be a deliberate choice and the best option in their situation. The men reported that they were sure they wanted to die, but for three of them ambivalence came into play when the pain became intolerable or right after the attempt, and they called for help themselves:

"When I did it, I was very clear; very conscious. But then I lost courage (...) So ... a part of you will die and a part of you will live and then you become very ambivalent and then you telephone and get things going. So, it is really about getting over the threshold that you are not afraid anymore: this time I make it" (middle-aged man).

The challenge for this middle-aged man was to get beyond the fear of death. Like the other two men who had second thoughts, he seemed unable to carry out his wish/intent to take his life. However, this inability appears in different shapes: whereas one had the telephone number of the emergency department ready before the suicidal act, the two others found it and called after the act. For one of them, it was the first time he had attempted suicide and he seemed ambivalent. For the other, it was his third suicide attempt and he called because he, in his own words, lost the courage after having swallowed sleeping pills. Another participant could not bear the pain after having drunk a diluent, which had also been the problem with his previous

(first) suicide attempt. Part of some of the stories was a regret at having disrupted the suicide attempt.

Discussion

In this study, we interviewed men after a suicidal act medically serious enough to require hospitalization. One-third of the men expressed that they actually had not wanted to die, while the rest had decided that death was the best option in their life situation. We compared these two groups on the two themes developed in the analysis, namely what they perceived as the main reason or trigger for their suicidal act and to whom/what they attributed responsibility for the act. All the men who did not want to die and half of the men who had wanted to die emphasized relationship problems as the main reason/trigger for the suicidal act. The elevated risk of suicidal behavior and ideation after breakdowns in intimate relationships has been known for some time [26]. Krysinska [5] has emphasized a male vulnerability to negative life events, while Lester, Gunn and Quinett [4] emphasized men's vulnerability specifically to relationship problems: "Men also appear to be more impacted by breakdowns in their marital and romantic relationships, perhaps because they benefit more from marriage and perhaps because men find it hard to meet the modern expectations for increased intimacy". In their systematic review of research on relationship breakdown and suicide risk, Evans et al. [8, 14] found 17 studies with higher risk for men, six with a higher risk for women, and six with no gender difference. Van Orden et al. [27] pointed out that women in general value family and being loved higher than men and then in the absence of these "... suffer greater emotional pain than do men in the same situations". This stands in contrast to Evans et al. [8, 9], who underline men's larger vulnerability under relationship breakups and suggest as explanations "... men's role inflexibility, the increasing importance of the care of the children, men's desire for control in relationships, and men's social network" [9].

In order to understand and target this vulnerability we need to know more about particularities, as we meet different reactions to problems based on men's masculine identity. Three quarters of our participants described relationship problems as the main reason or trigger for their suicidal act, though they were related to different underlying feelings such as feeling betrayed, abandoned, ashamed, or being a failure in terms of inability to take responsibility for the wife. The individual emotional reactions must be understood on the background of their history and context and their relationship with those. Several publications and anthologies [2, 4, 28] have contributed significantly to the contextualized understanding of gendered suicide scripts, while suicide among men in the specific Norwegian context still is mainly unexplored. With the exception of Rasmussen et al. [29], who have contributed with their psychological autopsy study on suicide among young men, where they found suicides to be signature acts of compensatory masculinity, we still do not know much about the particularities among men in Norway.

In the present study, the main trigger for the suicidal act among our participants was in line with other countries a variety of problems related to close relationships. In fact, three quarters of them mentioned such problems that covered many different issues and the men also felt hurt in different ways as their actual background and context was different. In addition, the age range was from 20 to 76 years, contributing even more to the complexity of the situation as their situation and psychological make-up might have differed significantly. The relationship problems mentioned were connected to the men's lived masculinity, ranging from shame, or tainted masculine honor, to taking responsibility as a man for the wife. Most of these problems could be interpreted in line with men's desire for control in relationships as a consequence of the traditional Norwegian masculinity norms as independence and self-sufficiency. The two oldest men stated that they had not wanted to be a burden to their wives, which could be interpreted as role inflexibility [9]. In 2017, Canetto, in her article "Suicide: Why are older men so vulnerable?" [30] convincingly showed that illness may lead men to suicide in a much higher degree than women. Her explanation is "Rigidity in coping and in sense of self, consistent with hegemonic-masculinity scripts, emerged as individual-level clues". The meanings and consequences of severe illness thus are highly dependent on gender values and the ideal of self-sufficiency and independence that traditionally were Norwegian masculine ideals. Except for this perceived burdensomeness, we could not find any trigger specific for the age groups (young adults, middle-aged, old).

Relationship problems and perceived burdensomeness draw the attention towards the *Interpersonal Theory of Suicide* (*IPTS*); a theory developed by Joiner [31] and further explicated by Van Orden and colleagues [27]. Judging from the recent systematic review and meta-analysis of the studies testing this theory to date conducted by Chu and colleagues [32], this theory currently seems to dominate the suicide research field. The *IPTS* posits that thwarted belongingness and perceived burdensomeness must be present *simultaneously* for a suicidal desire to emerge.

Certainly, some of the (relationship) problems found above may be interpreted as thwarted belongingness, but this does not seem to be accompanied by feelings of burdensomeness. The men who explicitly said that they felt like a burden (to their wives), expressed this in a context of long lasting, stable relationships, indicating that this had nothing to do with thwarted belongingness. In his

book outlining the *IPTS*, Joiner [31] claims that this theory is able to explain suicidality "worldwide, across cultures" and in their meta-analysis of all the 122 studies testing the *IPTS* to date (all quantitative), Chu et al. [32] on the one hand claim that the findings support the theory, but on the other admit that the evidence is mixed, and that effect-sizes are small to medium, indicating huge variations. Qualitative studies like the present one, are able to present more nuanced and contextualized pictures of what lies behind suicidal behavior compared to what quantitative risk factor research is able to. In qualitative studies, some of the complexity and individual variability involved in suicidal behavior becomes apparent [20]. Such studies contribute to question the relevance of reductionist theories like the *IPTS*, which posits that suicide can be explained by three factors only (acquired capability to enact lethal self-harm in addition to thwarted belongingness and perceived burdensomeness). However, (masculine) identity always is contextual and dynamic, developed and maintained in an ongoing interplay with other people and the surrounding society. Consequently, the prominent approach to suicide prevention seems to require a dynamic and systemic perspective instead of a pure individualistic approach.

In keeping with Fleischer [33] and Staples & Widger [34], we found suicidality to be clearly relational. During the last 60 years this relational aspect of suicidality repeatedly has been described in communicative terms as 'symbol' [35], 'appeal' [36], 'manipulation' [37] or 'cry for help' [38], and hence defined suicide as a communicative act. Men's hesitance to express distress and seek help might be an additional argument to study their suicidal behavior as their specific form for communication in order to understand why it seemed necessary to turn from verbal communication to suicidal acts. It might therefore be fruitful to view suicidal acts as relational, communicative acts and thus to interpret them within the framework of communication theory [33, 39].

In this study we found an interesting difference in attribution of responsibility between the "not to die" and "to die" group. Only one in the "not to die" group took full responsibility for the suicidal act, whereas all but one did the same in the "to die" group. The men who did not want to die described the suicidal act as involuntary because of either alcohol or blackout. This attribution of responsibility goes beyond classical attribution theory [40], as the men who renounced their own responsibility for the suicidal act, did not attribute it externally to someone else, but to forces that were beyond their power within themselves. For three men, the explanations seemed to offer a way of distancing themselves from the act without feelings of guilt or shame. This mechanism enabled them to sympathize with those close to them and create a shared project to deal with the problems. The other two participants who did not take responsibility, felt betrayed by their family and did not want to talk with them, and only reluctantly with health personnel. The denial thus did not create a constructive platform for these men. The only man in the "not to die" group taking full responsibility for his suicidal act was ashamed, did not want to talk to either family or professionals and just wanted to "pull himself together".

In the "to die" group, all but one took full responsibility and the one not doing so described the suicidal act as a "failure", as he was determined to die. His ashamed reaction to the 'failed' attempt can be understood in line with Canetto and others' work on gendered cultural scripts of suicidal behavior [2, 4], as a failure of the masculine ideal of being in full control.

The differences in attribution of responsibility might indicate the level of determination or a way of ascribing meaning to the suicidal act at the same time as maintaining their masculinity. They described the suicidal act as a deliberate act; an act they had thought extensively about for a longer or shorter period of time. An important question might be whether their attribution of responsibility and thus level of determination and meaning-making might be an indicator of the prognosis for their future and their proneness to repeat the suicidal act, with or without lethal intent. This has implications for suicide prevention.

The diversity of the stories speaks heavily against standardized efforts, including categorizing patients in relation to the level of suicide risk. The time should rather be spent listening to patients' stories. This is in line with comprehensive research, which shows that clinicians should stop categorizing patients in relation to the level of suicide risk, and that health authorities should withdraw guidelines that require this [41]. The diversity of stories and needs of the patients rather calls for time to build up strong meeting-points with health personnel [42, 43]. Professionals must be given space, time and trust to apply their health professional skills when meeting the individual patient [44]. This requires the health professionals to be provided with suicidological competence that far exceeds a biomedical understanding of suicidality [45]. Not taking responsibility for a suicidal act might for example be an important message for health professionals to explore why the men renounce responsibility and which psychological function this may have. This should be addressed in the follow-up of suicide attempts by men and should also be studied in depth in further context sensitive research.

Conclusion
Relationship problems were the main reason or trigger of the suicidal act for most participants, but in very different ways, mirroring lived masculinity. As relationship problems cover a vast variety of issues that are irrefutably intertwined with their specific history and context, standardized efforts in terms of suicide prevention might not be the way forward. Besides a variety of relationship problems, some men also described ennui and physical pain as main reason/trigger of the suicidal act. The most striking finding of our study, however, is the uniqueness of each story.

Authors' contributions
HH made all interviews, while the BLK did the initial analysis of the data. The analysis was then discussed extensively with HH. Based on the modified analysis BLK wrote the first draft of the article, which then was revised by HH. Through a series of revisions done by both authors consensus on the final manuscript was reached. Both authors have read and approved the final manuscript.

Consent for publication
Not applicable.

Competing interests
The authors declare that they have no competing interests.

References
1. Canetto SS, Sakinovsky I. The gender paradox in suicide. Suicide Life Threat Behav. 1998;28:1–23.
2. Canetto SS, Cleary A. Men, masculinities and suicidal behavior. Soc Sci Med. 2012;74:461–5.
3. Samaritans Research report. Men, Suicide and Society. Why disadvantaged men in mid-life die by suicide. 2012, https://www.samaritans.org/about-us/our-research/research-report-men-suicide-and-society
4. Lester D, Gunn JF III, Quinnett P. Suicide in men: how men differ from women in expressing their distress. Springfield: Charles C Thomas Publisher; 2014.
5. Krysinska K, Andriessen K, Corveleyn J. Religion and spirituality in online suicide bereavement: an analysis of online memorials. Crisis. 2014;35(5):349–56.
6. Cleary A. Suicidal action, emotional expression, and the performance of masculinities. Soc Sci Med. 2012;74:498–505.
7. Möller-Leimkühler AM. The gender gap in suicide and premature death or: why are men so vulnerable? Eur Arch Psychiatry Clin Neurosci. 2003;253:1–8.
8. Evans R, Scourfield J, Moore G. Gender relationship breakdown, and suicide risk: a review of research in western countries. J Fam Issues. 2016;37(16):2239–64.
9. Scourfield J, Evans R. Why might men be more at risk of suicide after a relationship breakdown? Am J Mens Health. 2015;9(5):380–4.
10. Seale C, Charteris-Black J. The interaction of class and gender in illness narratives. Sociology. 2008;42(3):453–69.
11. Gunnell D, Rasul F, Stansfeld SA, Hart CL, Davey Smith SG. Gender differences in self-reported minor mental disorder and its association with suicide. A 20-year follow-up of the Renfrew and paisley cohort. Soc Psychiatry Psychiatr Epidemiol. 2002;37(10):457–9.
12. Stack S. Suicide: a 15-year review of the sociological literature. Part I: cultural and economic factors. Suicide Life Threat Behav. 2000;30(2):145–62.
13. Agerbo E. Midlife suicide risk, partner's psychiatric illness, spouse and child bereavement by suicide or other modes of death: a gender specific study. J Epidemiol Community Health. 2005;59:407–12.
14. Evans R, Scourfield J, Moore G. Gender, relationship breakdown and suicide risk: a systematic review of research in western countries. In: Samaritans Research report. Men, Suicide and Society. Why disadvantaged men in mid-life die by suicide. 2012:37–47, https://www.samaritans.org/about-us/our-research/research-report-men-suicide-and-society.
15. Courtenay W. Key determinants of the health and the well-being of men and boys. Int J Mens Health. 2003;2(1):1–30.
16. Brownhill S, Wilhelm K, Barclay L, Schmied V. 'Big build': hidden depression in men. Aust N Z J Psychiatry. 2005;39:921–31.
17. Qin P, Agerbo E, Westergård-Nielsen N, Eriksson T, Mortensen PM. Gender differences in risk factors for suicide in Denmark. Br J Psychiatry. 2000;177:546–50.

18. Lease SH, Montes SH, Baggett LR, Sawyer RJ II, Fleming-Norwood KM, Hampton AB, Ovrebo E, Coftci A, Boyraz G. A cross-cultural exploration of masculinity and relationships in men from Turkey, Norway and the United States. J Cross-Cult Psychol. 2013;44(1):84–105.

19. Døving R. Mannskap for likestilling [Male struggle for equality]. Aftenposten. 2006;14:6.

20. Hjelmeland H, Knizek BL. Time to change direction in suicide research. In: O'Connor R, Pirkis J, editors. The International Handbook of Suicide Prevention. 2nd ed. Chichester: Wiley Blackwell; 2016. p. 696–709.

21. Franklin JC, Ribeiro JD, Fox KR, Bentley KH, Kleiman EM, Huang X, Musacchio KM, Jaroszewski AC, Chang BP, Nock MK. Risk factors for suicidal thoughts and behaviors: a meta-analysis of 50 years of research. Psychol Bull. 2017; 143(2):187–232.

22. Canetto SS. Suicidal behaviors among Muslim women. Patterns, pathways, meanings, and prevention. Crisis. 2015;36(6):447–58.

23. Bengtsson M. How to plan and perform a qualitative study using content analysis. NursingPlus Open. 2016;2:8–14.

24. Hsieh HF, Shannon S. Three approaches to qualitative content analysis. Qual Health Res. 2005;15(9):1277–188.

25. Graneheim UH, Lindgren BM, Lundman B. Methodological challenges in qualitative content analysis: a discussion paper. Nurse Educ Today. 2017; 56:29–34.

26. Judd F, Jackson H, Komiti A, Bell R, Fraser C. The profile of suicide: changing or chanable? Soc Psychiatry Psychiatr Epidemiol. 2012;47(1) https://doi.org/ 10.1007/S00127-010-0306-z.

27. Van Orden KA, Cukrowicz KC, Witte TK, Braithwaite SR, Selby EA, Joiner TE. The interpersonal theory of suicide. Psychol Rev. 2010;117(2):575–600.

28. Culture, Medicine and Psychiatry. Special issue: Ethnographies of Suicide, 2012, vol.36,2. Springer.

29. Rasmussen ML, Haavind H, Dieserud G. Young men, masculinities, and suicide. Arch Suicide Res. 2017; https://doi.org/10.1080/1311118.20171340855.

30. Canetto SS. Suicide: why are older men so vulnerable? Men Masculinities. 2017;20(1):49–70.

31. Joiner T. Why people die by suicide. Cambridge Massachusetts: Harvard University Press; 2005.

32. Chu C, Tucker RP, Patros CHG, Buchman-Schmitt JM, Stanley IH, Hom MA, Hagan CR, Rogers ML, Podlogar MC, Chiurliza B, Ringer FB, Michaels MS, Joiner TE. The interpersonal theory of suicide: A systematic review and meta-analysis of a decade of cross-national research. Psychol Bulletin. 2017; https://doi.org/10.1037/bul0000123.

33. Fleischer E. Den talende tavshed. Selvmord og selvmordsforsøg som talehandling. Viborg: Odense universitetsforlag; 2000.

34. Staples J, Widger T. Situating suicide as an anthropological problem: ethnographic approaches to understanding self-harm and self-inflicted death. Cult Med Psychiatry. 2012;36:183–203.

35. Menninger K. Man against himself. New York: Harcourt; 1938.

36. Stengel E. Suicide and attempted suicide. Oxford England: Penguin Books; 1964.

37. Sifneos PE. Manipulative suicides. Psychiatry Q. 1966;40(3):525–37.

38. Farberow NL, Shneidman ES. The cry for help. New York: McGraw-Hill Book Company; 1965.

39. Knizek BL, Hjelmeland H. A theoretical model for interpreting suicidal behaviour as communication. Theory Psychol. 2007;17(5):697–720.

40. Heider F. The psychology of interpersonal relations. New York: Wiley; 1958.

41. Large MM, Ryan CJ. Suicide risk categorisation of psychiatric inpatients: what it might mean and why it is of no use. Australas Psychiatry. 2014; 22:390–2.

42. Hagen J, Hjelmeland H, Knizek BL. Connecting with suicidal patients in psychiatric wards: Therapist challenges. Death Stud. 2017;41(6):360.

43. Hagen J, Hjelmeland H, Knizek BL. Relational Principles in the Care of Suicidal Inpatients: Experiences of Therapists and Mental Health Nurses. Issues Ment Health Nurs. 2017;38(2):99.

44. Straume S. Selvmordsforebyggingens pris. Tidsskr Nor Psykol foren. 2014;51:242–51.

45. Hjelmeland H, Hagen J, Espeland K, Nygaard TU, Knizek BL. Tidsskr Nor Legeforen 2018. doi: https://doi.org/10.4045/tidsskr.18.0349.

3

The relationship between college students' alexithymia and mobile phone addiction: testing mediation and moderation effects

Songli Mei[1], Gang Xu[1], Tingting Gao[1], Hui Ren[1] and Jingyang Li[2*]

Abstract

Background: To explore the relationship between college students' alexithymia and mobile phone addiction as well as the mediating effects of mental health and the moderating role of being a single child or not.

Methods: A total of 1034 college students from Changchun were assessed with the Toronto Alexithymia Scale (TAS-20), General Health Questionnaire (GHQ) and Mobile Phone Addiction Index (MPAI).

Results: Alexithymia was positively correlated with mental health and mobile phone addiction. Alexithymia had not only a direct impact on mobile phone addiction but also an indirect impact via mental health. For college students who were not only children, higher levels of alexithymia led to an increase in mobile phone addiction, whereas the influence of alexithymia on mobile phone addiction was much weaker among only children.

Conclusion: Mental health has a partial mediating effect on the relationship between alexithymia and mobile phone addiction, and the relationship was significantly moderated by whether students were only children or not.

Keywords: Alexithymia, Mental health, Mobile phone addiction, Only child

Background

The term alexithymia originates from Greek and literally means "lacking words for emotions" [1]. Alexithymia is a multifaceted construct associated with difficulties in identifying, analyzing and verbalizing feelings, constricted imagination, and a concrete, externally oriented way of thinking [2]. Individuals with alexithymia have limited ability to understand their own feelings and others' emotions and cannot regulate emotions properly in interpersonal contexts [3]. Research on the absolute and relative stability of alexithymia has shown that alexithymia is a personality trait instead of a state-dependent phenomenon that is secondary to other clinical problems [4]. The most widely used self-reported measure of alexithymia is the 20-item Toronto Alexithymia Scale (TAS-20) [5]. There are three factors for this scale: (1) difficulty in identifying feelings (DIF), (2) difficulty in describing feelings (DDF), and (3) externally oriented

thinking (EOT). The prevalence of alexithymia has been shown to range from 13 to 19% [6]. The significant percentage of 24.1% of young people is observed to have high levels of alexithymia [7].

Alexithymia is very common in individuals with psychiatric disorders [8] and is a sign of negative emotion in psychiatric populations [9]. Alexithymia may restrict the control of emotional states and may lead to negative affect, including depression and anxiety [10]. Individuals who suffer from intolerable psychological disease sometimes cannot express themselves by suitable words [11]. It is generally accepted that alexithymia has profound effects on mental health. Compared with non-individuals with alexithymia, individuals with alexithymia were prone to report more mental health-related problems [12]. There was an inverse and strong relationship between alexithymia and mental health; that is, mental health may be strengthened by interventions targeting alexithymia [13].

The mobile phone has gained a strong position in modern life and human society and is regarded as an indicator of communication technology [14]. Despite its convenience for many people, the problems derived from overuse

* Correspondence: lijingyang@126.com
[2]Department of Mental Health, The First Hospital of Jilin University, NO. 71 Xinmin Street, Changchun, Jilin Province, China
Full list of author information is available at the end of the article

of the mobile phone are a subject of much concern. Mobile phone addiction is characterized by uncontrolled mobile phone use that leads to adverse consequences on an individual's physical and mental health and social functioning [15]. Individuals with symptoms of mobile phone addiction tend to bring their phone with them wherever they are and think about their phone even if they cannot use it, which ultimately influences daily tasks [16]. Of all applications, instant messaging receives the highest use among mobile phone users in China (92.1%), with 11.0% higher use than the second most common use, the search engine [17]. This shows that individuals use the mobile Internet for social needs more than for other functions. Some users believe that mobile phone instant messaging not only can help them build deeper friendships but also is more comfortable than face-to-face interactions [18]. However, people who overuse mobile phones are more likely to have difficulties expressing their emotions than the general population is [19]. Individuals with mobile phone dependence may have deficient facial expression recognition and take more time to identify types of emotion. Alexithymia is significantly correlated with dysregulation of emotions and affects, which makes it difficult to guide one's own behavior [20]. Mobile phone addiction among university students could result from pre-existing factors [21]. Alexithymia is considered a high-risk factor for mobile phone addiction [22].

There is a significant negative correlation between mental health and the level of addiction to mobile phone use [23]. Mobile phones can be used to avoid negative emotions, which may magnify such affects because of negative emotional responses and unresolved fundamental problems [24]. Students who have poor mental health and are psychologically unbalanced are more susceptible to engaging in addictive mobile phone behaviors because they attempt to decrease their intense negative emotions by communicating with others [25].

The literature review showed that alexithymia, mental health and mobile phone addiction are correlated with each other. A previous study has shown that alexithymia could mediate the association between self-awareness and anxiety as well as depression [26]. Alexithymia is closely and positively correlated with chronic pain, and negative affects, including depression and anxiety symptoms, mediate this relationship [27]. Mental health might be a mediator in the association between alexithymia and mobile phone addiction.

China has relaxed its more than three-decade-old family planning policy. The implementation of the universal two-child policy is intended to actively address the country's aging trend. Only children represent a certain proportion in China. Whether one is an only child or not has an influence on alexithymia, and the alexithymia scores of children with a sibling were higher than those

of children without [28]. A Chinese study also found that the level of mobile phone dependence among college students who were only children was significantly higher than that among those who were not only children [29]. However, these studies investigated differences in alexithymia and mobile phone addiction only in only children.

The aim of the present study was to determine the potential mechanisms underlying the relationship between alexithymia and mobile phone addiction. Specifically, we will examine how alexithymia influences mobile phone addiction through mental health and differences in the association between alexithymia and mobile phone addiction among only children and children with a sibling. Based on the literature review, we propose the following two hypotheses:

Hypothesis 1: Mental health will mediate the association between alexithymia and mobile phone addiction.

Hypothesis 2: Being an only child or not will moderate the association between alexithymia and mobile phone addiction.

Method
Participants
A cross-sectional survey was conducted from April to May 2015. A convenience cluster sampling method was employed to produce a sample of college students. All participants were recruited from Jilin University, a comprehensive university in Northeast China. Everybody involved in this study will be rewarded with credits of some certain courses and told to participant voluntarily and could withdraw at any time. The participants answered a traditional paper-and-pencil questionnaire with the guidance of well-trained researchers during school classes. It took the respondents approximately 30 min to complete the anonymous questionnaire. A small gift was given to make up for the time spent on the survey.

The prevalence of mobile phone addiction among Chinese undergraduates was 21.3%, so $\pi = 21.3\%$. A relative error of 15% was allowed in the present study. The absolute error can be calculated by $\delta = 0.15\pi = 0.15 \times 21.3\%$. We adopt 95% confidence intervals; thus, $\mu_a = 1.96$. According to the following equation for the sample size, we calculated the minimum sample size: n $= [1.96^2 \times 21.3\% \times (1-21.3\%)]/(0.15 \times 21.3\%)^2 \approx 631$. Considering the invalid cases, the desired sample size should increase by 10%: $631 \times (1 + 10\%) \approx 695$.

$$n = \left(\frac{u_a^2 \pi(1-\pi)}{\delta^2} \right)$$

A total of 1200 college students participated in this survey. After the subjects with missing data were excluded, the sample included 1034 subjects.

Measures
Toronto alexithymia scale (TAS-20)

The Toronto Alexithymia Scale-20 (TAS-20) is a self-report scale for the assessment of alexithymia [5]. The instrument consists of 20 items rated using a five-point Likert scale. The total score ranged from 20 to 100, with higher scores indicating a higher level of alexithymia traits. Research suggests that TAS-20 is appropriate for use with the Chinese population [30]. According to a categorical approach [31], a total of 57 points or more indicates a high level of alexithymia, while the range of values from 40 to 57 indicates a moderate level of alexithymia, whereas and 40 points or below indicates a low level of alexithymia. The Cronbach's alpha in this study was 0.81.

General health questionnaire (GHQ-12)

Mental health was measured with the General Health Questionnaire (GHQ-12) [32]. The GHQ-12 includes 12 items describing mood states over the previous 4 weeks. The original GHQ rating method (0–0–1-1) was used in the questionnaire. The total score ranged from 0 to 12 points, with higher scores indicating poor psychological well-being. Research suggests that the GHQ-12 is appropriate for use with the Chinese population [33].The Cronbach's alpha in this study was 0.76.

Mobile phone addiction index (MPAI)

Mobile phone addiction was measured by the Chinese version of the Mobile Phone Addiction Index (MPAI) [34], which was developed by Leung [35]. This is a self-report questionnaire with 17 items, which rated on a 5-point Likert scale. It contains four subscales: inability to control craving, feeling anxious and lost, withdrawal or escape and productivity loss. Higher scores indicated higher levels of mobile phone addiction. The Cronbach's alpha in this study was 0.87.

Data analysis

The descriptive analysis was used to determine the demographic characteristics of the participants. Pearson correlation analyses of the study variables were conducted. We adopt independent-samples T-test to examine differences in mobile phone addiction and mental health between individuals with high and low alexithymia. The structural equation model (SEM) was used to study the effects of alexithymia on mobile phone addiction through mental health. The bootstrapping method was used to verify mediation effects. In this study, we bootstrapped 5000 samples from the data, and 95% bootstrap confidence intervals (CI) were calculated. A hierarchical multiple linear regression was conducted to verify whether being an only child moderated the relationship between alexithymia and mobile phone addiction. Statistical analysis was conducted using the SPSS 18.0 version program and Amos 17.0 software.

Results
Sample characteristics

The mean age of the participants was 19.97 years (SD = 1.22). The sample consisted of 1034 college students, of whom 52.7% ($n = 545$) were women. Five hundred forty-three (52.5%) participants were only children. Over half (57.4%, $n = 594$) were from urban areas. A total of 534 individuals (51.6%) had moderate income, and 286 individuals (27.7%) had low family income, while the remainder had high income (20.7%, $n = 214$). Table 1 shows the detail of demographic characteristics of participants.

Bivariate statistics

Means, standard deviations and correlations between all the study variables are presented in Table 2. All the dimensions of alexithymia, mobile phone addiction and poor mental health were positively correlated with each other, while externally oriented thinking was not correlated with withdrawal or escape.

Comparison for mobile phone addiction and mental health by alexithymia

The results showed that there were significant differences in mobile phone addiction and mental health between individuals with high and low alexithymia ($P < 0.001$).The mobile phone addiction and mental health scores of individuals with high alexithymia were

Table 1 Demographic characteristics of the college students

Variables	n	%
Gender		
Male	489	47.3
Female	545	52.7
Single child		
Yes	543	52.5
No	491	47.5
Area of family residence		
Urban	594	57.4
Rural	440	42.6
Grade		
One	348	33.7
Two	563	54.4
Three	123	11.9
Family income status		
Low income	286	27.7
Moderate income	534	51.6
High income	214	20.7

Table 2 Means, standard deviations and correlations for all variables ($n = 1034$)

Variables	$M \pm SD$	1	2	3	4	5	6	7	8
1. Difficulty in Identifying Feelings	17.28 ± 5.14	1							
2.Difficulty in Describing Feelings	13.23 ± 3.22	0.68^{**}	1						
3. Externally Oriented Thinking	20.05 ± 3.94	0.28^{**}	0.31^{**}	1					
4. Inability to Control Craving	14.89 ± 4.85	0.32^{**}	0.27^{**}	0.19^{**}	1				
5. Feeling Anxious and Lost	12.11 ± 4.87	0.19^{**}	0.16^{**}	0.07^{*}	0.47^{**}	1			
6. Withdrawal or Escape	7.57 ± 3.11	0.20^{**}	0.15^{**}	0.05	0.37^{**}	0.43^{**}	1		
7. Productivity Loss	5.24 ± 2.20	0.29^{**}	0.24^{**}	0.13^{**}	0.59^{**}	0.37^{**}	0.39^{**}	1	
8. Mental Health	3.20 ± 2.60	0.44^{**}	0.37^{**}	0.23^{**}	0.30^{**}	0.22^{**}	0.15^{**}	0.30^{**}	1

Note:$^{**}P<0.01$, $^{*}P<0.05$

significantly higher than those of individuals with lower alexithymia. The higher level of alexithymia an individual had, the greater the possibility of mental health problems and mobile phone addiction (Table 3).

Mediation analysis of alexithymia on mobile phone addiction

To determine the relationship between alexithymia, mental health and mobile phone addiction, we first created a direct model of alexithymia on mobile phone addiction according to the stepwise regression method. Second, we created mental health as the mediator variable and built the mediation model of mental health on the relationship between alexithymia and mobile phone addiction. The results of the hierarchical regression on the mediation model test were as follows. After controlling for gender and being an only child, the path coefficient of alexithymia on mobile phone addiction was 0.316 ($t = 10.694$, $P < 0.001$) in the direct path model, and the explanation rate was 10.9% ($R^2 = 0.109$). After mental health was included as the mediator variable, the direct path coefficient of alexithymia on mobile phone addiction was reduced to 0.218 ($t = 6.749$, $P < 0.001$). The explanation rate of the mediation model for mobile phone addiction variance increased by 14.7% ($R^2 = 0.147$). This result indicated that the mediation model was superior to the direct path model. The inclusion of mental health (mediator variable) can explain the greater variance in mobile phone addiction,

Table 3 Comparison of mobile phone addiction and mental health by alexithymia

Variables	High alexithymia	Low alexithymia	t
Inability to Control Craving	17.36 ± 5.30	12.74 ± 4.20	-9.44^{***}
Feeling Anxious and Lost	13.65 ± 5.12	11.55 ± 5.17	-4.15^{***}
Withdrawal or Escape	8.25 ± 3.30	6.78 ± 3.36	-4.46^{***}
Productivity Loss	6.12 ± 2.20	4.31 ± 2.30	-8.16^{***}
Mobile Phone Addiction	45.38 ± 12.16	35.39 ± 11.53	-8.46^{***}
GHQ	5.08 ± 2.97	1.96 ± 1.80	-11.95^{***}

Note:$^{***}P<0.001$

which can better explain the relationship between alexithymia and mobile phone addiction and play a partial mediating role in the relationship.

Alexithymia was used as the predictor variable, mobile phone addiction as the outcome variable, and mental health as the mediating variable to build the SEM by Amos 17.0 software. The fit indices of the model yielded satisfactory results ($\chi^2/df = 1.384$, NFI = 0.992, TLI = 0.995, CFI = 0.998, RESEA = 0.019). The result of the path coefficients is presented in Fig. 1.

To gain an improved understanding of the mediation effects, we performed the mediation tests by applying the bootstrapping procedure. We drew 5000 bootstrapping samples and computed 95% confidence intervals (95%CI). We made alexithymia the predictor variable, mobile phone addiction the outcome variable and mental health the mediating variable. Then, we included the study variables in the PROCESS macro for SPSS. The results demonstrated that the total effect of the model was 0.115. The confidence interval was excluding zero (LLCI = 0.075, ULCI = 0.157), which showed that a reasonable mediation model was established. The mediation effects of mental health could explain 13.7% ($R^2 = 0.137$) of the total variance. Thus, alexithymia exerted a significant indirect effect on mobile phone addiction via mental health.

Moderation analysis of being an only child

A hierarchical multiple linear regression was conducted to verify whether being an only child moderated the relationship between alexithymia and mobile phone addiction. Because only children belonged to two categorical variables and alexithymia was a continuous variable, we needed to apply grouping regression analysis to test the moderation analysis, according to the suggestion of Wen [36]. Above all, alexithymia as the continuous predictor was centered. A dummy variable represented whether children were only children. The interaction term of alexithymia and being an only child or not was obtained at the same time. Then, mobile phone addiction was used as the outcome variable through

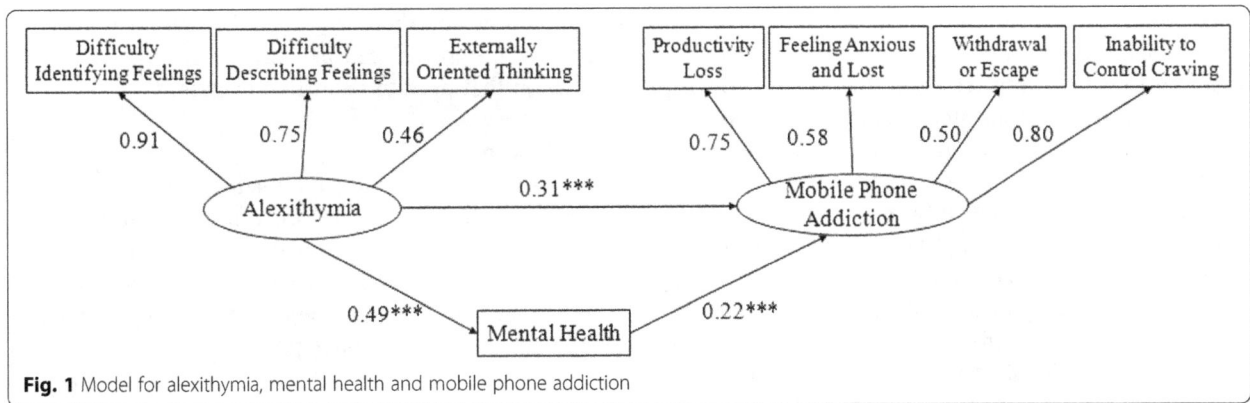

Fig. 1 Model for alexithymia, mental health and mobile phone addiction

hierarchical multiple linear regression. First, alexithymia and being an only child or not were entered in Step 1. Second, the interaction term of alexithymia and being an only child or not was entered in Step 2. The results showed that R_1^2 was significantly higher than R_2^2 ($\triangle R^2 = 0.006$, $\triangle F = 6.818, P < 0.01$), which explains the moderation effect of whether being an only child or not was significant. To investigate the improved mechanism of the mediation effects, we performed a regression analysis of alexithymia and mobile phone addiction for only children and for not only children. The results showed that alexithymia was positively associated with mobile phone addiction among college students who were only children ($\beta = 0.259$, $R^2 = 0.067$, $F = 39.295$, $P < 0.001$) and those who were not children ($\beta = 0.372$, $R^2 = 0.139$, $F = 79.105$, $P < 0.001$). Simple slope tests showed that for college students who were not only children, higher levels of alexithymia led to an increase in mobile phone addiction ($\beta = 0.482$, $P < 0.001$). However, for college students who were only children, the effect of alexithymia on mobile phone addiction was much weaker ($\beta = 0.304$, $P < 0.001$) (Fig. 2).

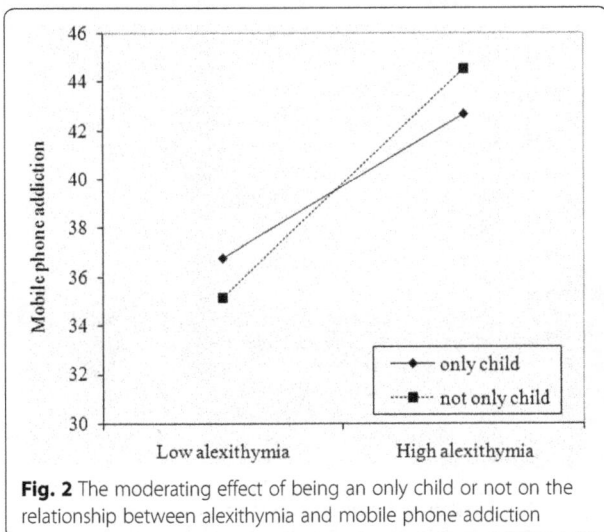

Fig. 2 The moderating effect of being an only child or not on the relationship between alexithymia and mobile phone addiction

Discussion

Our finding of a positive relationship between alexithymia, poor mental health and mobile phone addiction is consistent with the existing literature [19, 37, 38]. The present study also extended previous work by showing that scores of mobile phone addiction and GHQ in high alexithymia was significantly higher than in low alexithymia. Compared to individuals without alexithymia, individuals with alexithymia were subject to a higher potential risk for Internet addiction [22]. The most obvious reason for this association is that individuals with alexithymia attempt to regulate their emotions by addictive behavior [39]. However, a previous study has argued that individuals with social relationship problems that might be caused by alexithymia showed less frequent mobile phone use [40]. In general, the mental health of individuals with alexithymia was poor when compared to that of individuals without alexithymia [41]. A meta-analysis indicated that alexithymia served as a critical path to different indicators of mental health [42]. Alexithymia has direct effects on the inability to experience emotions, leading to poor mental health. The hierarchy of needs theory proposed by Maslow holds that an individual's mental health is closely related to the satisfaction of a need. If an individual's needs are not met, negative mentality may be more easily generated and cause psychological problems [43]. Based on the associated expectations of anonymity, convenience and avoidance, individuals use the mobile phone to obtain psychological and physiological satisfaction. According to the theory of use and gratification, long-term mobile phone use will form mobile phone addiction.

According to the results of the mediation test, mental health mediated the relationship between alexithymia and mobile phone addiction, which supports Hypothesis 1. To our knowledge, this is the first study to investigate the mechanism among alexithymia, mental health, and mobile phone addiction in a sample of college students. Alexithymia had not only a direct impact on mobile phone addiction but also an indirect impact via mental health. College students are in a period of the rapid development of social consciousness. They pay more attention to their own values and inner world, and hope to receive attention from others and integrate into their peer groups. When these needs are not met, mobile phones, the Internet and other new media can help students achieve the impression of communication and share their feelings. Mobile phones are a convenient and popular tool for contacting others [40]. An increasing body of studies has provided evidence of the association between alexithymia and Internet addiction [44]. Individuals with alexithymia may use the Internet to express their feelings as a compensatory, nonverbal strategy [1]. The opportunity to gain better control over the communication process can help individuals with alexithymia manage their moods, regulate their emotions during social interactions and find a more effective means of communication that suits them [45]. Individuals with alexithymia have difficulty gaining enough resources to face stressful life events, which causes highly negative evaluations of coping style. Individuals with alexithymia may seek to relieve the poor mental health due to alexithymia by turning to mobile phones and therefore may be more prone to excessive use of mobile phones.

In addition, our results showed that the association between alexithymia and mobile phone addiction was moderated by being an only child or not, which supports Hypothesis 2. More specifically, for college students who were not only children, higher levels of alexithymia led to an increase in mobile phone addiction, whereas the effect of alexithymia on mobile phone addiction was much weaker among only children. This may be because children with siblings face competition for all types of resources from their brothers and sisters. To attract their parents' attention, it is easy to establish an inappropriate defense mechanism and then avoid inner emotional cognition. The basic function of the mobile phone makes the phone a better means to seek peer recognition and improve one's sense of belonging. When only children grow up in a relatively relaxed and wealthy economic condition, they are more willing to express and examine their inner feelings, and the risk that they will depend on mobile phones to meet their emotional demands is low.

Limitations
Because the present study was based on a self-reported questionnaire, there might be many associated confounding factors. In addition, a cross-sectional survey cannot be used to draw a definitive conclusion. Thus, further study requires a longitudinal design. In addition, only one university was involved in this study, which could affect the generalizability of the findings. Lastly, in addition to the influence of mental health and being an

only child or not, there must be other variables affecting the relationship between alexithymia and mobile phone addiction that need to be further discussed.

Conclusion
The present study verified the mediating effect of mental health and the moderating effect of being an only child or not between alexithymia and mobile phone addiction. Mental health and individual characteristics should be considered when relevant departments design strategies for the prevention of mobile phone addiction.

Abbreviations
CI: Confidence intervals; SEM: Structural equation model

Acknowledgements
We would like to thank all the participants at Jilin University for their assistance in the study.

Funding
This research has received support from the Science and Technology International Cooperation Project of Jilin Province 20160414035GH.

Authors' contributions
TG, SM and JL designed the study. GX, TG and HR performed the study. GX analyzed the data and drafted the manuscript. SM and JL participated in revising the manuscript. All authors approved the final manuscript.

Consent for publication
Not applicable.

Competing interests
The authors declare that they have no competing interest.

Author details
[1]Department of Social Medicine and Health Management, School of Public Health, Jilin University, NO. 1163 Xinmin Street, Changchun, Jilin Province, China. [2]Department of Mental Health, The First Hospital of Jilin University, NO. 71 Xinmin Street, Changchun, Jilin Province, China.

References
1. Nemiah JC, Freyberger H, Sifneos P. Alexithymia: A view of the psychosomatic process. Mod Trends Psychosom Med. 1976;3:430–9.
2. Sifneos PE. The prevalence of 'alexithymic' characteristics in psychosomatic patients. Psychother Psychosom. 1973;22:255–62.
3. Hesse C, Floyd K. Affectionate experience mediates the effects of alexithymia on mental health and interpersonal relationships. J Soc Pers Relat. 2008;25:793–810.
4. De Timary P, Luts A, Hers D, Luminet O. Absolute and relative stability of alexithymia in alcoholic inpatients undergoing alcohol withdrawal: Relationship to depression and anxiety. Psychiatry Res. 2008;157:105–13.

5. Bagby RM, Parker JD, Taylor GJ. The twenty-item Toronto Alexithymia Scale - I. Item selection and cross-validation of the factor structure. J Psychosom Res. 1994;38:23–32.

6. Lee YJ, Yu SH, Cho SJ, Cho IH, Koh SH, Kim SJ. Direct and indirect effects of the temperament and character on alexithymia: A pathway analysis with mood and anxiety. Compr Psychiatry. 2010;51:201–6.

7. Galván EL. Alexithymia: Indicator of communicative deficit in emotional health. Procedia Soc Behav Sci. 2014;132:603–7.

8. De Panfilis C, Rabbaglio P, Rossi C, Zita G, Maggini C. Body image disturbance, parental bonding and alexithymia in patients with eating disorders. Psychopathology. 2003;36:239–46.

9. Marchesi C, Ossola P, Tonna M, De Panfilis C. The TAS-20 more likely measures negative affects rather than alexithymia itself in patients with major depression, panic disorder, eating disorders and substance use disorders. Compr Psychiatry. 2014;55:972–8.

10. De Berardis D, Campanella D, Gambi F, La Rovere R, Sepede G, et al. Alexithymia, fear of bodily sensations, and somatosensory amplification in young outpatients with panic disorder. Psychosomatics. 2007;48:239–46.

11. Pompili M. Exploring the phenomenology of suicide. Suicide Life Threat Behav. 2011;40:234–44.

12. Pandey R, Saxena P, Dubey A. Emotion regulation difficulties in alexithymia and mental health. Eur J Psychol. 2013;7:604–23.

13. Atari M, Yaghoubirad M. The big five personality dimensions and mental health: The mediating role of alexithymia. Asian J Psychiatr. 2016;24:59–64.

14. Biglu MH, Ghavami M. Factors influencing dependence on mobile phone. J Anal Res Clin Med. 2016;4:158–62.

15. Walsh SP, White KM, Cox S, Young RM. Keeping in constant touch: The predictors of young Australians' mobile phone involvement. Comput Hum Behav. 2011;27:333–42.

16. Dziurzyńska E, Pawłowska B, Potembska E. Coping strategies in individuals at risk and not at risk of mobile phone addiction. Curr Probl Psychiatry. 2016;17:250–60.

17. China Internet Network Information Center (CNNIC). The 41st China Statistical Report on Internet Development. http://cnnic.net.cn/hlwfzyj/hlwxzbg/hlwtjbg/201803/P020180305409870339136.pdf. Accessed 26 Mar 2018.

18. Kamibeppu K, Sugiura H. Impact of the mobile phone on junior high-school students' friendships in the Tokyo metropolitan area. Cyberpsychol Behav. 2005;8:121–30.

19. Ha JH, Chin B, Park DH, Ryu SH, Yu J. Characteristics of excessive cellular phone use in Korean adolescents. Cyberpsychol Behav Soc Netw. 2008;11:783–4.

20. Taylor GJ, Bagby RM, Parker JD. Disorders of affect regulation: Alexithymia in medical and psychiatric illness. Cambridge: Cambridge University Press; 1997.

21. Hong FY, Chiu SI, Huang DH. A model of the relationship between psychological characteristics, mobile phone addiction and use of mobile phones by Taiwanese university female students. Compu Hum Behav. 2012;28:2152–9.

22. De Berardis D, D'Albenzio A, Gambi F, Sepede G, Valchera A, et al. Alexithymia and its relationships with dissociative experiences and Internet addiction in a nonclinical sample. Cyberpsychol Behav. 2009;12:67–9.

23. Beydokhti A, Hassanzadeh R, Mirzaian B. The relationship between five main factors of personality and addiction to SMS in high school students. Curr Res J Biol Sci. 2012;4:685–9.

24. Roser K, Schoeni A, Foerster M, Roosli M. Problematic mobile phone use of Swiss adolescents: Is it linked with mental health or behaviour? Int J Public Health. 2016;61:307–15.

25. Babadi-Akashe Z, Zamani BE, Abedini Y, Akbari H, Hedayati N. The relationship between mental health and addiction to mobile phones among university students of Shahrekord, Iran. Addict Health. 2014;6:93–9.

26. Rutten EA, Bachrach N, van Balkom AJ, Braeken J, Ouwens MA, Bekker MH. Anxiety, depression and autonomy-connectedness: The mediating role of alexithymia and assertiveness. Psychol Psychother. 2016;89:385–401.

27. Shibata M, Ninomiya T, Jensen MP, Anno K, Yonemoto K, et al. Alexithymia is associated with greater risk of chronic pain and negative affect and with lower life satisfaction in a general population: The Hisayama Study. PloS One. 2014:9, e90984.

28. He X, Zhang Y, Xu X. The influence of alexithymia on subjective well-being among college students (in Chinese). Chin J School Health. 2013;34:534–6.

29. Wang C, Wang S, Li W, Dong X, Chi G. Study on the mobile phone dependence syndrome and its distribution among 2213college students in Guangzhou (in Chinese). Chin J Epidemio. 2013:949–52.

30. Zou Z, Huang Y, Wang J, He Y, Min W, et al. Association of childhood trauma and panic symptom severity in panic disorder: Exploring the mediating role of alexithymia. J Affect Disord. 2016;206:133–9.

31. Zhu X, Yi J, Yao S, Ryder AG, Taylor GJ, Bagby RM. Cross-cultural validation of a Chinese translation of the 20-item Toronto Alexithymia Scale. Compr Psychiatry. 2007;48:489–96.

32. Goldberg DP, Hillier VF. A scaled version of the general health questionnaire. Psychol Med. 1979;9:139–45.

33. Yang TZ, Huang L, Wu ZY. The application of Chinese health questionnaire for mental disorder screening in community settings in mainland China. Chin J Epidemio. 2003;24:769–73.

34. Huang H, Niu LY, Zhou CY, Wu HM. Reliability and validity of mobile phone addiction index for Chinese college students (in Chinese). Chin J Clinl Psychol. 2014;22:835–8.

35. Leung L. Linking psychological attributes to addiction and improper use of the mobile phone among adolescents in Hong Kong. J Child Media. 2008;2: 93–113.

36. Wen Z, Hau KT, Chang L. A comparison of moderator and mediator and their applications (in Chinese). Acta Psychologica Sinica. 2005;37:268–74.

37. Gilanifar M, Delavar MA. The relationship between alexithymia and general symptoms of pregnant women. Rom J Intern Med. 2017;55:14–8.

38. Elhai JD, Levine JC, Dvorak RD, Hall BJ. Fear of missing out, need for touch, anxiety and depression are related to problematic smartphone use. Compu Hum Behav. 2016;63:509–16.

39. Taylor GJ, Bagby RM, Parker JD. The alexithymia construct: A potential paradigm for psychosomatic medicine. Psychosomatics. 1991;32:153–64.

40. Mattila AK, Luutonen S, Ylinen M, Salokangas RK, Joukamaa M. Alexithymia, human relationships, and mobile phone use. J Nerv Ment Dis. 2010;198:722–7.

41. Posse M, Hällström T, Backenrothohsako G. Alexithymia, social support, psycho-social stress and mental health in a female population. Nord J Psychiatry. 2002;56:329–34.

42. Li S, Zhang B, Guo Y, Zhang J. The association between alexithymia as assessed by the 20-item Toronto Alexithymia Scale and depression: A meta-analysis. Psychiatry Res. 2015;227:1–9.

43. Maslow AH. Toward a psychology of being. New York: Nostrand; 1968.

44. Kandri TA, Bonotis KS, Floros GD, Zafiropoulou MM. Alexithymia components in excessive internet users: A multi-factorial analysis. Psychiatry Res. 2014;220:348–55.

45. McKenna KYA, Bargh JA. Plan 9 from cyberspace: The implications of the internet for personality and social psychology. Pers Soc Psychol Rev. 2000;4:57–75.

4

Prevalence of orthorexia nervosa in university students and its relationship with psychopathological aspects of eating behaviour disorders

María-Laura Parra-Fernández[1], Teresa Rodríguez-Cano[2], María-Dolores Onieva-Zafra[1]* iD, María José Perez-Haro[3], Víctor Casero-Alonso[4], Elia Fernández-Martinez[1] and Blanca Notario-Pacheco[5]

Abstract

Introduction: Orthorexia nervosa (ON) is characterized by an obsession with healthy eating, which may lead to severe physical, psychological and social disorders. It is particularly important to research this problem in populations that do not receive clinical care in order to improve early detection and treatment.

Objective: The aim of this study was to research the prevalence of ON in a population of Spanish university students and to analyze the possible associations between ON and psychological traits and behaviors that are common to ED.

Method: A cross-sectional study with 454 students from the University of Castilla La Mancha, Spain. In total, 295 women and 159 men participated, aged between 18 and 41 years. The ORTO-11-ES questionnaire and the Eating Disorder Inventory (EDI-2) were used for this study. The chi squared test was used to compare the homogeneity among the different groups.

Results: The scores on the ORTO-11-ES suggested that 17% of students were at risk of ON. The scores on the EDI-2 for the group at risk of ON were significant, compared to the remaining individuals, regarding their drive for thinness (17.1% vs 2.1%), bulimia (2.6% vs 0%), body dissatisfaction (26.3% vs. 12.4%), perfectionism (14.5% vs 4.8%), interoceptive awareness (13.2% vs 1.3%), asceticism (15.8% vs 3.7%) and impulsiveness (9.2% vs 1.9%).

Discussion and conclusion: These findings suggest that many of the psychological and behavioral aspects of ED are shared by people who are at risk of ON. Future research should use longitudinal data, examining the temporal relationship among these variables or other underlying variables that may contribute to the concurrence of ED and ON.

Keywords: Orthorexia nervosa, Eating disorders, University students, Psychological traits, Behavioral traits

Introduction

The term 'eating disorders' (EDs) encompasses a variety of disorders characterized by abnormal eating behaviors associated with emotional difficulties. The EDs described in the fifth edition of the diagnostic and statistical manual of mental disorders (DSM-5) [1] may not be entirely applicable to specific populations due to the wide variability in the frequency, the time-period and the characteristics of each individual, limiting the application of available diagnostic criteria.

Orthorexia nervosa (ON) is described as an obsession for healthy food. This term was used for the first time by Bratman in 1997 [2]. People who suffer from this eating fixation undergo a monomania for healthy food without artificial additives and are more concerned with the quality of food than the quantity [3]. This extreme concern for food can lead to a disorder with many different levels of severity. These patients

* Correspondence: MariaDolores.Onieva@uclm.es
[1]Faculty of Nursing , University of Castilla-La-Mancha, Ciudad Real, Spain
Full list of author information is available at the end of the article

have important dietary restrictions, which are related to medical disorders that are potentially mortal associated with malnutrition, affective instability and social isolation [3].

To date, neither the diagnostic criteria published for ON [4, 5], nor the different studies available have given enough clarity to include this disorder in the DSM-5 [1], nor in the tenth edition of the International Classification of Diseases (ICD-10) [6]. Furthermore, some studies have related ON with obsessive compulsive disorders (OCD) [7–10]. Donini et al. performed a study, in which they developed and validated a questionnaire to detect the risk of suffering ON: the ORTO-15 [11]. The same study reported an association between ON and OCD. In addition, most of the literature consulted by the authors of this study, reveals clinical characteristics of ON that are common in EDs, in particular in anorexia nervosa (AN) [12–15]. A study by Brytek—Matera found that the participants who displayed a great level of concern with healthy foods also showed a positive correlation with satisfaction and/or the appearance of their body, and therefore this is one of the characteristics that is also found in patients with AN [16]. A study developed by Vandereycken et al. showed that ON is a disorder that is often referred and acknowledged by patients with ED. According to this study, 67% of professionals in charge of the treatment of these patients observed this phenomenon in their clinical practice, and 69% considered that the disorder warranted greater attention [17]. Both ED and ON are characterized by a lack of pleasure related with eating food and show a need for controlling the intake of food as a tool for improving their self-esteem and/or self-fulfillment, granting them a sense of control over their own life [18]. The difference between these two disorders is that, while people with orthorexia are focused on eating healthy and pure foods, preoccupied by quality, those who suffer from anorexia and/or bulimia are more concerned with the quantity of the foods they eat, rather than the quality of the same [19]. Vargas et al. point out that although the difference between both effectively resides in the final motivation, i.e. weight loss in AN or feeling healthy in the case of ON, similar social and psychological consequences may exist in both disorders [20]. Furthermore, some authors attempt to identify or clarify the existing relationship between some EDs and mental disorders [21]. Dell'Osso et al. propose the hypothesis that people at risk of suffering ON, besides sharing some traits with people who suffer autism spectrum disorders (ASDs) such as for example ritual-like behaviors when preparing food, may also share consequences such as the risk for social isolation [22].

Among the different studies available on the prevalence of ON, several questionnaires [11, 23, 24] have been used to determine the presence of the disorder. Most of these are based on the proposal by Donini et al., i.e. the ORTO-15 [11]. Depending on the instrument used and the populations in which the study is performed, the results of the prevalence rates vary. One of the first studies performed in Italy by Donini et al. in 2004 using the ORTO-15 demonstrated a prevalence of 6.9% in a population of 404 students [25]. Kinzl et al. used the original test by Bratman in a sample of 283 dieticians, and found that 34.9% of the population had a high risk of ON [10]. In a study involving 446 German university students conducted by Depa et al. employing the Düsseldorfer Orthorexie Skala (DOS) [23], a 3.3% estimated prevalence of ON was reported, together with a 9.0% prevalence for the risk of developing ON [26]. It is important to consider that most studies have been performed in non-clinical settings, and mainly on university students [8, 13, 19, 23, 26, 27].

Lifestyle habits and food consumption are developed since infancy and begin to establish themselves in adolescence and youth. The diet of youth, and especially that of university students is an important challenge, as it may involve important lifestyle changes [28]. The university population is an especially vulnerable group from the nutritional point of view, as they are beginning to take responsibility for their own dietary habits and they undergo a critical period in the consolidation of eating habits and behaviors [29]. Young adulthood (19–24 years) is an important developmental period for exploring and establishing our relationship with health habits, beliefs and eating norms, as well as for body image development [30]. Considering that many of the conditions and behaviors established during teenage years persist throughout life, adolescence and adulthood, these periods represent powerful developmental opportunities for evaluating predictors and risk factors for ED. These behaviors should be addressed due to their adverse consequences such as metabolic risks later on in adulthood. Improving our understanding of populations who do not receive clinical care such as people with a risk of ED is particularly important for early detection and treatment of ON [31, 32].

To date there is no data available on prevalence in the Spanish university population, or regarding the possible relations with characteristics that appear in other EDs.

Therefore, the aims of this study were to estimate the prevalence rate of ON in a Spanish university population with a tool that has been validated for this purpose and to determine the possible correlation of ON with psychological and behavioral aspects that appear in other EDs. The present study has considered indicators which are commonly associated with EDs: the body mass index

(BMI) and sex, which will help us to clarify and further our understanding regarding this phenomenon.

Method
Study design and subjects
This cross-sectional study was planned and performed between January and May 2017, in Ciudad Real, Spain. We invited 800 university students from different faculties (Nursing, Law, Chemistry, Computer Science and Education), of which 454 university students participated (response rate: 56.75%) including 295 women and 159 men, aged between 18 and 51 years (mean age, 21.74 ± 4.73 years). The participants were recruited through informative talks delivered during university lectures in different faculties.

Data collection was performed via a questionnaire prepared by the researchers. The revised questionnaire was divided into three sections: (1) Sociodemographic characteristics; (2) the Eating Disorder Inventory-2 questionnaire (EDI-2) [33, 34]; and (3) the ORTO-11-ES [35, 36].

The University students voluntarily signed up to the study and they were asked to complete an online survey developed using the JotForm platform. It was assumed that the students who did not respond were within the same range of conditions as those who did. For ethical reasons, we were unable to research the causes which made these students decide not to participate.

Ethical considerations
The participants did not receive any financial incentive to take part in the study. Participants were informed that their information was to be kept confidential and would only be used for scientific purposes, obtaining the written informed consent of participants. The ethical committee of the Castilla-La Mancha University Hospital approved the study (Number C-45), according to the ethical principles for medical research gathered in the Declaration of Helsinki [37].

Measurements
Demographic information
The sociodemographic forms gathered information on the age, gender, height and weight of participants. The BMI of each participant was calculated based on the self-reported height and weight.

Eating disorder inventory (EDI-2)
This is a self-reported 91-item questionnaire, answered on a 6-point Likert-Type scale using a 3-point system where 'sometimes', 'rarely', and 'never', are assigned zeros while 'often', 'usually' and 'always' are assigned a score of 1, 2 and 3, respectively. The questionnaire is used to assess eating-disorder symptoms, attitudes and behaviors. It contains 11 subscales: drive for thinness, body satisfaction, bulimia, effectiveness, perfectionism, interpersonal disruption, interoceptive awareness, maturity fears, asceticism, impulse regulation and social insecurity. The sub-scale scores can be calculated by simply adding the scores of all the items of each specific sub-scale. The EDI-2 total score ranges from 91 to 546. We used a Spanish version of the scale validated by Corral, González, Pereña & Seis dedos (1998), which showed an internal consistency of 0.83–0.92 [34].

The EDI-2 is widely used in Spain and it has been demonstrated to be a valid instrument for the accurate diagnosis and detection of the risk of ED [38–40] in the Spanish population. We chose to use the EDI-2 based on its good psychometric properties, in both clinical settings and non-clinical samples [33] as well as the possibility it offers for separately assessing different dimensions [41].

ORTO-11- ES questionnaire
The ORTO-15 questionnaire was originally developed in Italian [11]. This tool consists of 15 self-report multiple-choice items using a 4-point Likert-type scale (always, often, sometimes, never) to measure three underlying factors related to eating behavior: cognitive-rational (items 1, 5, 6, 11, 12 and 14), clinical (items 3, 7, 8, 9 and 15) and emotional aspects (items 2, 4, 10 and 13). It is used to investigate obsessive behavior related to the selection, preparation, habits of food consumption and attitudes towards healthy food. The lower the score, the higher the indication of a behavior or attitude related to orthorexia. The Italian group [11] suggested a cut-off score of 40 points, whereby scores below this figure indicate ON related behavior.

For the present study, we have used the ORTO-11-ES [35] as a tool for assessing ON. This tool is based on a structure of three factors for the abbreviated 11-item version, and has demonstrated an appropriate internal consistency (Cronbach's alpha = 0.80). Furthermore, the test has demonstrated a good predictive capacity for a threshold value of < 25 (79.5% effectiveness, 75% sensitivity and specificity 79.6%).

Statistical analyses
An exploratory statistical analysis of all the demographic variables and the ON-tendencies was carried out. Quantitative features were described by the median and the inter-quartile range (IQR) and qualitative variables were described using frequencies and percentages.

To identify the score differences among the different groups (individuals with ON tendencies and individuals without ON tendencies) and without an assumption of normality for scores and small sample sizes ($N < 30$) for some of the subgroups, the Wilcoxon-Mann-Whitney

(W-M-N) and Kruskal-Wallis (K-W) tests for independent samples were performed.

For each feature (gender, smoker and BMI), the prevalence of ON was calculated as the proportion of individuals of a certain population that are under risk of suffering ON in this period.

This analysis has also been performed for each sub-scale of the Eating Disorder Inventory-2, i.e. for Drive for Thinness, Bulimia, Body Dissatisfaction, Ineffectiveness, Perfectionism, Interpersonal Distrust, Interoceptive Awareness, Maturity Fears, Asceticism, Impulse Regulation and Social Insecurity. Moreover, a correlation analysis was performed between the scores of the sub-scales of the EDI-2 and the scores of the ORTO-11-ES, using the Spearman coefficient.

The significance level was established at $p < .05$ for all cases. The R statistical software was used to perform all the statistical analyses [42].

Results

The sample included 454 students recruited from the Castilla-La Mancha University, and who voluntarily answered the questionnaire. A summary of the demographic variables is shown in Table 1.

The mean score obtained by the total participants regarding the ORTO-11-ES questionnaire was 27.78 and the standard deviation was ±3.34. The cut-off score was established at < 25 [35] ranging from 16 to 36 points, with 76 (17%) participants under risk of suffering ON.

The location parameter for the age, in those who were under a true risk of suffering ON, was not significantly different from those who were not under a real risk (W-M-N = 12,917, p = .16), neither was it significant for gender (W-M-N = 22,916, p = .69). The BMI variable was categorized into three groups, 1) below 18.5 (thinness); 2) 18.5, 24.9 (normal weight); 3) 25–41 (obesity). The differences of the ORTO-11-ES scores among the three groups were also non-significant (K-W $\chi2(2)$ = 1.9466 p = .38). On the other hand, statistical differences were found for smokers (W = 13,462, p = .00).

Table 1 Descriptive analysis of the sample

Qualitative variable		Frequency
Smoker	Yes	92 (20.30%)
	No	362 (79.70%)
Sex	Female	295 (65.00%)
	Male	159 (35.00%)
Marital Status	Single	444 (97.8%)
	Married	10 (2.20%)
Quantitative variable		Median (IQR)
Age		20.00 (19.00–22.00)
Body Mass Index		22.21 (20.31–24.50)

Prevalence and features of orthorexia nervosa

The prevalence of ON is significantly higher in women, as reported in the Italian population. [43]. There are no significant differences among the other groups. (See Table 2).

Concerning the ED, the analysis suggests that the individuals at risk of suffering ON have a higher prevalence rate of drive for thinness (17.1% vs 2.1%, $\chi2(1)$ = 32.22, p = .00), bulimia (2.6% vs 0%, $\chi2(1)$ = 9.99, p = .00), body dissatisfaction (26.3% vs. 12.4%, $\chi2(1)$ = 9.6, p = .00), perfectionism (14.5% vs 4.8%, $\chi2(1)$ = 9.98, p = .00), interoceptive awareness (13.2% vs 1.3%, $\chi2(1)$ = 27.74, p = .00), asceticism (15.8% vs 3.7%, $\chi2(1)$ = 17.12, p = .00) and impulse regulation (9.2% vs 1.9%, $\chi2(1)$ = 11.46, p = .00) than people who are not at a risk of suffering this disorder (see Table 3).

In addition, a correlation analysis of the ED sub-scale scores and the ON scores has been carried out (see Table 4). Due to the lack of normality in all the scores, the Spearman correlation coefficient was calculated. All of these tests were negative and statistically significant ($p < 0.05$). The negative sign indicates that, in general, high values of the ED subscales correspond to low values for the ON scores. The highest (negative) correlation coefficient (– 0.564, p = 0.00) was found between drive for thinness and the ON score.

Discussion and conclusion

The aim of the present study was to determine the prevalence of suffering ON and its possible relation with psychological and behavioral aspects of ED in a population of Spanish university students. We used the ORTO-11-ES [35], our findings reveal that 17% (76 students) of the sample presented a high risk of suffering from ON. This percentage is far from that obtained in the unique study on ON conducted on a sample of the Spanish population, where the results showed a prevalence of 86% [44]. However, this pilot study did not use a validated translation of the original ORTO-15 [11], rather it used the English version on a sample of 136 ex-students of Ashtanga yoga. Moreover, the age range of participants in the aforementioned study was higher than the age of university students [44]. Dunn et al. [45] found that 1.0% of students in

Table 2 Prevalence of Orthorexia for each feature

Feature	Prevalence of ON (%)	χ^2	DF	p-value
Male	11.9	4.03	1	**.04**
Female	19.3			
Smoker	18.0	1.89	1	.17
Non-smoker	12.0			
BMI: Thinness	25.0	1.95	2	.38
BMI: Normal weight	16.2			
BMI: Obesity	15.4			

Bold data indicates statistically significance ($p < .05$) indicated bold data

Table 3 Prevalence of eating disorders in a population at risk of ON and in a healthy population

Dimension EDI-2	Orthorexia Nervosa		χ^2	df	p-value
	Yes (%)	No (%)			
Drive for thinness	17.1	2.1	32.22	1	**.00**
Bulimia	2.6	0.0	9.99	1	**.00**
Body Dissatisfaction	26.3	12.4	9.69	1	**.00**
Ineffectiveness	9.2	4.0	3.77	1	.05
Perfectionism	14.5	4.8	9.98	1	**.00**
Interpersonal Distrust	6.6	8.7	0.38	1	.54
Interoceptive Awareness	13.2	1.3	27.74	1	**.00**
Maturity Fears	22.4	14.3	3.13	1	.08
Asceticism	15.8	3.7	17.12	1	**.00**
Impulse regulation	9.2	1.9	11.46	1	**.00**
Social Insecurity	11.8	8.5	0.88	1	.35

Bold data indicates statistically significance ($p < .05$) indicated bold data

the United States suffered from ON and suggested that 10.0% of the population was at risk of developing this disorder. In Italian populations, different studies place the prevalence of ON in a range of between 6.9 to 57.6% [25, 46]. In Turkey, a validated adaptation of this tool, the ORTO-11, showed a prevalence of approximately 45% in different studies with samples of university healthcare students [8, 13]. The greatest prevalence, 74.2%, was reported in a study conducted in Hungary, also using a translated and validated version of ORTO-11-Hu in a sample of university students [19]. Considering the varying results obtained across different countries, in part, some of these differences may be explained by socio-cultural factors, being closely related with the eating habits linked to the culture of each country [7, 47]. However, other authors attribute these differences to the structure of the questionnaire itself rather than cultural problems [48]. Furthermore, when interpreting these results, it is important to

Table 4 Correlation analysis of the EDI-2 sub-scales scores and the ON scores

Dimension EDI-2	Spearman coefficient	p-value
Drive for thinness	−0.564	0.00
Bulimia	−0.260	0.00
Body Dissatisfaction	−0.347	0.00
Ineffectiveness	−0.228	0.00
Perfectionism	−0.248	0.00
Interpersonal Distrust	−0.147	0.00
Interoceptive Awareness	−0.344	0.00
Maturity Fears	−0.113	0.02
Asceticism	−0.168	0.00
Impulse regulation	−0.210	0.00
Social Insecurity	−0.148	0.00

consider that the prevalence is linked to the interpretation of different versions of a self-reported questionnaire, which have used different cut-off points [11, 36, 49, 50] .

A significant correlation between ON and the psychopathological characteristics of other EDs, was observed based on the variables included in the EDI-2 subscales: drive for thinness, bulimia symptoms, body dissatisfaction, perfectionism, interoceptive awareness, asceticism and impulsiveness. These findings highlight the possible relation between the risk of suffering ON and the diagnosis of ED. Some of our results reinforce findings from previous studies [51, 52]. In a sample of 220 university students, Barnes et al. [51] concluded that there was a positive relation between ON and other ED, regarding the body image attitude and the perfectionist personality of these individuals. Also, having a personal history of having suffered an ED was found to be a strong predictor for ON. Another study, also along these lines, performed with 459 university students in the United States, showed a positive correlation between ON and perfectionism [52]. Two further clinical studies also highlighted the close relation between ED and ON [23, 53]. One of these, conducted in Germany with a sample of 1122 hospitalized patients with psychiatric diagnoses found positive correlations between ON and the dimensions drive for thinness, interoceptive awareness and asceticism in patients diagnosed with ED [53]. The second study was performed with another tool for the detection of ON: the Dußßdorfer Orthorexie "DOS" scale [23]. This study included a sample of 1340 participants and found positive correlations with the EDI-2 subscales of thinness, bulimia and body dissatisfaction, suggesting proximity between ON and ED [23]. Currently, there is much debate surrounding the relationship between AN and ON, ranging from how to classify and differentiate these disorders, in some cases considering ON as a new disorder, or a subset of AN [53]. It is well known that undertaking weight-loss diets can lead certain individuals towards adopting extreme eating habits. There is a large coincidence between supposedly 'healthy' foods and generally 'slimming' foods which can lead individuals towards a confusion that is difficult to manage [23]. At times, this may lead to an obsession with healthy eating, until individuals adopt a more severe pathology, such as AN [17]. On the other hand, the opposite hypothesis can lead us to affirm that an orthorexic behavior can be interpreted as a phase or a tendency in patients who have been previously diagnosed with ED and are in a recovery phase, and who, displaying an improvement of symptoms, can end up developing orthorexic behaviors [18, 41]. These findings emphasize how concerns regarding healthy eating can act as a predisposing factor for developing AN or Bulimia nervosa (BN), and as a key residual symptom which may potentially favor relapses of the illness [54, 55]. Only with further research studies on clinical samples can we reveal the relationship between these two pathologies, and determine whether ON may be a factor that predicts the development of AN or viceversa.

Another aim of our study was to explore the relationship of ON with variables such as gender, age, weight, and body mass index. We found significant differences for the mean score on the ORTO-11-ES [35] scale in the female population. If we compare this with other studies, this result is striking as in most studies no differences were found regarding gender [8, 44, 52, 56]. In the study by Donini et al., they concluded that men are more sensitive to suffering from this problem [11]. This result has been repeated in one other study performed on a sample of Turkish students [13, 25]. However, there are other studies, which, like ours, report a greater proportion of women at risk of developing ON [7, 13, 57]. Although the gender difference of ON is harder to detect, in part, due to the lack of research in clinically diagnosed individuals [58], undoubtedly, gender is a critical factor in many aspects of life, including the attitudes and perceptions of one's body image [59]. Indeed, there are a series of characteristics related to the internalization and externalization of emotions which may explain the different prevalence rates by gender in many mental illnesses [60].

Regarding the BMI, our results failed to find a significant correlation of the same with ON, a finding that supports most previous studies performed in different populations [56, 61]. In a study conducted by Aksoydan et al. in a population of 94 Turkish artists, no differences were found between the mean ORTO-15 score and the BMI [56]. Also, another study performed in Poland with 400 participants aged between 18 and 35 years failed to find a significant correlation with the BMI [61]. Varga et al. found that the association between the ON scores and the BMI was statistically significant, albeit insignificant [19]. Some authors suggest that the BMI can predict orthorexic behaviors in combination with other variables such as medical reasons, diet and healthy nutrition [7]. In contrast, another study also performed in Turkey on 878 medical students with a mean age of 21.3 ± 2.1 years found that, as the BMI increased, the ON score decreased, and, therefore, the risk of orthorexia nervosa increased [27]. Some authors justify this on the basis that overweight and obesity can expose the individual to humiliation and force the person to diet and consume healthy foods [13] .

Although this study is one of the first to examine the prevalence of ON in Spain, there are several limitations worth considering. First, the results do not provide information on the mechanisms that underlie the relationship between ON and EBD; for example, by considering other underlying factors such as biological factors, and personality, which could contribute to the high concurrence of these behaviors. Due to the cross-sectional design of this study, we cannot determine the time course of the development of EDs and ON. Therefore, by considering ON as a potential risk factor for developing an ED, a more complete longitudinal study is necessary in the future. Despite these limitations, the current study focuses on a gap in the literature regarding ON and EBD, broadly demonstrating the relationship between these.

Our results highlight the long path ahead for the scientific community, in order to recognize that ON can be included as another diagnosis within eating disorders. Additional studies are needed to describe the behavior of people with orthorexia (i.e. their etiology, diagnosis, treatment and the prevention of the same). On the other hand, studies on these subjects provide the health professional with the information necessary to be able to identify individuals with orthorexic behavior and thus provide appropriate treatment to derive the patient towards the most appropriate resource.

Abbreviations

AN: Anorexia nervosa; BMI: Body mass index; BN: Bulimia nervosa; DOS: Düsseldorf Orthorexie Skala; DSM-5: Diagnostic and statistical manual of mental disorders; ED: Eating disorder; EDI-2: Eating Disorder Inventory; ICD-10: International Classification of Diseases; IQR: Inter-quartile range; OCD: Obsessive compulsive disorders; ON: Orthorexia nervosa; ORTO-11-ES: Spanish version Test for the diagnosis of Orthorexia nervosa; ORTO-15: Test for the diagnosis of orthorexia

Acknowledgements

The authors thank the students who took part in this study and generously granted us their time and provided us details about their experiences in clinical practice.

Funding

The authors did not receive any funding for this paper.

Authors' contributions

Study conception and design: P-F ML, R-C T, O-Z MD, F- M E, N-P B. Data collection, statistical expertise, analysis and interpretation of data: P-H MJ, C-A V, P-F ML, O-Z MD. Manuscript preparation, supervision, administrative support and critical revision of the paper. P-F ML, R-C T, O-Z MD, F- M E, N-P B. All authors read and approved the final manuscript.

Consent for publication

"Not applicable"

Competing interests

The authors declare that they have no competing interests.

Author details
[1]Faculty of Nursing , University of Castilla-La-Mancha, Ciudad Real, Spain.
[2]Head of Mental Health, Castilla la Mancha Health Services, Ciudad Real,
Spain. [3]Biostatech Advice, Training and Innovation in Biostatistics, S.L
Santiago de Compostela, A Coruña, Spain. [4]School of Industrial Engineers,
University of Castilla-La Mancha, Ciudad Real, Spain. [5]Faculty of Nursing,
University of Castilla-La-Mancha, Cuenca, Spain.

References
1. American Psychiatric Association. Guía de consulta de los criterios
    diagnósticos del DSM-5® [Internet]. American Psychiatric Publishing; 2013.
2. Bratman S. Health food junkie. Bratman S Heal Food Junkie Yoga J. 1997:
    42–50 Available: https://www.google.es/?gws_rd=ssl.
3. Brytek-Matera A. Orthorexia nervosa-an eating disorder, obsessive-
    compulsive disorder or disturbed eating habit? Arch Psychiatry Psychother.
    2012;1:55–60.
4. Moroze RM, Dunn TM, Craig Holland J, Yager J, Weintraub P. Microthinking
    about micronutrients: a case of transition from obsessions about healthy
    eating to near-fatal "orthorexia nervosa" and proposed diagnostic criteria.
    Psychosomatics. 2015. https://doi.org/10.1016/j.psym.2014.03.003.
5. Dunn TM, Bratman S. On orthorexia nervosa: a review of the literature and
    proposed diagnostic criteria. Eat Behav. 2016;21:11–7. https://doi.org/10.
    1016/j.eatbeh.2015.12.006.
6. World Health Organization. The ICD-10 classification of mental and
    behavioural disorders : clinical descriptions and diagnostic guidelines.
    [Internet]. World Health. Organization; 1992. Available: www.who.int/
    classifications/icd/en/.
7. Arusoğlu G, Kabakçi E, Köksal G, Merdol TK. Orthorexia nervosa and
    adaptation of ORTO-11 into Turkish. Turk Psikiyatri Derg. 2008;19: 283–91.
    Available. http://www.ncbi.nlm.nih.gov/pubmed/18791881.
8. Tuïay Bag˘ Ci Bosi A, Derya C-A, Atay Guïer C-A. Prevalence of
    orthorexia nervosa in resident medical doctors in the faculty of
    medicine (Ankara, Turkey). Appetite. 2007;49: 661–666.
    doi:https://doi.org/10.1016/j.appet.2007.04.007
9. Kinzl JF, Hauer K, Traweger C, Kiefer I. Orthorexia nervosa in
    dieticians. Psychother Psychosom Karger Publishers. 2006;75:395–6.
    https://doi.org/10.1159/000095447.
10. Mathieu J. What is orthorexia? J am diet Assoc. Elsevier. 2005;105:1510–2.
    https://doi.org/10.1016/J.JADA.2005.08.021.
11. Donini LM, Marsili D, Graziani MP, Imbriale M, Cannella C. Orthorexia
    nervosa: validation of a diagnosis questionnaire. Eat Weight Disord. 2005;10.
    https://doi.org/10.1007/BF03327537.
12. Bartrina AJ. Ortorexia o la obsesion por la dieta saludable. Arch Latinoam
    Nutr. 2007;57:313–5 Available: https://www.alanrevista.org/ediciones/2007/4/
    art-2/.
13. Fidan T, Ertekin V, Işikay S, Kirpinar I. Prevalence of orthorexia among
    medical students in Erzurum. Turkey Compr Psychiatry. 2010;51:49–54.
    https://doi.org/10.1016/j.comppsych.2009.03.001.
14. Kummer A, Dias FMV, Teixeira AL. On the concept of orthorexia nervosa:
    letter to the editor. Scand J Med Sci Sport. 2008;18:395–6. https://doi.org/10.
    1111/j.1600-0838.2008.00809.x
15. Gramaglia C, Brytek-Matera A, Rogoza R, Zeppegno P. Orthorexia and
    anorexia nervosa: two distinct phenomena? A cross-cultural comparison of
    orthorexic behaviours in clinical and non-clinical samples. BMC Psychiatry.
    BioMed Central. 2017;17:75. https://doi.org/10.1186/s12888-017-1241-2.
16. Brytek-Matera A, Donini LM, Krupa M, Poggiogalle E, Hay P. Orthorexia
    nervosa and self-attitudinal aspects of body image in female and male
    university students. J Eat Disord. 2015;3:2. https://doi.org/10.1186/
    s40337-015-0038-2.
17. Vandereycken W. Media hype, diagnostic fad or genuine disorder?
    Professionals' opinions about night eating syndrome, orthorexia, muscle
    dysmorphia, and emetophobia. Eat Disord. 2011;19:145–55. https://doi.org/
    10.1080/10640266.2011.551634.
18. Segura-Garcia C, Ramacciotti C, Rania M, Aloi M, Caroleo M, Bruni A, et al. The
    prevalence of orthorexia nervosa among eating disorder patients after
    treatment. Eat Weight Disord. 2015. https://doi.org/10.1007/s40519-014-0171-y.
19. Varga M, Thege BK, Dukay-Szabó S, Túry F, van Furth EF, Bratman S, et al.
    When eating healthy is not healthy: orthorexia nervosa and its

    measurement with the ORTO-15 in Hungary. BMC Psychiatry. BioMed
    Central. 2014;14:59. https://doi.org/10.1186/1471-244X-14-59.
20. Varga M, Dukay-Szabó S, Túry F, van Furth EF, van Furth Eric F. Evidence
    and gaps in the literature on orthorexia nervosa. Eat Weight Disord. 2013;18:
    103–11. https://doi.org/10.1007/s40519-013-0026-y.
21. Dell'Osso L, Carpita B, Gesi C, Cremone IM, Corsi M, Massimetti E, et al.
    Subthreshold autism spectrum disorder in patients with eating disorders.
    Compr Psychiatry WB Saunders. 2018;81:66–72. https://doi.org/10.1016/J.
    COMPPSYCH.2017.11.007.
22. Pini S, Abelli M, Carpita B, Dell'Osso L, Castellini G, Carmassi C, et al. Historical
    evolution of the concept of anorexia nervosa and relationships with orthorexia
    nervosa, autism, and obsessive-compulsive spectrum. Neuropsychiatr Dis Treat.
    2016;12:1651–60. https://doi.org/10.2147/NDT.S108912.
23. Barthels F, Meyer F, Pietrowsky R. Die Düsseldorfer Orthorexie Skala–
    Konstruktion und Evaluation eines Fragebogens zur Erfassung ortho-
    rektischen Ernährungsverhaltens. Z Klin Psychol Psychother. 2015;44:97–105.
    https://doi.org/10.1026/1616-3443/a000310.
24. Bauer SM, Fusté A, Andrés A, Saldaña C. The Barcelona Orthorexia Scale
    (BOS): development process using the Delphi method. Eating and Weight
    Disorders. 3 Aug 2018. https://doi.org/10.1007/s40519-018-0556-4
25. Donini LM, Marsili D, Graziani MP, Imbriale M, Cannella C. Orthorexia
    nervosa: a preliminary study with a proposal for diagnosis and an attempt
    to measure the dimension of the phenomenon. Eat Weight Disord. 2004;9:
    151–7. https://doi.org/10.1007/BF03325060.
26. Depa J, Schweizer J, Bekers S-K, Hilzendegen C, Stroebele-Benschop N.
    Prevalence and predictors of orthorexia nervosa among German students
    using the 21-item-DOS. Bulim Obes: Eat Weight Disord - Stud Anorexia;
    2016. https://doi.org/10.1007/s40519-016-0334-0.
27. Asil E, Sürücüoğlu MS. Orthorexia nervosa in Turkish dietitians. Ecol Food
    Nutr. 2015;54:303–13. https://doi.org/10.1080/03670244.2014.987920.
28. Cervera Burriel F, Serrano Urrea R, Vico García C, Milla Tobarra M, García
    Meseguer MJ. Hábitos alimentarios y evaluación nutricional en una
    población universitaria. Nutr Hosp. Grupo Arán S.L. 2013;28:438–46. https://
    doi.org/10.3305/NH.2013.28.2.6303.
29. Sánchez Socarrás V, Aguilar Martínez A. Food habits and health-related
    behaviors in a university population. Nutr Hosp. 2014;31:449–57. https://doi.
    org/10.3305/nh.2015.31.1.7412.
30. Nelson MC, Story M, Larson NI, Neumark-Sztainer D, Lytle LA. Emerging
    adulthood and college-aged youth: an overlooked age for weight-related
    behavior change. Obesity. 2008;16:2205–11. https://doi.org/10.1038/oby.
    2008.365.
31. Becker AE, Franko DL, Nussbaum K, Herzog DB. Secondary prevention for
    eating disorders: the impact of education, screening, and referral in a
    college-based screening program. Int J Eat Disord. 2004;36:157–62. https://
    doi.org/10.1002/eat.20023.
32. Tavolacci MP, Grigioni S, Richard L, Meyrignac G, Déchelotte P, Ladner J.
    Eating Disorders and Associated Health Risks Among University Students. J
    Nutr Educ Behav. Elsevier. 2015;47:412–420.e1. https://doi.org/10.1016/J.
    JNEB.2015.06.009.
33. Garner D. Eating Disorder Inventory –2,EDI-2.Proffesional Manual. odessa:
    Psychological Assessment. Resources. 1991.
34. Corral S, González M, Pereña J SN. Adaptación española del Inventario de
    trastornos de la conducta alimentaria. EDI-2: Inventario de Trastornos de la
    Conducta Alimentaria. [Internet]. Madrid:TEA; 1998.
35. Parra-Fernandez ML, Rodríguez-Cano T, Onieva-Zafra MD, Perez-Haro MJ,
    Casero-Alonso V, Muñoz Camargo JC, et al. Adaptation and validation of the
    Spanish version of the ORTO-15 questionnaire for the diagnosis of
    orthorexia nervosa. Manalo E, editor. PLoS One. 2018;13: e0190722. https://
    doi.org/10.1371/journal.pone.0190722
36. Parra-Fernandez ML, Rodríguez-Cano T, Perez-Haro MJ, Onieva-Zafra MD,
    Fernandez-Martinez E, Notario-Pacheco B. Structural validation of ORTO-11-ES for
    the diagnosis of orthorexia nervosa. Bulim Obes: Spanish version. Eat Weight
    Disord - Stud Anorexia; 2018. https://doi.org/10.1007/s40519-018-0573-3.
37. Declaración de Helsinki - WMA - The World Medical Association [Internet].
    [cited 26 Feb 2018]. Available: https://www.wma.net/what-we-do/medical-
    ethics/declaration-of-helsinki/
38. Castro-Zamudio S, Castro-Barea J. Impulsividad y búsqueda de sensaciones:
    factores asociados a síntomas de anorexia y bulimia nerviosas en
    estudiantes de secundaria. Escritos Psicol / Psychol Writings Escritos de
    Psicologia. 2016;9:22–30. https://doi.org/10.5231/psy.writ.2016.2706.

Prevalence of orthorexia nervosa in university students and its relationship with psychopathological...

31

39. Rojo-Moreno L, Iranzo-Tatay C, Gimeno-Clemente N, Barber-Fons MA, Rojo-Bofill LM, Livianos-Aldana L. Genetic and environmental influences on psychological traits and eating attitudes in a sample of Spanish schoolchildren. Rev Psiquiatr y Salud Ment (English Ed. Elsevier). 2017. https://doi.org/10.1016/j.rpsmen.2017.05.006.

40. Fernández-Delgado A, Jáuregui-Lobera I. Variables Psicológicas Y psicopatológicas Asociadas a los trastornos de la conducta alimentaria (TCA) Variables psicológicas y psicopatológicas asociadas con trastornos de la alimentación (ED). J Negat No Posit Results. 2016;1:71–80 Available: http://revistas.proeditio.com/jonnpr/article/view/1011/pdf1011.

41. Barthels F, Meyer F, Huber T, Pietrowsky R. Orthorexic eating behaviour as a coping strategy in patients with anorexia nervosa, Eat Weight Disord - Stud Anorexia, Bulim Obes. Springer International Publishing. 2016:1–8. https://doi.org/10.1007/s40519-016-0329-x.

42. Rosseel Y. lavaan: An R Package for Structural Equation Modeling. J Stat Softw. 2012;48:1–36. https://doi.org/10.18637/jss.v048.i02.

43. Dell'Osso L, Abelli M, Carpita B, Massimetti G, Pini S, Rivetti L, et al. Orthorexia nervosa in a sample of Italian university population. Riv Psichiatr. 51:190–6. https://doi.org/10.1708/2476.25888.

44. Herranz Valera J, Acuña Ruiz P, Romero Valdespino B, Visioli F. Prevalence of orthorexia nervosa among ashtanga yoga practitioners: a pilot study. Eat Weight Disord - Stud Anorexia, Bulim Obes. 2014;19:469–72. https://doi.org/10.1007/s40519-014-0131-6.

45. Dunn TM, Gibbs J, Whitney N, Starosta A. Prevalence of orthorexia nervosa is less than 1%: data from a US sample. Eat Weight Disord. 2016;22:185–92. https://doi.org/10.1007/s40519-016-0258-8.

46. Bo S, Zoccali R, Ponzo V, Soldati L, De Carli L, Benso A, et al. University courses, eating problems and muscle dysmorphia: are there any associations? J Transl Med. 2014;12:221. https://doi.org/10.1186/s12967-014-0221-2.

47. Varga M, Dukay-Szabo S, Túry F. orthorexia nervosa and it's background factors. Ideggyogy Sz, Available. 2013;66:220–7 http://www.ncbi.nlm.nih.gov/pubmed/23971352.

48. Missbach B, Hinterbuchinger B, Dreiseitl V, Zellhofer S, Kurz C, König J. When Eating Right, Is Measured Wrong! A Validation and Critical Examination of the ORTO-15 Questionnaire in German. Manalo E, editor. PLoS One. 2015;10: e0135772. https://doi.org/10.1371/journal.pone.0135772

49. Hyrnik J, Janas-Kozik M, Stochel M, Jelonek I, Siwiec A, Rybakowski JK. The assessment of orthorexia nervosa among 1899 polish adolescents using the ORTO-15 questionnaire. Int J Psychiatry Clin Pract. 2016;20:199–203. https://doi.org/10.1080/13651501.2016.1197271.

50. Ramacciotti CE, Perrone P, Coli E, Burgalassi A, Conversano C, Massimetti G, et al. Orthorexia nervosa in the general population: a preliminary screening using a self-administered questionnaire (ORTO-15). Eat weight Disord, Available. 2011;16:e127–30 http://www.ncbi.nlm.nih.gov/pubmed/21989097.

51. Barnes MA, Caltabiano ML. The interrelationship between orthorexia nervosa, perfectionism, body image and attachment style. Eat weight Disord - stud anorexia, Bulim Obes. Springer International Publishing. 2017; 22:177–84. https://doi.org/10.1007/s40519-016-0280-x.

52. Oberle CD, Samaghabadi RO, Hughes EM. Orthorexia nervosa: assessment and correlates with gender, BMI, and personality. Appetite Academic Press. 2017;108:303–10. https://doi.org/10.1016/J.APPET.2016.10.021.

53. Andreas S, Schedler K, Schulz H, Nutzinger DO. Evaluation of a German version of a brief diagnosis questionnaire of symptoms of orthorexia nervosa in patients with mental disorders (Ortho-10). Eat weight Disord - stud anorexia, Bulim Obes. Springer International Publishing. 2018;23:75–85. https://doi.org/10.1007/s40519-017-0473-y.

54. Koven NS, Abry AW. The clinical basis of orthorexia nervosa: emerging perspectives. Neuropsychiatr Dis Treat Dove Press. 2015;11:385–94. https://doi.org/10.2147/NDT.S61665.

55. Dell'Osso L, Carpita B, Muti D, Cremone IM, Massimetti G, Diadema E, et al. Prevalence and characteristics of orthorexia nervosa in a sample of university students in Italy. Eat Weight Disord - Stud Anorexia, Bulim Obes. Springer International Publishing. 2017:1–11. https://doi.org/10.1007/s40519-017-0460-3.

56. Aksoydan E, Camci N. Prevalence of orthorexia nervosa among Turkish performance artists. Eat Weight Disord. 2009;14:33–7 doi:6158 [pii].

57. Koven NS, Senbonmatsu R. A neuropsychological evaluation of orthorexia nervosa. Open J Psychiatry Scientific Research Publishing. 2013;03:214–22. https://doi.org/10.4236/ojpsych.2013.32019.

58. Brytek-Matera A, Rogoza R, Gramaglia C, Zeppegno P. Predictors of orthorexic behaviours in patients with eating disorders: a preliminary study. BMC Psychiatry. BioMed Central. 2015;15:252. https://doi.org/10.1186/s12888-015-0628-1.

59. Blashill AJ. Gender roles, eating pathology, and body dissatisfaction in men: a meta-analysis. Body Image. 2011;8:1–11. https://doi.org/10.1016/J.bodyim.2010.09.002.

60. Wills TA, Simons JS, Sussman S, Knight R. Emotional self-control and dysregulation: a dual-process analysis of pathways to externalizing/internalizing symptomatology and positive well-being in younger adolescents. Drug Alcohol Depend Elsevier. 2016;163:S37–45. https://doi.org/10.1016/J.DRUGALCDEP.2015.08.039.

61. Brytek-Matera A, Krupa M, Poggiogalle E, Donini LM. Adaptation of the ORTHO-15 test to polish women and men. Eat Weight Disord. 2014;19:69–76. https://doi.org/10.1007/s40519-014-0100-0.

5

BEATVIC, a body-oriented resilience therapy using kickboxing exercises for people with a psychotic disorder

Bertine de Vries[1*], Elisabeth C. D. van der Stouwe[2,3], Clement O. Waarheid[4], Stefan H. J. Poel[4], Erwin M. van der Helm[5], André Aleman[1,3], Johan Arends[4], Gerdina H. M. Pijnenborg[1,4] and Jooske T. van Busschbach[2,6]

Abstract

Background: People with a psychotic disorder have an increased risk of becoming the victim of a crime. To prevent victimization a body-oriented resilience therapy using kickboxing exercises was developed. This study aims to explore the feasibility of the therapy, to improve the therapy protocol and to explore suitable outcomes for a RCT.

Methods: Twenty-four adults with a psychotic disorder received 20 weekly group sessions in which potential risk factors for victimization and strategies for dealing with them were addressed. Sessions were evaluated weekly. During pre and post assessment participants completed questionnaires on, among other, victimization, aggression regulation and social functioning.

Results: The short recruitment period indicates the interest in such an intervention and the willingness of clients to participate. Mean attendance was 85.3 and 88% of the participants completed fifteen or more sessions. The therapy protocol was assessed as adequate and exercises as relevant with some small improvements to be made. The victimization and aggression regulation questionnaires were found to be suitable outcome measurements for a subsequent RCT.

Conclusion: The results support the feasibility of the BEATVIC therapy. Participants subjectively evaluated the intervention as helpful in their attempt to gain more self-esteem and assertiveness. With some minor changes in the protocol the effects of BEATVIC can be tested in a RCT.

Keywords: Psychotic disorder, Psychomotor, Nonverbal therapy, Kickboxing, Victimization, Assertiveness, Social cognition, Self-esteem

Background

With psychotic disorder having a median global prevalence of 4.6 per 1000 persons [1], and this leading to a four to six times higher risk of becoming a victim of a crime [2, 3], the prevention of victimization in these already vulnerable people is an important public health concern [4]. However, currently there is no evidence-based intervention which aims to decrease the risk of victimization for people with a psychotic disorder.

To prevent victimization of people with a psychotic disorder, a body-oriented resilience therapy with kickboxing exercises was developed, henceforward referred to as BEATVIC [5]. This therapy is based on principles of what is called body-oriented psychotherapy in Anglo Saxon countries [6], or what in European countries is referred to as psychomotor therapy (PMT) [7]. PMT is an experience-based approach, which combines physical activity with body and emotional awareness [8].

* Correspondence: bertine.de.vries@gmail.com
[1]Department of clinical psychology and experimental psychopathology, faculty of behavioral and social sciences, University of Groningen, Grote Kruisstraat 2/1, 9712 TS Groningen, Netherlands
Full list of author information is available at the end of the article

The intervention addresses several important risk factors that are assumed to be associated with victimization in individuals with a psychotic disorder, and which are amenable to change (see Fig. 1). First of all, social cognitive impairments are common in people with a psychotic disorder and may lead to difficulties in social functioning [9, 10] which is associated with victimization [11]. Another potential risk factor is poor insight. A lack of clinical and/or cognitive insight is associated with aggressive behaviour [12], which itself could elicit aggression in others [13], leading indirectly to victimization. Accordingly, another factor that is addressed in BEATVIC concerns problems in aggression regulation. Self-stigma, e.g. as a result of earlier victimization [14] could result in low self-efficacy [15], low self-esteem and reduced empowerment [16]. Consequently, people may experience difficulties standing up for themselves in social situations which makes them more prone to become victimized [17]. For people with psychosis, as for anyone else, the traumatic experience of being a victim may lead to hyper arousal including an increased physiological arousal [18] and emotion dysregulation. This could impair the ability to adequately detect or respond to risks and for this reason it may be associated with revictimization [19]. Victimized people often get revictimized, suggesting a vicious cycle, which is included in the model as well. For a more comprehensive explanation of risk factors see an earlier published paper [5].

A suitable intervention should address several of the suggested risk factors and encompass ways to deal with the underlying deficits and inadequate responses. From this perspective BEATVIC was developed. In this psychomotor intervention, positive effects of physical exercise (e.g. improve physical and psychological functioning) [20, 21], were combined with those of assertiveness training (e.g. increase self-esteem, assertiveness) [22, 23] and martial arts (e.g. positive effect on aggression regulation, empowerment and social interactions) [24–26]. To provide an activating, challenging and possibly destigmatizing context kickboxing was used as the basic form of exercise.

The current feasibility study was set up in preparation for a multicentre randomized controlled trial (RCT), aimed at investigating the effectiveness of BEATVIC. The aim of the current study was threefold: (1) to explore the feasibility of the intervention and application of a RCT; (2) to improve the intervention protocol; (3) to explore suitable outcome measures for a possible subsequent RCT.

Methods

This feasibility study had a pretest-posttest quasi-experimental design without a control group.

Participants

Twenty-four participants were recruited from five teams from both in- and outpatient facilities of the department of psychotic disorders of GGZ-Drenthe in Assen, in the Netherlands. In order to be eligible to participate in this study, the participants had to meet the following criteria: (1) a diagnosis in the psychotic spectrum according to DSM-IV-TR criteria, verified by the Mini-SCAN; (2) age of 18 years or older; (3) ability to give informed consent. Exclusion criteria were as follows: (1) PANSS mean positive symptoms ≥5; (2) substance dependence (not substance abuse), verified by Mini-SCAN; (3) IQ < 70,

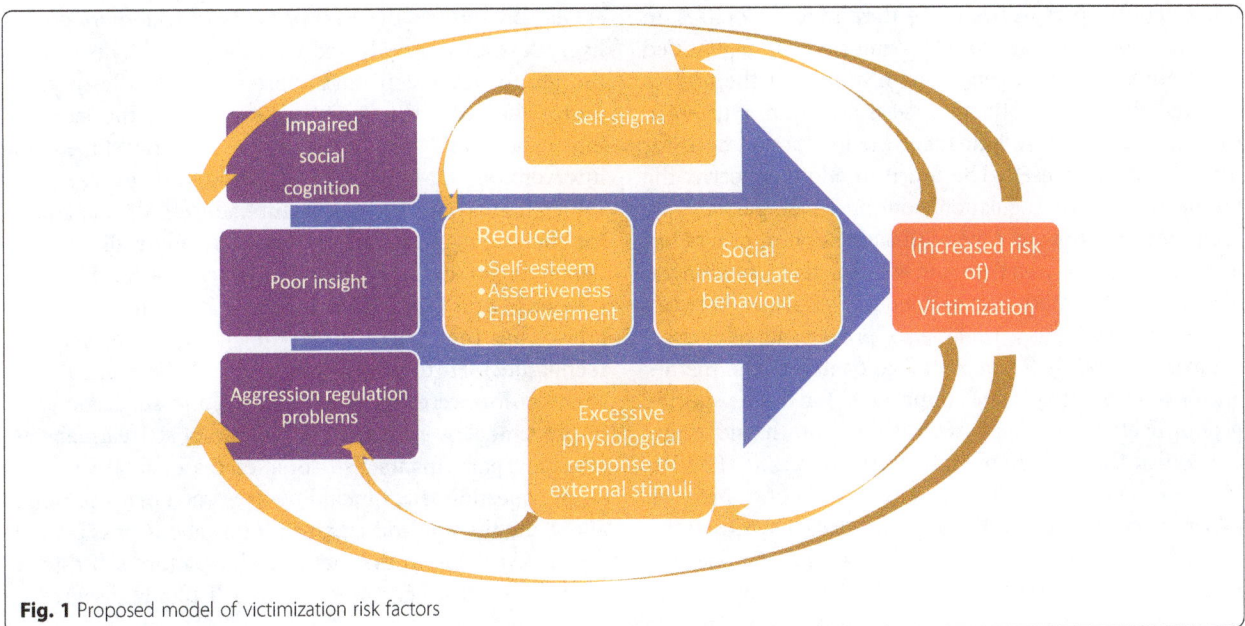

Fig. 1 Proposed model of victimization risk factors

estimated by the onsite therapist who was treating the client; (4) pregnancy; (5) co-morbid personality disorder or co-morbid neurological disorder, both verified by onsite therapist.

Procedure

Eligible clients were initially informed about the intervention by their case managers or clinicians. Subsequently, the research team provided interested clients with more information by telephone, mail and/or through open information meetings. After two weeks clients were contacted again for their final decision. When they agreed to participate, a screening interview was planned to obtain written informed consent and to assess whether the study criteria were met. Three therapy groups of eight participants each were scheduled. Before and after BEATVIC pre and post assessments were performed.

Intervention

BEATVIC consists of 20 weekly group sessions of 75 minutes. All sessions are led by a psychomotor therapist and an expert by experience. The intervention contains five modules each targeting specific risk factors (see Fig. 1). Every session starts with a warming-up followed by kickboxing exercises and one or two thematic (kickboxing) exercises. The first module focusses on self-stigma and is an introductory module during which participants get to know each other and are introduced to kickboxing techniques. The focus of the second module, entitled "recognizing dangerous behaviour", lies on social cognition and participants practice identifying threatening non-verbal signals. They are stimulated to share and verify their own perception of situations and to consider other people's perspectives. The third module focuses on insight and again on social cognition and is entitled "how others see me": people learn to look at themselves through the eyes of others. Special attention is given to the way body posture influences the interaction both for others and for oneself. The fourth module concerns the theme "aggression regulation", during which participants learn not only how to cope with aggression of others but also to recognize, regulate and control their own anger. The aim of this module is to adequately balance between improving resilience, while also preventing aggressive behaviour. Module five repeats and combines the themes and exercises that were important for each specific group. Each session ends with cooling-down and a discussion of the risk factors that were addressed. The latter will help people to make a connection between experiences during the therapy and daily life situations. In addition, after and during each session the participants check their arousal level and do a calming breathing exercise. Furthermore, participants are stimulated to continue kickboxing or to engage in other sports after the intervention. A group visit to a training center in the region and/or a guest lesson from a local trainer are offered to facilitate this.

Measures
Screening interview

During the screening interview the DSM diagnosis and the absence of alcohol and drug addiction were verified by the *mini Schedules for Clinical Assessment in Neuropsychiatry* (miniSCAN; 2011 Dutch version) [27]. The *Positive and Negative Syndrome Scale (PANSS)*, which consists of a 30 item rating scale based on a semi-structured interview, was administered during pre and post assessment, first to verify the absence of florid psychosis and, second as an outcome measure indicating the change in severity of the symptoms [28]. Finally, demographic variables including gender, age, family contact, living situation and daily activities were collected.

Feasibility of the intervention and application of an RCT

To gain knowledge about the feasibility of the intervention, the willingness of the therapists to refer participants and the willingness of the clients to participate were explored. In a logbook adherence, drop-outs and time schedules were registered. After each session and during the final evaluation, trainers and participants were asked whether they observer or experienced any adverse events at home or during a session, this was also registered in a logbook. In addition, the clinicians and case managers were asked to report possible negative side effect of the intervention in their client.

Evaluation and improvement of the intervention protocol

Every session was evaluated with the participants (during the group discussion) and subsequently by the psychomotor therapist, the expert by experience, the kickboxing expert and the researchers who developed the intervention. All exercises were reviewed with regard to the content (were the risk factors addressed?), suitability for the target group (e.g. mentally or physically not too demanding?), arousal levels (was stress increased or decreased?), and learning curve (how often should the exercise be repeated before the group managed the technique?). Furthermore, outcomes of the evaluation of each session were registered in a log and suggestions for improvement were discussed. In the post treatment assessment participants also completed a qualitative evaluation questionnaire including eleven open questions about the therapy and eighteen items about possible outcomes (e.g. 'Due to the therapy: I have more self-esteem', 'I can prevent a fight', rated from 1 'I totally disagree' to 7 I totally agree).

Exploration of outcome measures

In general, the aim of a feasibility study was to explore some of the important outcome measures for the RCT, not to test all risk factors as the effect on those will be investigated in the RCT [29]. In our study two different victimization and perpetration questionnaires were explored, as well as one questionnaire on social behaviour and two on aggression regulation.

Victimization and perpetration

Three subscales of the *Dutch crime and victimization survey* (Integrale veiligheidsmonitor IVM [30], an adaptation of the international crime and victimization survey, were used: personal crimes, property crimes and perpetration.

For comparison, there is IVM data available on 1729 people from the general population who live in the same region as the study participants and who were interviewed at the time of this study [30]. While the IVM has been used in large surveys with people with Severe Mental Illness [31] and in studies with people with psychosis [14] no psychometric information is available. However, there are no indications of invalidity of the response in these groups. Since the examined time period is one to 5 years, the instrument was not thought to be sensitive to changes over the intervention period of 5 months. Moreover, as the incidence of crime is low, in this feasibility study no changes in victimization were expected after the intervention period. Therefore, the IVM was not included in the post measurement.

The revised *Conflict Tactics Scale (CTS2)* [32], assesses whether a respondent was involved in various types of psychological or physical conflicts and their reactions. The following subscales are distinguished: psychological aggression, physical assault, sexual coercion, physical injury and negotiation. Since victims not always see themselves as having experienced abuse, participants are asked not about attitudes, emotions and cognitive behaviours, but to indicate whether 39 forms of conflict related behaviours applied to themselves or their partner in a given time period. In our study we were interested in a broader range of social interactions and thus changed the word 'partner' to 'someone'. Besides the prevalence, it is possible to calculate the frequency (or chronicity) in which an incident occurs. Frequency was categorized as once, twice, 3–5, 6–10, 11–20 or > 20 times in the previous 5 months [33]. As the CTS2 measures more subtle forms of victimization than the IVM, prevalence rates were calculated at baseline and the frequency of incidents at both pre and post measurement were used to explore possible changes. The internal consistency, reliability and construct validity of the CTS2 is good [32].

Social behaviour

The Inventory of Interpersonal Situations (IIS) measures social anxiety [34]. Respondents need to report on the frequency of occurrence and the level of discomfort they experience in 35 different social situations, ranging from 1 'no discomfort' to 5 'very much discomfort'. Five subscales are distinguished: giving criticism, expressing opinions, giving compliments, initiating contacts, and positive self-evaluation. This questionnaire has been proven to be sensitive to change in social anxiety resulting from social interventions for people with a severe mental illness [35] and the reliability and validity are good [34]. The ISS has a Dutch norm group from the general population (n = 580) and the scaled scores are divided on a 7-point scale ranging from 'very low' to 'very high' [36].

Aggression regulation

To assess aggression regulation we used the Dutch translation of The *State Trait Anger Expression Inventory (STAXI)* [37]. This instrument measures to what extent participants internalize or externalize feelings of anger and assesses their control over expression and containment of these feelings of anger. Participants respond by rating 40 items on a scale ranging from 1 'almost never' to 4 'almost always'. The STAXI has been proven to be sensitive to changes in aggression regulation resulting from a dance/movement therapy in people with schizophrenia [38], has good to high psychometric properties [39]. The STAXI has a Dutch norm group from het general population (n = 464) [40],

The *Novaco Anger Scale-Provocation Inventory (NAS-PI)* was added to gain insight in how people experience anger and what kind of situations provoke anger. A total score for anger disposition is calculated with 48 items divided into three domains (cognitive, arousal and behavioural). Participant rate the items on a 3-point scale ranging from 1 'never true' to 3 'always true'. The second part is the provocation inventory, with 25 items on anger-eliciting situations to be rated on a 4-point scale ranging from 1 'not at all angry' to 4 'very angry'. The NAS-PI has previously been used for people with a psychotic disorder [41] and has good reliability and validity [42]. The NAS-PI has a Dutch norm group of 160 male preparatory secondary vocational education students [43].

Possible influential risk factors

To monitor alcohol and drug use a screening list to check for the risk of substance dependence (in Dutch *Screening Risico op Verslavingsproblemen*; [44] was applied. The instrument consists of eleven questions to determine the amount of alcohol and drugs the participant uses in 1 week or month. To examine whether participants have experienced trauma and potential trauma related symptomatology the *Trauma Screening Questionnaire (TSQ)* was administered. The TSQ is a short screening instrument that contains five re-experiencing and five arousal items from the DMS-IV PTSD criteria (e.g. "upsetting dreams about the event" and "difficulty falling or staying asleep") participants were asked to state whether they experienced these trauma related symptoms twice in the past week (yes/no). Both sensitivity and specificity of the TSQ are high [45]. The PANSS (see screening interview) was also used to measure possible influential risk factors. Video-recorded PANSS interviews were rated by independent and trained screeners, who were blind to the moment, pre or post, of assessment.

Statistical analyses

To explore the outcome measures, pre and post treatment outcomes on each instrument were compared separately using a paired sample t-test (two sided). Alpha was set at 0.05 and no Bonferroni corrections were made due to the explorative nature of the feasibility study. We tested two sided because we wanted to explore both sides of the distribution just in case of unexpected results, for example, if kickboxing leads to more aggression instead of less aggression. In order to check the assumptions we used boxplots, QQ-plots and the Shapiro Wilk test. When assumptions were violated the Wilcoxon Signed Rank test was used. All tests were executed with the SPSS package for IBM statistics version 23.0.

As attendance varied between participants, it might be possible that some of the participants, who missed multiple sessions, obtained less information and exercise and therefore differ from high attenders. Therefore, pre-post analyses were performed twice: once including all completers and again including only the high attenders who participated in at least 75% of the sessions. The results of all completers are reported unless the description in the results says otherwise.

Results

Feasibility of the intervention and application of an RCT

After the therapists and case-managers received detailed information about the intervention and the feasibility study, all teams agreed to participate and were willing to refer clients. In four of the five teams the case load was screened immediately for eligible patients while one team started a month later due to shortage of staff. It took approximately two months, and 155 invitations to clients to include 24 clients. The main reasons for not participating were lack of time, not feeling the need for resilience therapy, no interest in kickboxing, or not willing to participate in the pre and post assessments. Sample characteristics are displayed in Table 1.

Table 1 Sample characteristics

	Completers	Drop-out
N	17	7
Age mean (SD)	35.9 (10.1)	31.0 (12.1)
Male n (%)	13 (76.5)	5 (71.4)
Living situation n (%)		
Alone	11 (64.7)	1 (14.3)
Partner	0 (0.0)	1 (14.3)
Friends	1 (5.9)	0 (0.0)
Family	2 (11.8)	0 (0.0)
Supported housing	3 (17.7)	5 (71.4)
Family contact n (%)		
1–7 times a week	14 (82.4)	5 (71.4)
1–3 times a month	3 (17.7)	2 (28.6)
Daily activity n (%)		
Part-time paid job	2 (11.8)	0 (0.0)
Student	1 (5.9)	1 (14.3)
Volunteer or other activities	8 (47.1)	2 (28.6)
Unemployed	6 (35.3)	4 (57.1)
Diagnosis n (%)		
Paranoid schizophrenia	7 (41.2)	0 (0.0)
Disorganized schizophrenia	0 (0.0)	3 (42.9)
Depression with psychotic features	1 (5.9)	0 (0.0)
Schizophreniform disorder	4 (23.5)	0 (0.0)
Delusion disorder	1 (5.9)	1 (14.3)
Brief psychotic disorder	1 (5.9)	2 (28.6)
Psychotic disorder NOS	3 (17.7)	1 (14.3)

During the intervention, seven participants dropped out: three persons never attended a session, three participants attended only one session, and one participant dropped out after four sessions. There were multiple reasons for dropout such as a lack of motivation, lack of time or physical or mental problems. Due to the small sample size we did not tested differences between characteristics of this dropout group and the completers statistically. However, compared to the completers, the dropout group consisted of relatively more young people, and more people living in supported housing facilities. Three out of seven dropouts were diagnosed with disorganized schizophrenia versus none in the group of completers (see Table 1). Dropouts and completers were comparable with regard to gender, alcohol and drug use, symptoms score of the PANSS, amount of family contact, victimization, trauma, social behaviour, and aggression regulation. The mean attendance was 85.3% (SD = 13.4, range 50–100%), and 88% of the participants completed 75% (fifteen sessions) or more of the twenty sessions. Attendance was highest during the first two modules and lowest during modules 3, 4 and 5 (see Fig. 2).

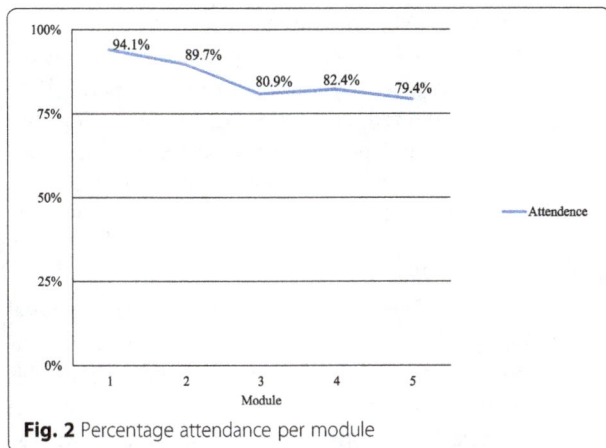

Fig. 2 Percentage attendance per module

Attendance was especially affected when the continuity of the sessions was interrupted due to holidays. In these cases participants reported to forgot to show up. Other reasons were no time, no transportation, mental problems or other obstacles like the flu or lack of motivation. No adverse advents considered to be related to the intervention were reported.

Evaluation of the intervention protocol

Of the seventeen participants who completed the evaluation form, ten persons indicated that 20 weekly sessions were sufficient, while five of them recommended more sessions (between 25 and 40 sessions), and two individuals preferred a more intense course of therapy with two sessions per week. Fourteen participants reported that the 75 min now set for each session was appropriate, two suggested longer sessions, and one thought 75 min was too long. Overall, participants enjoyed the therapy

and thought it was helpful and informative. The sequence order and structure of the modules were positively evaluated and the (thematic) exercises within each session were rated as relevant.

The kickboxing exercises were reported to be doable for all participants, regardless of weight, strength, stamina or flexibility. Within-group differences with regards to strength or stamina were not a problem; everyone found themselves participating at their own level with exercises adapted in case of physical problems. Table 2 shows the outcomes of the qualitative evaluation questionnaire. According to the participants the intervention especially had a positive effect on identifying and setting boundaries, recognizing those of others, self-esteem, faith in own strength, confidence, recognizing dangerous situations, feelings of safety, and people though they had a lower change of becoming a victim. Most mean scores increased when only the high attenders, who attended 75% or more of the sessions, were included in the analysis.

Although it was not a goal of the intervention, some of the participants did notice that they had lost weight, improved their stamina and endurance, and were drinking less alcohol at the end of the intervention. None of the participants reported alarming arousal levels during or at the end of a session. Several participants noticed that their arousal level was lower after a session and that they felt more relaxed.x

Improvement of the intervention protocol

Based on the information gathered by means of the evaluation questionnaire and feedback from participants, trainers, expert by experience, kickboxing expert and researchers, several adaptations in the intervention protocol

Table 2 Outcomes qualitative evaluation questionnaire

Due to the therapy	Completers Mean (SD) N = 17	High attenders Mean (SD) N = 13[a]	Due to the therapy	Completers Mean (SD) N = 17	High attenders Mean (SD) N = 13[a]
I enjoy social contacts more	4.59 (0.80)	4.54 (1.04)	I experience less self-stigma	4.47 (1.59)	5.00 (1.00)
I have more social contacts (outside therapy)	4.18 (1.33)	4.31 (0.63)	I have more self-esteem	5.24 (1.56)	5.46 (1.27)
I recognize other people's boundaries better	5.29 (0.85)	5.38 (0.87)	I am more assertive	4.76 (1.35)	5.08 (0.95)
I can identify my own boundaries better	5.59 (1.06)	5.77 (0.93)	I have more faith in my own strength	5.47 (1.18)	5.46 (1.05)
I can set my own boundaries more easily	5.35 (1.06)	5.54 (0.88)	I have more confidence	5.44 (0.96)	5.42 (1.08)
I recognize dangerous situations better	5.18 (0.95)	5.23 (0.60)	I feel safer on the street	5.35 (1.00)	5.38 (1.04)
I can prevent a fight	4.76 (0.97)	4.77 (0.83)	I have more respect for others	4.81 (0.83)	4.67 (0.78)
I recognize when I become angry or agitated	4.35 (1.37)	4.69 (0.86)	Others have more respect for me	4.63 (0.81)	4.42 (0.67)
I have more control over my emotions	4.53 (1.01)	4.62 (0.87)	I am less likely to become a victim	5.35 (1.00)	5.54 (0.97)

[a]Attended to 75% or more of the sessions; Scoring range: 1 totally disagree, 2 disagree, 3 somewhat disagree, 4 neutral, 5 somewhat agree, 6, agree, 7 totally agree

for the RCT were made after this pilot. First of all, it was noticed that in general more time than expected was needed for the participants to fully understand a theme, manage a technique or to make a kickboxing combination routine. For this reason multiple repetitions of important themes and techniques were added to the protocol, in combination with the advice to explain and practice complex kickboxing combinations in small steps. Secondly, more challenging exercises (e.g. high kick, sparring) were included in the protocol as the participants liked the challenge and it created theme-related learning opportunities. Thirdly, an intensive work-out on kickboxing pads was added to every session because participants emphasized that they enjoyed such an intensive exercise because this in particular provided positive experiences of strength and acquired kickboxing skills. Finally, although BEATVIC is a body-oriented therapy, participants positively evaluated the opportunity to talk and reflect on the therapy in the end of the session. For this reason, time was reserved for discussion at the end of each session. After the therapy ended, nine out of seventeen participants continued kickboxing at a local gym. One year later six participants still attended weekly training sessions.

Exploration of outcome measures
Victimization
Table 3 shows that based on the IVM, at baseline 75% of the participants had been a victim of at least one crime in the previous five years. Both, personal and property crimes were reported by 58% of the participants. Compared to the five year rate, with 21%, the one-year victimization prevalence was approximately between three times lower, and sexual harassment or assault were not reported at all. Prevalence of victimization in the general population living in the same region was half of that in participants with all events taken into account, and only 25% in case of personal crime.

Baseline measures of the CTS2 showed that 24% of the participants had experienced physical assault in the preceding five months. Psychological aggression was reported by 47% of the participants with no one reporting sexual coercion or physical injury. Pre and post measures revealed that the experienced frequency (or chronicity) of psychological aggression towards the participants had increased after the intervention (p 0.048). No such changes were found for the other victimization subscales.

On the negotiation items of the CTS2 only one participant reported negatively. After the intervention, the frequency of negotiation during conflict had increased ($p < 0.01$) compared to baseline.

Perpetration
Seventeen percent of the participants indicated that they had been the perpetrator of a crime themselves in the previous year (IVM), measured at baseline. The CTS2 results showed that 41% had used psychological aggression, 24% had used physical assault and two participants (12%) had physically injured someone in the preceding five months. None of the participants reported to have used sexual coercion. No differences between pre and post measurements were found on perpetration scores (see Table 3).

Aggression regulation
Compared to a Dutch norm group from the general population, participants scored one decile higher on 'internal anger' (mean 22.5, sd 7.0) scale and two deciles lower on 'external anger' (mean 21.2, sd 5.6) on the STAXI at baseline. 'Control of internal anger' was as high in participants as in the norm group (mean 26.0, sd 6.8) and 'control of external anger' was two deciles higher (mean 27.4 sd 6.4). At post measurement the mean score on control of internal anger was one decile higher than at baseline but this increase was not significant (p 0.071). The three other subscales did not show a significant change over time (see Table 4).

At pre and post measurement the participants scored both one decile lower on the NAS total score compared to the norm group (mean 89.7, sd 14.2). In accordance no significant difference was found between pre and post scores for the NAS total score as well as for the PI score. However, when only the high attenders were included in the analyses the 'arousal' subscale of the NAS-PI showed a significant decrease over time (p 0.033) (see Table 4).

Social behaviour
At baseline, the median score of the participants was 'above average' on the ISS compared to the norm group on the 'total social discomfort' scale. After therapy this decreased to 'average' discomforts however this change was statistically nonsignificant. At baseline the median frequency of 'total social contacts' scale was 'below average' compared to the norm group. At post measurement the median frequency of the 'total social contacts' scale was still 'below average' but again nonsignificant (see Table 4).

Possible influential risk factors
No differences between pre and post measurement were found on all scales of the PANSS, or on the screening risk of substance dependence questionnaire. Most participants did not experience symptoms of trauma at pre or post measurements (see Table 5).

Discussion
To our knowledge, BEATVIC is the first body-oriented resilience therapy that aims to decrease victimization risk in people with a psychotic disorder. The goal of this study was to evaluate its feasibility in order to evaluate

Table 3 Number, percentage and chronicity of victimization and perpetration

	Participants N = 24		General population N = 1729
IVM	Previous year % (n)[a]	Previous five years % (n)[a]	Previous year % (n)[a]
Property crime[b]	12.5 (3)	58.3 (14)	8.6 (149)[c]
Attempted burglary	4.2 (1)	16.7 (4)	
Burglary	4.2 (1)	25.0 (6)	
Bicycle theft	8.3 (2)	20.8 (5)	
Theft (other)	4.2 (1)	12.5 (3)	
Vandalism	4.2 (1)	25.0 (6)	3.6 (62)
Pick-pocketing	0.0 (0)	4.2 (1)	
Robbery	0.0 (0)	8.3 (2)	
Personal crime[d]	8.3 (2)	58.3 (14)	1.9 (33)
Sexual harassment or assault	0.0 (0)	8.3 (2)	
Threats of violence	8.3 (2)	41.7 (10)	
2003Physical assault	4.2 (1)	16.7 (4)	
Other victimization incidents	12.5 (3)	12.5 (3)	
Total victimization[e]	20.8 (5)	75.0 (18)	12.5 (216)
Perpetration[f]	16.7 (4)		

CTS2 Towards participant (victimization)	Completers N = 17					
	Previous five months % (n)[a]	Pre Mdn (IQR)[h]	Post Mdn (IQR)[h]	Z	r	p
Psychological aggression[g]	47.1 (8)	0.00 (2.00)	2.00 (2.00)	−1.98	0.48*	0.048
Physical assault[g]	29.4 (5)	0.00 (1.00)	0.00 (1.00)	−0.85	0.21	0.40
Sexual coercion[g]	0.0 (0)	0.00 (0.00)	0.00 (0.00)	−1.00	0.24	0.32
Physical injury[g]	0.0 (0)	0.00 (0.00)	0.00 (0.00)	−1.34	0.33	0.18
		Pre Mean (SD)	Post Mean (SD)	Paired Diff. (95% CI)	t	p
Negotiation[i]	94.1 (16)	6.94 (6.04)	6.69 (3.81)	0.06 (−2.44–2.56)	0.05	0.96

CTS2 Towards someone (perpetration)		Pre Mdn (IQR)[h]	Post Mdn (IQR)[h]	Z	t	p
Psychological aggression[g]	41.2 (7)	0.00 (2.00)	1.00 (3.00)	0.92	0.22	0.36
Physical assault[g]	4 (23.5)	0.00 (1.00)	0.00 (0.50)	−0.17	0.04	0.86
Sexual coercion[g]	0.0 (0)	0.00 (0.00)	0.00 (0.00)	−1.00	0.24	0.32
Physical injury[g]	11.7 (2)	0.00 (0.00)	0.00 (0.00)	−0.97	0.24	0.33
		Pre Mean (SD)	Post Mean (SD)	Paired Diff. (95% CI)	t	p
Negotiation[i]	100.0 (17)	2.76 (1.56)	7.65 (4.40)	−4.88 (−6.91- -2.85)	−5.10	< 0.01

[a] At least one incident n > 0; [b]Consists of burglary, attempted burglary, bicycle theft, theft (other), vandalism, pick-pocketing, robbery; [c]Consists of property crime without vandalism; [d] Consists of sexual harassment or assault, threats of violence, physical assault. [e] Consists of property crime, personal crime and other victimization incidents; [f] Consists of threats of violence, physical assault, sexual assault or other crimes (only previous year was examined); [g] Wilcoxon Signed Rank test; [h] Frequency; [i] Paired sample t-test. IVM = Dutch crime and victimization survey; CTS2: revised Conflicts Tactics Scale

the usefulness of a larger RCT that can shed light on efficacy of BEATVIC.

Feasibility of the intervention and application of an RCT
Our findings support the feasibility of BEATVIC. The mental health professionals were willing to refer to BEATVIC and a relatively large group of clients (one out of every six invited) was willing to participate. The mean age of the participants was 36 years. The oldest included participant was 51 years old, which indicates that BEATVIC appeals to a wide variety of people.

Table 4 Pre and post treatment aggression regulation and social behaviour scores

	Pre Mean (SD)	Post Mean (SD)	Paired Diff. (95% CI)	t	p
STAXI[a] N = 17					
Internalizing anger	24.94 (6.69)	24.65 (6.86)	0.29 (−1.77–2.36)	0.30	0.77
Externalizing anger	17.00 (4.46)	18.24 (4.19)	−1.24 (−2.84–0.37)	−1.64	0.12
Control of internalizing	27.53 (7.75)	29.53 (4.46)	−2.00 (−4.20–0.20)	−1.93	0.071
Control of externalizing	30.35 (5.99)	30.29 (4.67)	0.06 (−2.12–2.24)	0.06	0.96
NAS-PI[a] N = 13*					
Cognition	31.00 (3.34)	29.85 (3.53)	1.15 (−0.32–2.63)	1.70	0.11
Arousal	29.62 (3.82)	28.508 (3.93)	1.54 (0.15–2.92)	2.42	0.033
Behaviour	23.85 (4.18)	23.15 (3.29)	0.69 (−1.51–2.89)	0.69	0.51
NAS total	84.46 (10.18)	81.08 (9.74)	3.38 (−0.43–7.19)	1.93	0.077
PI total	55.90 (10.68)	54.62 (9.91)	1.31 (−2.30–4.91)	0.79	0.45
IIS[b] N = 17	Pre Mdn (IQR)	Post Mdn (IQR)	Z	r	p
Discomfort					
Giving Criticism	21.00 (5.00)	19.00 (6.00)	−1.80	0.44	0.072
Expressing Opinions	14.00 (6.00)	14.00 (4.00)	−0.86	0.21	0.39
Giving Compliments	6.00 (3.00)	5.00 (3.00)	−1.03	0.25	0.30
Initiating contacts	11.50 (7.00)	11.00 (7.00)	−0.54	0.13	0.59
Positive self-evaluation	8.00 (3.00)	8.00 (2.50)	−0.56	0.14	0.58
Total Discomfort	77.00 (24.00)	75.00 (11.00)	−1.04	0.25	0.30
Frequency					
Giving Criticism	17.00 (4.00)	16.00 (4.50)	−0.26	0.06	0.80
Expressing Opinions	17.00 (5.00)	16.00 (2.50)	−1.67	0.41	0.09
Giving Compliments	16.00 (4.50)	15.00 (4.00)	−0.23	0.06	0.81
Initiating contacts	14.00 (6.50)	17.00 (5.50)	−0.61	0.15	0.54
Positive self-evaluation	12.00 (6.00)	13.00 (4.50)	−0.38	0.09	0.70
Total Frequency	104.00 (30.25)	101.00 (26.00)	−0.02	0.01	0.98

[a]Paired sample t-test; [b] Wilcoxon Signed Rank test; * high attenders who attended 75% or more of the sessions; *STAXI* State Trait Anger Expression Inventory, *NAS-PI* Novaco Anger Scale-Provocation Inventory, *IIS* Inventory of Interpersonal Situations

Table 5 Pre and post PANSS, substance abuse and TSQ scores

N = 17	Pre Mdn (IQR)	Post Mdn (IQR)	Z	r	p
PANSS[a]					
Positive symptoms	11.00 (4.50)	11.00 (5.00)	−0.64	0.16	0.53
Negative symptoms	10.00 (5.00)	10.00 (3.50)	−0.27	0.07	0.90
General symptoms	24.00 (9.00)	25.00 (9.00)	−0.33	0.08	0.74
Total score	44.00 (19.00)	45.00 (17.50)	−0.57	0.14	0.60
Substance abuse[a]	20.00 (7.00)	19.00 (10.50)	−0.15	0.04	0.88
TSQ[a]	0.00 (2.00)	0.00 (3.00)	−0.34	0.08	0.73

[a]Wilcoxon Signed Rank test; *PANSS* Positive and Negative Syndrome Scale, *TSQ* Trauma Screening Questionnaire

The dropout rate of 29% was as could be expected based on previous studies: the estimated dropout rate of physical activity interventions for people with schizophrenia lies between the 20 and 35% [46]. Six out of seven dropouts attended none or only one session. It is possible that, despite all the provided information, these participants were not fully aware beforehand of what the treatment would entail and how much time would be involved. To prevent dropout it is recommended to verify whether the client received and understood all the information.

Overall attendance was good compared to other interventions [47, 48]. This finding is particularly relevant as high attendance is important because of the intensity of BEATVIC and its hierarchical structure where the kickboxing exercises are concerned. Non-attendance of two or more sessions means that important exercises are missed and participants fall behind in the group. In accordance, the high attenders who were present at more than 75% of the sessions reported that they had improved more on the addressed risk factors, compared to the low attenders. This is in line with a study of Scheewe et al. [49] who only found significant improvements in people who attended more than 50% of the exercise sessions. In line with these experiences, it was decided that to measure effectiveness in the RCT, we will not only use an intention-to-treat analysis but also perform a per-protocol analysis.

Evaluation and improvement of the intervention protocol
The BEATVIC therapy was positively evaluated by the trainers and the participants. Overall, the number, duration and sequence order of the sessions were seen as adequate, and the (thematic) exercises were rated as relevant. In the results section, an overview of implemented improvements was presented regarding the number of repetitions, the right amount of challenge and intensity of exercises, and total discussion time. Participants enjoyed the exercises and they subjectively reported positive effects on several factors.

Some of the participants noted that they had lost weight and felt that their stamina and endurance was improved. To objectively measure this, we will include physical outcomes in the RCT as this is particular relevant for the target group who also faces increased metabolic risks [50, 51]. This study has shown that it is appropriate to use kickboxing in a body-oriented therapy. The exercises were at a feasible level for all participants and people enjoyed learning the techniques which was confirmed by the fact that half of the group continued kickboxing at a local gym.

Exploration of suitable outcome measures
To find suitable instruments for the RCT we explored some of the important outcome measures.

Victimization and perpetration
The IVM and the CTS2 showed to be adequate instruments to detect victimization incidents. Although there is some overlap in subscales, both can be used complementary because of their specific characteristics. With the IVM the victimization prevalence can be compared to the general population who live in the same neighbourhood while the instrument also shows international comparability [52]. The IVM also provides information on victimization both in the preceding year (in our case 21%) and the preceding 5 year (75%). Subsequently, some types of victimization (e.g. sexual assault, robbery) were only reported during the 5 year period and not during the 1 year period. This indicates the importance for a follow-up in the RCT. Preferably more than 1 year to capture the less frequent victimization types.

The CTS2 measures more subtle forms of victimization and takes into account the frequency in which an incident occurs. In our study more people reported physical assault on the CTS2 (29%) than on the IVM (4.2%). A possible explanation might be that the CTS2 asks more specific assault questions which may elicit higher recall of incidents. The CTS2 showed to be sensitive to change: more psychological aggression was reported after the intervention than before and participants more often used negotiation as a communication technique.

Aggression regulation
The NAS-PI and the STAXI were used to explore whether these tests could capture changes in aggression regulation induced by the intervention. Only a significant improvement on the arousal subscale of the NAS-PI for the high attenders, but no other significant changes were found. At baseline on average the STAXI and NAS-PI scores did not indicate that the participants had aggression regulations problems and there may not have been much room for improvement. In the future it is recommended to perform a subgroup analysis for participants who have aggression regulation problems at the start of the treatment.

Social functioning
In this study the IIS was used to explore whether this test could capture changes in interpersonal situations. No significant changes were found and therefore we decided to use another test for the RCT. Besides a lack of power due to the small sample size, it is possible that the participants did not significantly improve on the IIS because it measures a broad spectrum of interpersonal situations. It is expected that the intervention can improve social functioning, as other studies that included martial arts found positive results on social behaviour [53, 54]. In the future it is recommended to measure aspects and/or underlying mechanisms of social functioning that are related to victimization, for example assertiveness and impaired social cognition.

Limitations of the study
First of all, because no control group was included no conclusions can be formulated as to whether the (subjective) improvements derive from the group meetings and time with the trainers or from BEATVIC. Secondly, since not all participants had been victimized at baseline, it was difficult to find improvements in this respect. These participants may have been appealed by the kickboxing-element of the therapy, rather than working on their resilience.

Conclusion

In this feasibility study BEATVIC was found to be a feasible intervention for people with a psychotic disorder. Both mental health professionals and clients gave positive evaluations and attendance was good. Trainers, participants and scientists gave suggestions for small improvements in the intervention protocol. Our results support the evaluation of BEATVIC in a RCT.

Abbreviations
CTS2: Conflict tactics scale; IIS: Inventory of interpersonal situations; IVM: Integrale Veiligheidsmonitor (Dutch crime and victimization survey); NAS-PI: Novaco anger scale-provocation inventory; PANSS: Positive and negative syndrome scale; PMT: Psychomotor therapy; STAXI: State trait anger expression inventory; TSQ: Trauma screening questionnaire

Acknowledgements
The authors like to acknowledge the participants and health care professionals of GGZ Drenthe who contribute to this study. Furthermore we like to thank students of the Rijks University of Groningen for conducting most of the measurements.

Funding
The study was funded by the Netherlands Organization for Scientific Research (NWO grant nr 432–12-807).

Authors' contributions
BV, JB, GP, CW, SP, JA, ES, AA and EH made substantial contribution to conception of the intervention and design of the study and/or were involved in acquisition of data. BV, JB, GP and ES made the first draft of the manuscript and CW, SP, AA and JA critically revised the manuscript. All authors read and approved the final manuscript.

Consent for publication
Not applicable.

Competing interests
The authors declare that they have no competing interests.

Author details
[1]Department of clinical psychology and experimental psychopathology, faculty of behavioral and social sciences, University of Groningen, Grote Kruisstraat 2/1, 9712 TS Groningen, Netherlands. [2]University of Groningen, University Medical Center Groningen, University Center of Psychiatry, Rob Giel Onderzoekcentrum, Hanzeplein 1, 9713 GZ Groningen, Netherlands. [3]Department of Neuroscience, BCN Neuroimaging Center, University of Groningen, University Medical Center Groningen, Antonius Deusinglaan 2, 9713 AW Groningen, Netherlands. [4]Department of Psychotic Disorders, GGZ-Drenthe, Dennenweg 9, 9404 LA Assen, Netherlands. [5]Helmsport, Vechtstraat 72B, 9725 CW Groningen, Netherlands. [6]Department of Human Movement and Education, Windesheim University of Applied Sciences, Campus 2-6, 8017 CA Zwolle, the Netherlands.

References
1. Moreno-Küstner B, Martín C, Pastor L. Prevalence of psychotic disorders and its association with methodological issues. A systematic review and meta-analyses. PLoS One. 2018;13(4):1–25.
2. Dean K, Moran P, Fahy T, Tyrer P, Leese M, Creed F, et al. Predictors of violent victimization amongst those with psychosis. Acta Psychiatr Scand. 2007;116(5):345–53.
3. Morgan VA, Morgan F, Galletly C, Valuri G, Shah S, Jablensky A. Sociodemographic, clinical and childhood correlates of adult violent victimisation in a large, national survey sample of people with psychotic disorders. Soc Psychiatry Psychiatr Epidemiol. Springer Berlin Heidelberg. 2016;51(2):269–79.
4. Choe JY, Teplin LA, Abram KM. Perpetration of Violence , Violent Balancing Public Health Concerns. Psychiatr Serv S2-Hospital Community Psychiatry. 2008;59(2):153–64.
5. Van der Stouwe ECD, De Vries B, Aleman A, Arends J, Waarheid C, Meerdink A, et al. BEATVIC, a body-oriented resilience training with elements of kickboxing for individuals with a psychotic disorder: study protocol of a multi-center RCT. BMC Psychiatry. 2016;16:1–11.
6. Röhricht F. Body psychotherapy for the treatment of severe mental disorders – an overview. Body Mov Danc Psychother. 2014;10(1):51–67.
7. Boerhout C, van Busschbach JT, Wiersma D, Hoek HW. Psychomotor therapy and aggression regulation in eating disorders. Body Mov Danc Psychotherapy. Boerhout, Cees, Lentis Center for Mental Health. Netherlands: Taylor & Francis. 2013;8(4):241–53.
8. Boerhout C, Swart M, Voskamp M, Troquete NAC, van Busschbach JT, Hoek HW. Aggression regulation in day treatment of eating disorders: two-Centre RCT of a brief body and movement-oriented intervention. Eur Eat Disord Rev. 2017;25(1):52–9.
9. Couture SM, Penn DL, Roberts DL. The functional significance of social cognition in schizophrenia: a review. Schizophr Bull. 2006;32(Suppl 1): S44–63.
10. Addington J, Girard TA, Christensen BK, Addington D. Social cognition mediates illness-related and cognitive influences on social function in patients with schizophrenia-spectrum disorders. J Psychiatry Neurosci. 2010; 35(1):49–54.
11. Chapple B, Chant D, Nolan P, Cardy S, Whiteford H, McGrath J. Correlates of victimisation amongst people with psychosis. Soc Psychiatry Psychiatr Epidemiol. 2004;39(10):836–40.
12. Ekinci O, Ekinci A. Association between insight, cognitive insight, positive symptoms and violence in patients with schizophrenia. Nor J Psychiatry. 2013;67(2):116-23.
13. Hiday V, Swartz M, Swanson J, Borum R, Wagner R. Impact of victimization on outpatient commitment among people with severe mental illness. Am J Psychiatry. 2002;159(8):1403–11.
14. Horsselenberg EMA, van Busschbach JT, Aleman A, Pijnenborg GHM. Self-Stigma and Its Relationship with Victimization, Psychotic Symptoms and Self-Esteem among People with Schizophrenia Spectrum Disorders. van Winkel R, editor. PLoS One. 2016;11(10):e0149763.
15. Kleim B, Vauth R, Adam G, Stieglitz R-D, Hayward P, Corrigan PW. Perceived stigma predicts low self-efficacy and poor coping in schizophrenia. J Ment Health. 2008;17(5):482–91.
16. Livingston JD, Boyd JE. Correlates and consequences of internalized stigma for people living with mental illness: a systematic review and meta-analysis. Soc Sci Med. Elsevier Ltd. 2010;71(12):2150–61.
17. Egan SK, Perry DG. Does low self-regard invite victimization? Dev Psychol. 1998;34(2):299–309.
18. Peri T, Ben-Shakhar G, Orr SP, Shalev AY. Psychophysiologic assessment of aversive conditioning in posttraumatic stress disorder. Biol Psychiatry. 2000; 47(6):512–9.
19. Iverson KM, Litwack SD, Pineles SL, Suvak MK, Vaughn RA, Resick PA. Predictors of intimate partner violence Revictimization: the relative Impact of distinct PTSD symptoms, dissociation, and coping strategies. J Trauma Stress. 2013;26(1):102–10.
20. Firth J, Carney R, Elliott R, French P, Parker S, McIntyre R, Yung A. Exercise as an intervention for first-episode psychosis: a feasibility study. Early Intervention in Psychiatry. 2016;12(3):307-15.
21. Firth J, Cotter J, Elliott R, French P, Yung AR. A systematic review and meta-analysis of exercise interventions in schizophrenia patients. Psychol Med. 2015;45(07):1343–61.
22. Seagull KL. How I learned to live with schizophrenia. Psychiatr Serv. 2014; 65(10):1192–3.
23. Temple S, Robson P. The effect of assertiveness training on self-esteem. Br J Occup Ther. 1991;54(9):329–32.
24. Elling AH, Wisse E, Berk vd H. Beloften van vechtsport: onderzoek in het kader van het programma "tijd voor vechtsport". Netherlands, Nieuwegein: Arko Sport Media, Opdr van KNKF. 2010.

25. Hasson-Ohayon I, Kravetz S, Roe D, Rozencwaig S, Weiser M. Qualitative assessment of verbal and non-verbal psychosocial interventions for people with severe mental illness. J Ment Health. 2006;15(3):343–53.

26. Twemlow SW, Biggs BK, Nelson TD, Vernberg EM, Fonagy P, Twemlow SW. Effects of participation in a martial arts-based antibullying program in elementary schools. Psychol Sch. 2008;45(10):947–59.

27. Damhuis N, Van Megen HJGM, Peeters CFW, Vollema MG. De MiniScan als psychiatrische interventie; pilotonderzoek naar de toegevoegde waarde van een gecomputeriseerd classificatiesysteem. Tijdschr Psychiatr. 2011;53(3):175–80.

28. Kay SR, Fiszbein A, Opler LA. The positive and negative syndrome scale (PANSS) for schizophrenia. Schizophr Bull. 1987;13(2):261–76.

29. Arain M, Campbell MJ, Cooper CL, Lancaster GA. What is a pilot or feasibility study? A review of current practice and editorial policy. BMC Med Res Methodol. 2010;10(1):67.

30. CBS. Integrale veiligheidsmonitor: Landelijk rapportage [safety monitor national report 2015]. Netherlands, Den Haag: Centraal Bureau voor Statistiek. 2015.

31. Kamperman AM, Henrichs J, Bogaerts S, Lesaffre EMEH, Wierdsma AI, Ghauharali RRR, et al. Criminal victimisation in people with severe mental illness: a multi-site prevalence and incidence survey in the Netherlands. PLoS One. 2014;9(3):1–13.

32. Straus MA, Hamby SL, Boney-McCoy S, Sugarman DB. The revised conflict tactics scales (CTS2). J Fam Issues. 1996;17(3):283–316.

33. Vega EM, O'Leary KD. Test-retest reliability of the revised conflict tactics scales (CTS2). J Fam Violence. 2007;22(8):703–8.

34. Van Dam-Baggen R, Kraaimaat F. Assessing social anxiety: the inventory of interpersonal\nSituations (IIS). Eur J Psychol Assess. 1999;15(1):25–38.

35. Van Dam-Baggen R, Kraaimaat F. Group social skills training or cognitive group therapy as the clinical treatment of choice for generalized social phobia? J Anxiety Disord. 2000;14(5):437–51.

36. Van Dam-Baggen R, Kraaimaat F. Inventaristatielijst Omgaan met Anderen. Handleiding. 2004.

37. Spielberger CD, Sydeman SJ, Owen AE, Marsh BJ. Measuring anxiety and anger with the state-trait anxiety inventory (STAI) and the state-trait anger expression inventory (STAXI). In: Maruish ME, editor. The use of psychological testing for treatment planning and outcomes assessment. 2nd ed. Mahwah: Lawrence Erlbaum Associates Publishers; 1999. p. 993–1021.

38. Lee H, Jang S, Lee S, Hwang K. The arts in psychotherapy effectiveness of dance / movement therapy on affect and psychotic symptoms in patients with schizophrenia. Arts Psychother. Elsevier Ltd. 2015;45:64–8.

39. Van Elderen T, Verkes RJ, Arkesteijn J, Komproe I. Psychometric characteristics of the self-expression and control scale in a sample of recurrent suicide attempters. Pers Individ Dif. 1996;21(4):489–96.

40. Van Elderen T, Maes S, Komproe I. The development of an anger expression and control scale. Br J Hralth Psychol. 1997;2:269–81.

41. Ringer JM, Lysaker PH. Anger expression styles in schizophrenia Spectrum disorders associations with anxiety, Paranoia, Emotion Recognition, and Trauma History. J Nerv Ment Dis. 2014;202(12):853–8.

42. Hornsveld RHJ, Muris P, Kraaimaat FW. The Novaco anger scale–provocation inventory (1994 version) in Dutch forensic psychiatric patients. Psychol Asses. 2011;23(4):937–44.

43. Hornsveld RHJ, Muris P, Kraaimaat FW. Drie zelfrapportage vragenlijsten voor de forensische psychiatrie; 2009.

44. Spijkerman R, Hendriks V, van der Gaag R. Screening risico op verslavingsproblemen [screening risk of substance dependance]; 2011.

45. Dekkers AMM, Olff M, Maring GWB. Identifying persons at risk for PTSD after trauma with TSQ in the Netherlands. Community Ment Health J. 2010;46(1):20–5.

46. Vancampfort D, Rosenbaum S, Schuch FB, Ward PB, Probst M, Stubbs B. Prevalence and predictors of treatment dropout from physical activity interventions in schizophrenia : a meta-analysis. Gen Hosp Psychiatry. Elsevier Inc. 2016;39:15–23.

47. Beebe LH, Tian L, Morris N, Goodwin A, Allen SS, Kuldau J. Effects of exercise on mental and physical health parameters of persons with schizophrenia. Issues Ment Health Nurs. 2005;26(6):661–76.

48. McGuire AB, Bonfils KA, Kukla M, Myers L, Salyers MP. Measuring participation in an evidence-based practice: illness management and recovery group attendance. Psychiatry Res. 2013;210(3):684–9.

49. Scheewe TW, Backx FJG, Takken T, Jörg F, van Strater AC, Kroes AG, et al. Exercise therapy improves mental and physical health in schizophrenia: a randomised controlled trial. Acta Psychiatr Scand. 2013;127(6):464–73.

50. Mitchell, AJ, Vancampfort D, Sweers K, van Winkel R, Yu W, De Hert M. Prevalence of metabolic syndrome and metabolic abnormalities in schizophrenia and related disorders--a systematic review and meta-analysis. Schizophrenia bulletin. 2011;39(2):306-18.

51. Gardner-Sood P, Lally J, Smith S, Atakan Z, Ismail K, Greenwood KE, et al. Cardiovascular risk factors and metabolic syndrome in people with established psychotic illnesses: baseline data from the IMPaCT randomized controlled trial. Psychol Med. 2015;45(12):2619–29.

52. De Vries B, van Busschbach JT, van der Stouwe ECD, Aleman A, van Dijk JJM, Lysaker PH, et al. Prevalence Rate and Risk Factors of Victimization in Adult Patients With a Psychotic Disorder: A Systematic Review and Meta-analysis. Schizophr Bull. 2018;(3):1–13. https://doi.org/10.1093/schbul/sby020.

53. Lakes KD, Hoyt WT. Promoting self-regulation through school-based martial arts training. J Appl Dev Psychol. 2004;25(3):283–302.

54. Movahedi A, Bahrami F, Mohammad S. Research in autism Spectrum disorders improvement in social dysfunction of children with autism spectrum disorder following long term Kata techniques training. Res Autism Spectr Disord. Elsevier Ltd. 2013;7(9):1054–61.

6

Prevalence and characteristics of suicidal ideation among 2199 elderly inpatients with surgical or medical conditions in Taiwan

Su-Jung Liao[1,2], Bo-Jian Wu[3], Tse-Tsung Liu[4], Chao-Ping Chou[5] and Jiin-Ru Rong[2*]

Abstract

Background: Worldwide, the elderly are at a greater risk of suicide than other age groups. There is a paucity of research exploring risk factors for suicide in hospitalized elderly patients. Therefore, a study designed to explore the prevalence and characteristic of suicidal ideation (SI), such as QOL (quality of life), a wish to die (WTD), and other factors in elderly inpatients with medical or surgical conditions in Taiwan was warranted.

Methods: A total of 2199 hospitalized elderly patients over age 65 were enrolled. Demographic data, 5-item Brief Symptom Rating Scale (BSRS-5), and the World Health Organization Quality of Life-BREF (WHOQOL-BREF) data were collected. Logistic regression models were used to find the SI-related factors for all participants and to investigate the covariates correlated with WTD in patients with SI. Receiver operating characteristic (ROC) curve analysis was used to find the most important items of the BSRS-5 predictive of SI in this population.

Results: SI was found in 3.1% (68/2199) of the elderly. The statistically significantly factors associated with SI were: BSRS-5 item 2 (depression) (odds ratio [OR] = 2.15, 95% confidence interval [CI] = 1.56–2.98), item 4 (inferiority) (OR = 1.62, 1.23–2.13), item 5 (insomnia) (OR = 1.52, 1.13–2.05), and physical domain of WHOQOL (OR = 0.84, 0.72–0.99). QOL15 (mobility) (OR = 0.64, 0.46–0.90) and QOL 16 (satisfaction with sleep) (OR = 0.62, 0.44–0.88) were also significantly associated with SI. The status of living alone (OR = 4.44, 1.24–15.87), QOL 26 (absence of negative feeling) (OR = 0.38, 0.15–0.98), and QOL 27 (being respected/accepted) (OR = 0.43, 0.20–0.92) were significantly associated with WTD among inpatients with SI. The ROC curve analysis revealed that depression, inferiority, and insomnia were the most important items in the BSRS-5 significantly associated with SI among the elderly inpatients.

Conclusion: To provide physical recovery and maintain mental health for physically ill elderly inpatients, setting up a multi-faceted approach targeting the aforementioned determinants of SI and WTD for reducing the risk of suicide attempt, and exploring other factors correlated with suicidal behaviors, are important topics and directions for clinical practice and further research.

Keywords: Elderly, Inpatients, Suicidal ideation, Wish to die, Quality of life, BSRS-5

* Correspondence: sujungliao@gmail.com
[2]Department of Nursing, National Taipei University of Nursing Health Science, No.365, Mingde Rd., Beitou Dist., Taipei City 112, Taiwan, Republic of China
Full list of author information is available at the end of the article

Background

The associated risk factors and prevalence for suicidal behaviors are diverse and are closely related to setting, measures, age groups, and different populations [1]. When compared with younger people, elderly adults are at a higher risk of suicide in most countries [2]. Concerning the risk of suicide, suicidal ideation (SI) usually plays an important role and paves the way to suicidal behaviors [3]. The prevalence of SI varies among the elderly, ranging from 0.7% in elderly primary care patients [4] to 26% in acute medically ill elderly inpatients [5].

Several studies have revealed multi-domain factors related to SI or suicidal behaviors. Quality of life (QOL) has been found to be associated with the risk of SI or suicidal behaviors in the elderly [6, 7]. In psychological autopsy, most of the cases with suicide death had a wish to die (WTD) [8], which was also found to be associated with all-cause mortality during five-year follow up in elderly primary care patients [9]. Furthermore, there are other risk factors related to SI and suicidal behaviors, which include clinical depression [5, 10–14], substance misuse [13, 15, 16], poor perception of health [11, 17], financial problems [12, 14], relationship problem [11, 14], poor social support [13, 15], living alone [18], marital status [15, 18], impaired cognition [19, 20], history of traumatic events [1], and the burden of physical illness [21].

More attention should be paid to elderly inpatients with physical illness because they are more likely to have a suicide attempt and suicide death because of old age, burden of physical diseases, and an increased concurrence of depression [5]. Thus, to single out elderly inpatients with SI at an early stage and provide timely adequate treatment in a general hospital, may decrease rates of suicidal behaviors and related mortality [5, 22]. Although this issue is important, only a small number of studies have explored the prevalence and characteristics of SI in elderly inpatients with medical or surgical conditions. One study in Iran revealed a high rate of SI in 650 hospitalized physically ill elderly patients, among whom 21.6% expressed SI, and 14.9% had a moderate to strong WTD [1]. In that study, regression models revealed that the presence of SI was significantly related to the history of traumatic events, length of hospital stay, severity of depression, and the level of social support. Another study in the UK also reported that a total of 36% had suicidal thoughts, and 22% expressed a WTD in 55 elderly patients who were admitted due to acute medical conditions [5]. Pessimism, previous deliberate self-harm, the severity of depression, and use of antidepressant were found to be significantly associated with the SI in the univariate analysis. There were some limitations in these prior studies: (1) a small sample size and use of univariate analysis to investigate SI-associated factors

[5]; (2) a lack of exploration of QOL [1, 5], which seemed to play a role in SI among the elderly [6, 7]; (3) WTD and its related factors among inpatients with SI was yet to be explored; (4) there seems to be very few similar studies focusing on physically ill hospitalized elderly in the Far East, let alone in Taiwan.

Regarding the instruments for screening SI, the Department of Health in Taiwan has been using the 5-item Brief Symptom Rating Scale (BSRS-5), which has been found to present with good psychometric properties to identify psychiatric morbidity in medical settings or the community [23], for suicide prevention programs on a large scale [24, 25]. The BSRS-5, which was designed for the early detection of minor mental disorders associated with depression and anxiety, is also a very useful tool to detect the presence of SI [23, 24]. It has been used by some hospitals for routinely screening inpatients with medical illness and people receiving regular physical check-ups. The proposed cut-off score of 5/6 for a total score of 5 items of the BSRS-5, which we called "model of 5/6 for BSRS-5" hereafter, was implemented to identify people with psychiatric comorbidity [26, 27]. In a case-control study for exploring suicide attempts in the elderly, those with BSRS-5 total scores greater than 5 were 17.8 times more likely to have a suicide attempt than those with scores less than or equal to 5 [10]. A study recruiting hospitalized medical inpatients in Taiwan found that depression, inferiority, insomnia, and hostility in BSRS-5 were significantly related to the presence of SI [24]. However, in that study, age distribution, such as mean, standard deviation or percentage across age groups was not specified, and subgroup analyses focusing on the elderly or comparisons between different age groups were not done. Hence, certain items of BSRS-5 in hospitalized elderly with medical or surgical conditions, remains unknown. Consequently, two important questions related to the BSRS-5 studies are worth exploring, i.e., (1) which items of BSRS-5 are predictive of SI in the physically ill elderly inpatients, and (2) is the predictive ability of a model made up of certain items of BSRS-5 in question 1 better than that of a model of 5/6 for BSRS-5? These answers may elucidate the most important factors related to SI for physically ill elderly inpatients and set up a parsimonious model to predict SI and build up more effective strategies mainly focusing on these characteristics to diminish rates of subsequent suicidal behaviors.

Thus, the aim of this study were: (1) to explore the prevalence of SI for physically ill elderly inpatients; (2) to find the association between QOL and SI; (3) to investigate the prevalence and the factors related to WTD; (4) to explore the association between the items of BSRS-5 and SI; (5) to find a parsimonious model predictive of SI from three models using items of the

BSRS-5 as predictor variables, i.e., certain items of BSRS-5 significantly associated with SI obtained from multivariate regression models, a single variable of BSRS-5 total scores greater than 5 (model of 5/6 for BSRS-5), and all five items of the BSRS-5.

Method

Study design and subjects

Since 2007, for maximizing the nationwide use of BSRS-5, which was called "Mood Thermometer" as a tool for mental health and suicide screening in Taiwan, the Taiwan Department of Health has been proposing a multi-site suicide prevention program with sufficient grants to hospitals. The suicide prevention program required that each grant-aided hospital should submit a research project using BSRS-5 alone rather than other SI screening instruments such as Columbia Suicide Screening [28] or Beck Scale for suicidal ideation (BSSI) [29] to single out community residents or patients with SI; subsequently, the program demanded that each subsidized hospital should refer the interviewees whose BSRS total scores were greater than 5 or those with the presence of SI to psychiatrists for further treatment. This study was a cross-sectional design. It was aided by grants and was conducted between February and December 2012 in Mennonite Christian Hospital in Hualien County, which is a referral hospital for a large area in the east of Taiwan. Subjects were selected by a convenience sampling from various medical services. A total of 2199 participants who were screened from a large pool of 2300 hospitalized elderly patients participated in this study. All of 101 patients were excluded because of reasons as follows: using antidepressants ($n = 54$, 53.4%), refusing to participate ($n = 19$, 18.8%), being admitted to wards which did not belong to the units defined in the inclusion criteria ($n = 11$, 10.9%), patients with acute critical conditions unfitted for participation ($n = 9$, 8.9%), schizophrenia patients admitted to the psychiatric ward ($n = 8$, 8%). Information was obtained from both the patients and families on the third day after admission by well-trained interviewers. Inclusion criteria included: (1) patients who were admitted to medical or surgical wards other than oncology, hospice, psychiatric wards or intensive care units; (2) patients over age 65; (3) patients who were able to communicate with interviewers. Exclusion criteria included: (1) patients who used antidepressants or mood stabilizers before admission; (2) patients had difficulty in communication due to sensory problems, or had significant cognitive impairment such as delirium or dementia. Sociodemographic information was obtained regarding sex, age, educational level (uneducated, primary school, junior high school, senior high school, or above), marital status (married, unmarried, which included single, divorced, or widowed), living situation (living alone, living with friends, or living with relatives), economic status (good, fair, or poor), and perceived health status (good or poor). The study design was reviewed by the Institutional Review Board (IRB) of Mennonite Christian Hospital. All the subjects provided informed consent before this study began.

Measures

Definition of suicidal ideation

A question in BSRS-5, "Do you have any suicide ideation?" was supplemented at the end of the questionnaire. If the subject answered "Yes", then the presence of SI was confirmed.

Quality of life

To measure the QOL, the Taiwanese version of the World Health Organization Quality of Life-BREF (WHOQOL-BREF TW) [30] was used to assess the global QOL of patients in medical settings. The WHOQOL-BREF TW includes 26 items (24 items that represent each of the 24 specific facets of the WHOQOL-100 and 2 global/general items). In addition, in the WHOQOL-BREF TW, two additional national items were generated and validated from the Taiwan version of the WHOQOL-100 [31]. The factor structure of the WHOQOL-BREF TW includes 4 domains, i.e., physical (QOL-PHY), psychological (QOL-PSY), social relationships (QOL-SR), and environmental (QOL-ENV). For a given item or domain of the WHOQOL-BREF, a higher score indicates a greater level of quality of life.

Wish to die

For those who had SI, each one should be assessed for the presence of a WTD, which was obtained using item 2 of the Beck Scale for SI (BSSI) that is a 19-item rating scale designed to evaluate the risk of suicidal intention [29]. We redefined item 2 in the BSSI, in which no wish or a weak WTD were categorized into a faint WTD (coded as 0), and a moderate or a strong WTD (MTS-WTD, coded as 1).

BSRS-5

The severity of distress and psychopathology were measured using the BSRS-5 [23] derived from the SCL-90-R [32]. The participants were asked to rate symptoms on a 5-point scale: 0, not at all; 1, a little bit; 2, moderately; 3, quite a bit; and 4, extremely, and a total score was calculated for each participant. A higher BSRS-5 total score indicates poorer mental health. The full scale included the following five items of psychopathology: (1) BSRS-5 item 1(anxiety): feeling tense or keyed up; (2) item 2 (depression): feeling low in mood; (3) item 3 (hostility): feeling easily annoyed or irritated; (4) BSRS-5 item 4 (inferiority): feeling inferior to others; and (5) item 5 (insomnia): having trouble falling asleep. A variable of a total score of BSRS-5 greater than 5 was formed because it represented significant psychiatric morbidity for an individual [26, 27], and it was highly associated with suicidal behavior in the elderly [10].

Cognitive function was assessed based on a Chinese version [33] of the Mini-Mental State Examination (MMSE) [34], in which the maximum score is 30, and a higher score indicates better cognition. Impaired cognition was defined for those who were uneducated and had MMSE scores less than 14, and the educated with the scores less than 24 [33].

Statistical analyses

SPSS version 19 (IBM company) was used to conduct statistical analyses. The significance level was set at a value of 0.05 (two-tailed). The rule for the selection of covariates in multivariate logistic regression models was as follows: for avoiding multi-collinearity, the covariates selected to be placed in the regression models in this study should be tested with the analysis of correlation in advance; Spearman rho for either or both of the covariates which were categorical variables or Pearson correlation coefficient for both which were continuous variables, were obtained. If the value of coefficients between two certain explanatory covariates was greater than 0.7, then the correlation coefficient between the dependent variable with these two explanatory covariates was examined. The covariate with greater absolute value of correlation coefficient between it and the dependent variable was put into the regression model.

Model 1: Multivariate logistic regression models to explore factors related to SI

For the reduction in the number of variables in the regression models, the univariate analyses were firstly used to explore the association between variables of interest and SI. Subsequently, the variables with statistically significant differences between groups were put into two multivariate logistic models. In the following description of different models, "A" denoted that "some or all items of BSRS-5" were included in the model, and "B" indicated that the model included the variable of "BSRS-5 total score greater than 5".

Model 1A Model 1A included independent variables, such as five items of BSRS-5, age, gender, and other covariates with statistically significant differences between groups.

Model 1B In Model 1B, except for the variable of BSRS-5 total scores greater than 5, which replaced the BSRS-5 item 1 through 5, other variables were the same as those in the Model 1A.

Model 2: Multivariate logistic models to explore the items of WHOQOL-BREF related to SI

For the reduction in the number of variables in the multivariate regression analysis, if some domains of WHOQOL-BREF were found to be statistically significantly associated with SI in Model 1A or Model 1B, then all items of these domains would be compared using a univariate analysis. The WHOQOL-BREF items with significant differences between groups were put into Model 2A and Model 2B.

Model 2A The independent variable of Model 2A included the WHOQOL-BREF items with significant differences after the univariate analysis, the same demographic factors included in Model 1A, and the items of BSRS-5 significantly related to SI in Model 1A.

Model 2B In Model 2B, except for the variable of BSRS-5 total scores greater than 5, which replaced the items of BSRS-5 in Model 2A, all independent variables were the same as those in Model 2A.

Model 3: Univariate logistic regression models exploring factors related to MTS-WTD in those who had SI

Univariate logistic regression models were used to explore the association between covariates and MTS-WTD because we expected the number of patients with MTS-WTD would be small in those who had SI. Except for the individual sum of four domains of WHOOQOL-BREF, all variables in Model 1A and 28 items of the WHOOQOL-BREF were put into univariate models as covariates.

Model 4: Comparison between different propensity score models of BSRS-5 predicting SI using Receiver Operating Characteristic (ROC) curve analysis

To get a parsimonious model predicting SI, we used a propensity score model (PSM), in which multiple variables were included and formed a propensity score (PS) (the value was between 0 and 1); the coefficients of covariates of the PSM were obtained from a multivariate logistic model [35]. The PS generated from different models was used as a state variable in the ROC curve analysis.

Model 4A The state variable in Model 4A was the PS generated from the PSM, which included certain BSRS-5 items found to be significantly associated with SI in Model 1A as predictor variables.

Model 4B Model 4B, i.e., the "model of 5/6 of BSRS-5", included a state variable, which was the PS generated from the PSM, and the covariate of BSRS-5 total scores greater than 5 as a predictor variable.

Model 4C In Model 4C, the state variable was the PS generated from the PSM, which included all items of BSRS-5 as predictor variables.

The difference in areas under the curve (AUCs) between each two models was compared [36]. We think a good model predicting SI should meet the following conditions: (1) the sensitivity, specificity, positive predictive value (PPV), negative predictive value (NPV), and accuracy, i.e., five indexes of ROC should be all greater than or equal to 0.8; (2) If two models met criteria 1, and the difference in AUCs between them did not reach a statistically significant level, then a parsimonious model was selected.

Results
Demographic data
The average age for all participants (n = 2199) was 76.4 ± 7.4. Male patients accounted for 55.4% (n = 1218). A total of 1195 (54.5%) were admitted to medical wards, in which most received the treatment from the team of pulmonary medicine (n = 276, 12.5%). For patients admitted to surgical wards (n = 908, 41.2%), most were under the care of general surgery (n = 249, 11.32%). Missed classification of ward accounted for 4.36% (n = 96). Table 1 presents the classification of subspecialty teams which took care of patients admitted to the general hospital. SI was found in 3.1% (68/2199) of the elderly, and 25.3% (557/2199) had BSRS-5 total scores greater than 5. Approximately one-fourth of participants with SI had a MTS-WTD (25.5%, 14/68). Sociodemographic variables are presented in Table 2. Table 3 shows the results of the comparison of characteristics between those with SI and those without. There were statistically

Table 1 Classification based on medical or surgical wards for participants admitted to the general hospital (n = 2199)

Classification of ward	Team	n	Percentage
Medical ward	–	1195	54.3%
	Cardiology	167	7.59%
	Nephrology	233	10.59%
	Neurology	206	9.36%
	Gastroenterology	247	11.23%
	Pulmonary medicine	276	12.55%
	Infectious disease	66	3.0%
Surgical ward	–	908	41.29%
	Neurosurgery	100	4.54%
	Urology	245	11.14%
	Orthopedics	235	10.68%
	Plastic surgery	79	3.59%
	General surgery	249	11.32%
Missed classification		96	4.36%

significant differences between the two groups in variables as follows: being unmarried, having poor economic status, perception of poor health, BSRS-5 item 1–5, BSRS-5 total scores greater than 5, physical domain of WHOOQOL-BRIEF(QOL-PHY), psychological domain of WHOOQOL-BRIEF(QOL-PSY), and environmental domain of WHOOQOL-BRIEF(QOL-ENV). Table 4 shows the illustration of different models in this current study.

Model 1: Factors related to SI in the multivariate analysis
The correlation analysis found that QOL-PSY and QOL-ENV was highly correlated (Pearson correlation coefficient = 0.74). Finally, QOL-ENV was deleted because the Spearman rho coefficient between QOL-PSY and SI was – 0.139, the absolute value of which was greater than that between QOL-ENV and SI (Spearman rho coefficient = – 0.09). In addition to age and gender, all those variables with statistically significant differences between those with SI and those without in Table 3 were put into regression models. Table 5 shows the factors statistically significantly related to SI in different models.

Model 1A
Model 1A included independent variables as follows: age, gender, economic status, perception of poor health, non-married, QOL-PHY, QOL-PSY, and five items of BSRS-5 item. Model 1A revealed factors statistically significantly associated with SI as follows: BSRS-5 item 2 (depression) (OR = 2.15, 95% CI = 1.56–2.98), item 4 (inferiority) (OR = 1.62, 95% CI = 1.23–2.13), item 5 (insomnia) (OR = 1.52, 95% CI = 1.13–2.05), and QOL-PHY (OR = 0.84, 95% CI = 0.72–0.99).

Model 1B
In Model 1B, BSRS-5 total scores greater than 5 (OR = 9.36, 95% CI = 4.86–18.0) and QOL-PHY (OR = 0.81, 95% CI = 0.69–0.94) were statistically significantly associated with the presence of SI.

Model 2: Items of QOL related to SI
Table 6 shows the items of WHOQOL-BREF that were related to SI. We put items of QOL-PHY into Model 2A and Model 2B because the scores of QOL-PHY were found to be related to SI in Model 1A and Model 1B.

Model 2A
Model 2A included the same demographic factors as those in Model 1A, BSRS-5 item 2 (depression), item 4 (inferiority), item 5 (insomnia), and all items of QOL-PHY except QOL11 (feeling of bodily appearance), which did not have statistically significant associations with SI in the univariate analysis, and QOL17 (level of daily activities), which was highly correlated with QOL15 (mobility) (Pearson

Table 2 Participant characteristics and demographic data

Variables		Minimum	Maximum	Mean	S.D.
Age (years)	–	65	101	76.4	7.4
Sex (n, %)	Male	–	–	1218	55.4
Marital status (n, %)	unmarried	–	–	1038	47.2
Education (n, %)	Uneducated	–	–	849	38.6
	Primary school	–	–	374	17.0
	Junior high school	–	–	688	31.3
	Senior high school or above	–	–	288	13.1
Living alone (n, %)	Alone	–	–	425	19.3
Economic status	Poor	–	–	341	15.5
(n, %)	Fair	–	–	1671	76.0
	Good	–	–	187	8.5
Perception of health status (n, %)	Poor	–	–	1281	58.3
Suicide ideation (n, %)		–	–	68	3.1
BSRS	Total scores	0	17	3.7	3.0
BSRS total score > 5 (n, %)		–	–	557	25.3
Quality of life subdomains	Total scores	26.4	77.4	52.4	7.3
	Physical health	5.1	19.4	12.5	2.5
	Social relationship	6.0	20.0	13.5	2.2
	Environmental	5.8	19.1	13.7	1.9
	Psychological	6.0	19.3	12.9	2.3
MMSE	Total scores	0	30	21.1	6.2
Impaired cognition (n, %)		–	–	850	38.7

Non-living alone: living with people including spouse, children, relatives, friends
Unmarried: current marital status including single, divorced, windowed
BSRS Brief Symptom Rating Scale
MMSE Mini-Mental State Examination

correlation coefficient = 0.73). The QOL17 was deleted in Model 2 because the Spearman rho coefficient between the QO15 and SI was – 0.11, the absolute value of which was greater than that between QOL 17 and SI (spearman rho coefficient = – 0.09). Model 2A revealed that QOL15 (mobility) was statistically significantly associated with SI (OR = 0.60, 95% CI = 0.42–0.85).

Model 2B
In Model 2B, except for the variable of BSRS-5 total scores greater than 5, which replaced BSRS-5 items 2, 4, and 5, all independent variables were the same as those in Model 2A. The Model 2B revealed that QOL15 (mobility) (OR = 0.64, 95% CI = 0.46–0.90) and QOL16 (satisfaction with sleep) (OR = 0.62 95% CI = 0.44–0.88) were statistically significantly associated with SI.

Model 3: Factors related to MTS-WTD
Table 7 presents the factors significantly related to MTS-WTD among participants with SI. A univariate model was used rather than a multivariate model due to a small number of participants with MTS-WTD ($n = $ 14), which might result in a low statistical power if a multivariate model were used. The results of Model 3 showed that living alone (OR = 4.44, 95% CI = 1.24–15.87), QOL 26 (absence of negative feeling) (OR = 0.38, 95% CI = 0.15–0.98) and QOL 27(being respected/accepted) (OR = 0.43, 95% CI = 0.20–0.92) were statistically significantly associated with MTS-WTD among inpatients with SI.

Model 4: Comparison between different models of BSRS-5 predicting SI
Table 8 shows the results of comparison between different models predicting SI.

Model 4A
Model 4A used a PSM to get a PS, in which predictor variables included BSRS-5 item 2 (depression), item 4 (inferiority), and item 5 (insomnia); these three items were obtained from Model 1A. In this model, for a given subject, if the PS > 0.0355, then it was predictive of SI.

Table 3 A comparison of characteristics between those with suicidal ideation and those who were without

Variables	Suicidal ideation	Non-suicidal ideation	p-value
Age (years)	76.0 (7.9)	76.4 (7.3)	0.68
Sex, male (n, %)	32 (47.1)	1186 (55.7)	0.16
Education (n, %)			0.23
Non-educated	30 (44.1)	819 (38.4)	
Primary school	12 (17.6)	362 (17.0)	
Junior high school	14 (20.6)	674 (31.6)	
More than senior high school	12 (17.6)	276 (13)	
Unmarried (n, %)	41(60.3)	997 (46.8)	0.03
Living alone (n, %)	17 (25.0)	408 (19.1)	0.23
Good economic support (n, %)	40 (58.8)	1395 (65.5)	0.26
Economic status (n, %)			0.001
Poor	25 (36.8)	316 (14.8)	
Fair	40 (58.8)	1631 (76.5)	
Good	3 (4.4)	184 (8.6)	
Perception of poor health (n, %)	56 (82.4%)	501 (23.5)	0.001
BSRS total score greater than 5 (n, %)	12 (17.6%)	1630 (76.5%)	0.001
BSRS-5 item 1 (anxiety)	1.54 (1.11)	0.67 (0.89)	0.001
BSRS-5 item 2 (depression)	2.19 (0.93)	0.87 (0.95)	0.001
BSRS-5 item 3 (hostility)	1.66 (1.16)	0.62 (0.85)	0.001
BSRS-5 item 4 (inferiority)	1.04 (1.2)	0.20 (0.56)	0.001
BSRS-5 item 5 (insomnia)	2.09 (1.04)	1.14 (1.01)	0.001
QOL-physical health	10.35 (1.19)	12.53 (2.46)	0.001
QOL-psychological	11.06 (1.83)	12.85 (2.2)	0.001
QOL-social relationship	13.07 (2.04)	13.54 (2.15)	0.07
QOL-environmental	12.51 (1.88)	13.63 (1.87)	0.001
Impaired cognition	21 (30.9%)	38.9 (38.9%)	0.18

Comparison analyses were used to compare the difference in variables between those with suicidal ideation and those without using independent t-test or chi-square test

Unmarried: current marital status including single, divorced, widowed

BSRS Brief Symptom Rating Scale, *QOL* quality of life rated with the WHOQOL-BREF

Model 4B
In Model 4B, i.e., the model of 5/6 for BSRS-5, for a given subject, if the PS > 0.0539, then it was predictive of SI.

Model 4C
Model 4C, in which predictor variables included all five items of BSRS-5, for a given subject, if the PS > 0.0386, then it was predictive of SI.

Figure 1 shows that the AUC of Model 4B was the least among three models. There were no statistically significant differences between the AUC of Model 4A and that of Model 4C (p = 0.785). However, the AUCs of both Model 4A and Model 4C were statistically significantly greater than that of Model 4B (p < 0.00001). Regarding the indexes of ROC, the specificity, PPV, and accuracy in the Model 4B were all below 0.8. Conversely,

five indexes of ROC of Model 4A and Model 4C were all greater than or equal to 0.8. In summary, Model 4A was the parsimonious model predictive of SI. In the BSRS-5, item 2 (depression), item 4 (inferiority), and item 5 (insomnia) were the most important items significantly associated with SI among the elderly inpatients in this study.

Discussion
The prevalence of SI
Our study found that the 3.1% of the elderly hospitalized patients with medical or surgical conditions had SI. Notably, the prevalence of SI in the current study was much lower than those of prior studies, i.e., 36% in the UK [5] and 21.6% in Iran [1]. The inconsistency might be explained by the following reasons. First, there were differences in the instruments assessing SI,

Table 4 Illustration of different models in this study

Model 1: Multivariate logistic regression models exploring factors related to SI	1A: Independent variables included age, gender, economic status, perception of poor health, unmarried, QOL-PHY, QOL-PSY, and five items of BSRS-5 item.
	1B: Independent variables included: variables were the same as those in the Model 1A except for the variable of BSRS-5 total scores greater than 5, which replaced the BSRS-5 item 1 through 5.
Model 2: Multivariate logistic models exploring the items of WHOQOL-BREF related to SI	2A: Independent variables included BSRS-5 item 2 (depression), item 4 (inferiority), item 5 (insomnia), and all items of QOL-PHY except QOL11 (feeling of bodily appearance) and QOL17 (level of daily activities).
	2B: Independent variables: all were the same as those in Model 2A except for the variable of BSRS-5 total scores greater than 5 replacing BSRS-5 item 2 (depression), item 4 (inferiority), item 5 (insomnia).
Model 3: Univariate logistic regression models exploring factors related to MTS-WTD in those who had SI	Independent variables: variables in Model 1A and 28 items of the WHOOQOL-BREF except for the individual sum of four domains of WHOOQOL-BREF, i.e., QOL-PHY, QOL-PSY, QOL-ENV, QOL-SR.
Model 4: Comparison between different propensity score models of BSRS-5 predicting SI using ROC curve analysis.	State variable in 4A-4C: propensity score from individual propensity score model
	4A: predictor variables included BSRS-5 item 2 (depression), item 4 (inferiority), and item 5 (insomnia)
	4B: predictor variable: the variable of BSRS-5 total scores greater than 5
	4C: predictor variables included all five items of BSRS-5

SI suicidal ideation, *BSRS* Brief Symptom Rating Scale, *WHOQOL-BREF* the World Health Organization Quality of Life-BREF, *QOL-PHY* physical domain of WHOQOL-BREF, *QOL-PSY* psychological domain of WHOQOL-BREF, *QOL-ENV* environmental domain of WHOQOL-BREF, *QOL-SR* the domain of social relationships of WHOQOL-BREF, *QOL* quality of life rated with the WHOQOL-BREF, *MTS-WTD* moderate to severe wish to die, *ROC* Receiver Operating Characteristic

i.e., the BSSI in both studies [1, 5] vs. the item 6 of BSRS-5 in this current study. One of the former studies used the total scores of 19 items of the BSSI; SI was coded if the total score for an individual was greater than 4 [1]. However, in this study, every interviewee was asked a present-tense-question: "Do you have any suicide ideation?" The definition of SI out of yes/no is different from those of the former studies. In addition, patients in the former studies had acute physical conditions, yet in our study, participants included acute or subacute patients who might be admitted for elective procedures, such as elective gastroscopy or elective operation. Finally, the discrepancy in the prevalence might be partly accounted for

Table 5 Multivariate logistic regression models exploring factors related to suicidal ideation

Independent variables	Model 1A[a]		Model 1B[b]	
	AOR	95% CI	AOR	95% CI
Age	1.002	0.96–1.04	0.98	0.94–1.02
Gender	1.11	0.63–1.93	0.99	0.58–1.70
Economic status (reference level = poor)				
Fair	0.74	0.41–1.35	0.61	0.35–1.08
Good	0.6	0.15–2.29	0.57	0.16–2.04
Single	1.44	0.80–2.58	1.42	0.82–2.48
Perception of poor health	1.14	0.55–2.36	1.08	0.54–2.15
BSRS-5 total scores > 5 (ref. level: ≤ 5)	–	–	9.36**	4.86–18.0
BSRS-5 item 1(anxiety)	1.25	0.93–1.68	–	–
BSRS-5 item 2(depression)	2.15**	1.56–2.98	–	–
BSRS-5 item 3(hostility)	1.22	0.91–1.64	–	–
BSRS-5 item 4(inferiority)	1.62**	1.23–2.13	–	–
BSRS-5 item 5(insomnia)	1.52**	1.13–2.05	–	–
QOL (physical health)	0.84*	0.72–0.99	0.81**	0.69–0.94
QOL (psychological)	0.93	0.79–1.09	0.89	0.77–1.04

*$p < 0.05$; **$p < 0.01$; *AOR* adjusted odds ratio, *BSRS* Brief Symptom Rating Scale, *QOL* quality of life rated with WHOQOL-BREF
[a]Model 1A: independent variables included age, gender, economic status, perception of poor health, non-married, QOL-physical health, QOL-psychological, QOL-environment and five items of BSRS-5
[b]Model 1B: except for BSRS total score greater than 5 which replaced five items of BSRS-5, other variables were the same as those in the Model 1A

Table 6 Multivariate logistic regression models exploring items of quality of life related to suicidal ideation

Independent variables	Suicidal ideation ($n = 68$)	
Model 2A for QOL related to SI [a]	AOR	95% CI
QOL Item 15 Mobility	0.60[**]	0.42–0.85
Model 2B for QOL related to SI [b]		
QOL Item 15 Mobility	0.64[*]	0.46–0.90
QOL Item 16 Satisfaction with sleep	0.62[**]	0.44–0.88

[*] $p < 0.05$; [**] $p < 0.01$; AOR adjusted odds ratio

SI suicidal ideation, QOL quality of life rated with WHOQOL-BREF, BSRS Brief Symptom Rating Scale

[a]Multivariate analysis: dependent variable: suicidal ideation; independent variables included demographic factors as those in Model 1, BSRS-5 item 2 (depression), BSRS-5 item4 (inferiority), BSRS-5 item5 (insomnia) and all items of QOL-physical health except item 11 and item 17-daily activities which was highly correlated with item 15-mobility (pearson correlation coefficient = 0.73) causing multi-collinearity. Only significant QOL variables were presented in this table

[b]Multivariate analysis: except BSRS total score greater than 5 which replaced BSRS-5 item 2, BSRS-5 item 4 and BSRS-5 item 5, all independent variables were the same as those in the Model 1A. Only significant QOL variables were presented in this table

Table 8 Comparison of indexes of receiver operation characteristic curve between different models

Model	△AUC	AUC	SEN	SPC	PPV	NPV	Accuracy
Model 4A[a]	△A-C	0.88	0.83	0.80	0.81	0.83	0.82
Model 4B[b]	△A-B[*]	0.79	0.82	0.76	0.77	0.81	0.79
Model 4C[c]	△B-C[*]	0.88	0.82	0.82	0.82	0.82	0.82

AUC area under curve, SEN sensitivity, SPC specificity, PPV positive predictive value, NPV negative predictive value

△AUC = difference in AUC between various models

△A-B[*]: significant difference in AUC between Model 4A and Model 4B ($p < 0.00001$); △B-C[*]: the same meaning as that of △A-B[*] ($p < 0.00001$); △A-C: no significant difference in AUC between Model 4A and Model 4C ($p = 0.785$)

[a]Model 4A

Propensity model:

$Y = 0.963*BSRS\text{-}5 \text{ item } 2 + 0.564*BSRS\text{-}5 \text{ item } 4 - 0.655*BSRS\text{-}5 \text{ item } 5 + 6.285$

propensity score = expY/(1 + expY);

For a given individual, if the propensity score > 0.0355, then the model was predictive of suicidal ideation

[b]Model 4B

BSRS-5 total score greater than 5 coded as 1, otherwise as 0

Propensity model:

$Y = 2.72*(BSRS\text{-}5 \text{ total score greater than } 5) - 4.911$

propensity score = expY/(1 + expY);

For a given individual, if the propensity score > 0.0539, then the model was predictive of suicidal ideation

[c]Model 4C

Propensity model:

$Y = 1.226*BSRS\text{-}5 \text{ item } 1 + 2.337*BSRS\text{-}5 \text{ item } 2 + 1.297*BSRS\text{-}5 \text{ item } 3 + 1.646*BSRS\text{-}5 \text{ item } 4 - 1.694*BSRS\text{-}5 \text{ item } 5 + 6.374$

propensity score = expY/(1 + expY);

For a given individual, if the propensity score > 0.0386, then the model was predictive of suicidal ideation

by the various sample sizes among three studies, i.e., 55 [5], 650 [1], and 2199 in our study.

Primary analysis of factors including demographic variables, BSRS-5, and four domains of QOL related to SI

Our study also found depression, inferiority, insomnia in BSRS-5, and the sum of physical domain of QOL were significantly associated with SI. As our result indicated, depression is a major determinant of SI or suicidal behavior among elderly people in the community [6, 10, 13] or inpatients [1, 5]. Although insomnia is highly associated with depression, after adjustment in the regression model, it was still significantly associated with SI. This finding is compatible with that of a study which found that poor sleep increases the risk of SI, but only among people with no or one mental health condition [37]. Total sleep time is an important predictor of suicidal behavior that requires particular attention [38], and changes in insomnia drive subsequent changes in suicidal ideation [39]. Therefore, it is important for physicians to detect insomnia as a sign of suicidal behavior, regardless of which illness a patient may suffer from [40]. Of interest, our study found that inferiority, which is seen as a lack of covert self-esteem [41], was correlated

with SI in elderly inpatients. This finding is compatible with that of a study which found that low self-esteem was associated with suicidal intent, independently of the severity of depression [42]. A study recruiting 2964 community members also found that low self-esteem is one of the major risk factors related to SI [43], and another study revealed that low self-esteem and low sense of self-efficacy may lead to a suicide attempt [44]. Two other studies in elderly inpatients [1, 5] revealed that factors related to SI were use of antidepressants, previous deliberate self-harm, pessimism, length of hospital stay, history of traumatic events, the level of social support, and the presence of depression, which was found to be a major determinant of SI in many studies [6, 10–14]. While clinical depression was found to be a common factor related to SI in previous research and this study, the dissimilarity of the results between both prior studies [1, 5] and current one may be

Table 7 Univariate logistic regression models exploring factors associated with a moderate to strong wish to die

Independent variables	Moderate to strong wish to die [a] ($n = 14$)	
Living alone	4.44[**]	1.24–15.87
QOL Item 26 Absence of negative feeling	0.38[*]	0.15–0.98
QOL Item 27 Being respected/accepted	0.43[*]	0.20–0.92

[*] $p < 0.05$; [**] $p < 0.01$

QOL quality of life rated with WHOQOL-BREF

[a]Univariate analysis: dependent variable: a moderate to strong wish to die; independent variables included all demographic factors, i.e., age, gender, economic status, economic resources, perception of poor health, single, living alone, impaired cognition, five items of the BSRS-5 and the variable of BSRS-5 total scores greater than 5 as well as QOL item 1–28

Prevalence and characteristics of suicidal ideation among 2199 elderly inpatients with surgical...

53

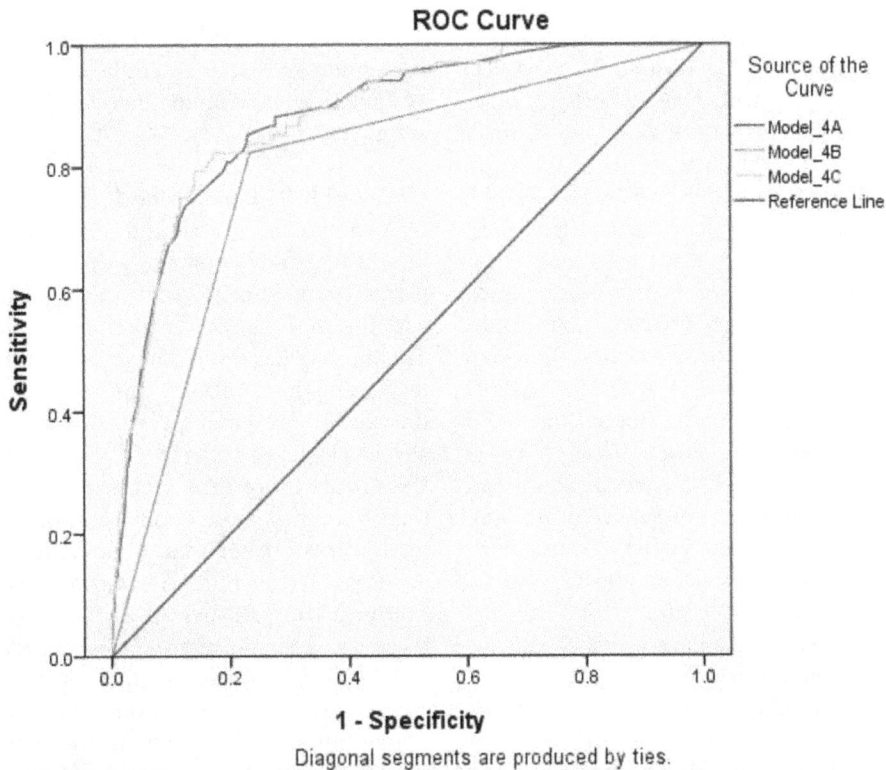

Fig. 1 Comparison of receiver operation characteristic curve between different models. Note. State variable in 4A-4C: propensity score from individual propensity score model. Model_4A: predictor variables included BSRS-5 item 2 (depression), item 4 (inferiority), and item 5 (insomnia). Model_4B: predictor variable: the variable of BSRS-5 total scores greater than 5. Model_4C: predictor variables included all five items of BSRS-5

caused by various sample sizes of inpatients identified with SI and different variables in the analysis, for example, the physical domain of QOL which was not explored in the other two studies but seemed to play a role in the presence of SI in our study.

The association of QOL and SI

Our finding is consistent with that of a study that revealed that a lower level of QOL was correlated with SI in the elderly [6]. A study that enrolled 4506 adults in the community aged 60 or above indicated an inverse relationship between the levels of QOL with SI [7]. After adjustment for covariates, our study found that the physical domain of WHOQOL-BREF was correlated with SI among elderly inpatients. In addition to "satisfaction with sleep", further analysis indicated "mobility" was the major determinants of QOL associated with SI. A large survey of 8500 adults over the age of 65, which found a moderate limitation in usual activities caused by arthritis and renal failure increased the risk of suicidal ideation and suicide attempt, supports our findings [45]. Additionally, a systematic analysis has shown the association between physical illness/functional disability and suicidal behavior [46].

Clinical implication based on the analysis of items of BSRS-5 and QOL-PHY related to SI

In short, the analysis of all factors revealed that depression, inferiority, insomnia in BSRS-5, and mobility in QOL-PHY were associated with the presence of SI. On the basis of findings from our study and prior research, it is important to screen elderly inpatients with depression, insomnia, or feelings of inferiority to others, and provide support for exploring the potentially effective treatment of these conditions to lessen the risk of SI and subsequent suicide attempt. In addition, it is necessary to remind the medical staff to improve the mobility and activities for physically ill elderly inpatients, particularly when they have presented with aforementioned BSRS-5 risk factors for SI. It is suggested that a suicide-intervention support team be setup in the hospital, especially focusing on inpatients with mobility limitations. Early screening and adequate intervention, such as using mobility aids, providing transport assistance, maximizing involvement in recreational activities, and arranging rehabilitation programs or surgical procedures improving mobility, such as arthroplasty for this population, are expected to decrease the suicidal ideation and suicidal behavior in the future.

Related factors of MTS-WTD in patients with SI

Among the elderly receiving primary care services, the prevalence of WTD was 6% [47]. Most strikingly, WTD was found to be associated with 5-year mortality independently of depressive status in the elderly in primary care patients who had a WTD without depression still had a higher mortality rate than those without WTD [9]. In other similar studies, the prevalence of inpatients with WTD seemed to be much lower than those with SI [1, 5]. Different from the analysis of prior studies, which evaluated the prevalence of all participants, our study, which revealed that 25.4% of patients with SI had a WTD, only assessed the presence of WTD for suicidal ideators. A study exploring the motives for suicide found that suicide attempts could be categorized into WTD and wish to change (WTC); the WTD group rather than the WTC group had a higher risk for suicide death [48]. Based on the observation of prior studies and our finding that only one-fourth of suicidal ideators had a MTS-WTD, it is reasonable to postulate that suicidal ideators who had a WTD might have a higher risk for subsequent suicidal behavior than those who had SI alone, although this hypothesis was not tested in the current study.

Our univariate analysis found that living alone, the level of negative feeling, and the level of being accepted/respected were associated with MTS-WTD in participants with SI. This observation is in accordance with that of a prior study, which revealed that depression and pessimism were related to WTD in medically ill elderly inpatients [5]. Likewise, other studies support our finding: the status of living was associated with suicide in the elderly [18]; perceived sense of belonging, substantial support, self-esteem, and chronic interpersonal problems were correlated with SI [49]; the factors related to WTD in the elderly were depression [50], hopelessness [51], social support, and subjective well-being [52]. The significant association between WTD and three variables in our study, i.e., living alone, negative feeling, and feelings of being accepted/respected suggest medical staff take proper measure in time; that is, when elderly inpatients are found to live alone before admission, or to present with negative feelings, such as hopelessness or a sense of being abandoned, they should be evaluated for the presence of WTD. If the above factors related to WTD are confirmed in an individual, for the purpose of preventing suicide, it should be recommended that they consult a social worker to provide sufficient social support, or a psychiatrist for proper evaluation and treatment, such as prescribing psychotropic agents, referral for psychological counseling, or administering cognitive behavior therapy. It is worth noting that WTD is an important issue in terminally ill patients in palliative care, although we did not address this topic here. There were many reasons when patients expressed a WTD [53]. It is of importance to broaden therapeutic options for suicide prevention and intervention by detecting the presence of WTD and appraising the motives for WTD statement in elderly inpatients.

Models of BSRS-5 predicting SI

Our study showed that the PSM including depression, inferiority, and insomnia was a parsimonious model predictive of SI compared to the 5/6 for BSRS-5 model and the other model including all five BSRS-5 items. This finding has double meanings: (1) depression, inferiority, and insomnia are the most important items of the BSRS-5, explaining the variance of SI in the physically ill elderly inpatients; (2) the predictive value of a PSM made up of three items of BSRS-5 on SI is better than that of a model using a single variable of BSRS total scores greater than 5 alone; this implies that not all items of the BSRS-5 contribute equally or significantly to the presence of SI. Our result revealed that there was a significant association between three items of BSRS-5, i.e. depression, inferiority, and insomnia and the presence of SI. However, limited by the cross-sectional design of this study, it does not necessary mean that SI causes the presence of these three items; it could also be that depression, inferiority, and insomnia are the results of SI. Of note, this finding highlights a fact that these three items of BSRS-5 are important markers for patients with SI. It is necessary to screen elderly inpatients presenting with these items and to tailor specific interventions for maximizing the effectiveness of suicidal prevention under the limited resources. A further implication is to use the PSM, including three items of the BSRS-5, to single out those with SI in this population (please download the calculator presented in the form of Excel [54]) although the calculation of the BSRS-5 total score for a cut-off point is seemingly easier to use.

This result is partly in line with that of a study also using the BSRS-5 which revealed that depression, inferiority, insomnia, and hostility were significantly related to the presence of SI in 969 hospitalized patients with general medical conditions in southern Taiwan [24]. Different from that study, hostility was not associated with SI in the current study. This disparity in results between the former study and our study may be due in part to dissimilarities in following factors: (1) age group: not specifying detail information of age in the former vs. elderly adults in our study, (2) the prevalence of SI: 12.7% (123/969) vs. 3.1% (68/2199), and (3) the mean score of hostility: 0.74 vs. 0.65. The most remarkable evidence indicating the characteristics of SI in elderly inpatients which differed from other age groups, is that the former study proposed a parsimonious model using BSRS-5 total scores 12/13 as a cut-off point predictive of SI (PPV = 0.92 and NPV = 0.88). However, this cut-off point tested in our study was found to be a statistically insignificant model for predicting SI in elderly inpatients (PPV = 0.95, NPV =0.52, AUC = 0.55, $p = 0.115$). This finding indicates that physically ill elderly inpatients have unique features regarding SI, which may be distinctly different from those of other age groups. More studies exploring the age effect on SI among inpatients with medical and surgical conditions are needed in the future.

Strength and limitation
To our knowledge, the strength of this study is that it is the first one recruiting a very large sample size of participants to explore SI, WTD, and QOL in physically ill elderly inpatients in East Asia. Second, a PSM was developed for more accurately predicting the presence of SI in this population. One possible limitation of this study is that the authors did not explore other factors related to the SI, such as the burden of physical illness, history of traumatic events, and substance misuse. Second, we only surveyed MTS-WTD in patients who had SI rather than all participants, and used univariate rather than multivariate analysis to explore the factors correlated to MTS-WTD owing to a small size of patients who had a MTS-WTD. Additionally, for establishing a predictive model, we did not have another large sample size of elderly inpatients as a validation group to retest the predictivity. Lastly, a very important limitation is that our study is cross-sectional; hence, causal inference between outcomes and risk factors should be made with caution.

In conclusion, in comparison with a traditional model using the BSRS-5 total score 5/6 as a cut-off point, we found that a propensity score model comprising three items of the BSRS-5, i.e., depression, insomnia, and inferiority are associated with the presence of SI among physically ill elderly inpatients. In addition to these three items, mobility in the WHOQOL-BREF is also correlated with SI. Approximately one-fourth of suicidal ideators had a MTS-WTD, which is associated with living alone, negative feelings, and feelings of not being accepted. WTD should be seen as a signal of a higher risk for subsequent suicidal behavior among those with SI. Careful appreciation of meanings and reasons for WTD for an individual is necessary to develop a mixture of effective therapeutic options for suicide prevention. To provide physical recovery and maintain mental health for physically ill elderly inpatients, setting up a multi-faceted approach targeting the aforementioned determinants of SI and WTD for reducing the risk of suicide attempts, and exploring other factors correlated with suicidal behaviors, are important topics and directions for clinical practice and further research.

Abbreviations
BSRS-5: The 5-item brief symptom rating scale; BSSI: The Beck Scale for suicidal ideation; MMSE: The mini-mental state examination; MTS-WTD: Moderate to strong wish to die; PS: Propensity score; PSM: Propensity score model; QOL: Quality of life; QOL-ENV: The domain of environment of the Taiwanese version of World Health Organization Quality of Life-BREF; QOL-PHY: The domain of physical health of the Taiwanese version of World Health Organization Quality of Life-BREF; QOL-PSY: Psychological domain of the Taiwanese version of World Health Organization Quality of Life-BREF; QOL-SR: The domain of social relationships of the Taiwanese version of World Health Organization Quality of Life-BREF; SI: Suicidal ideation; WHOOQOL: The World Health Organization Quality of Life; WHOQOL-BREF TW: The Taiwanese version of World Health Organization Quality of Life-BREF; WTD: Wish to die

Acknowledgements
The authors thank Shing-Rong Lin and Mennonite Christian Hospital psychiatric doctors for the assistance of conducting this study.

Funding
This work was supported by the Ministry of Health and Welfare.

Authors' contributions
Authors SJL and JRR designed the study and wrote the protocol. Authors BYW, TTL and CPC managed the literature searches and analyses. All authors contributed to and have approved the final manuscript.

Consent for publication
Not applicable.

Competing interests
The authors declare that they have no competing interests.

Author details
[1]Department of Nursing, Ministry of Health and Welfare, Yuli Hospital, 448 Chung-Hua Road, Yuli Township, Hualien County 981, Taiwan, Republic of China. [2]Department of Nursing, National Taipei University of Nursing Health Science, No.365, Mingde Rd., Beitou Dist., Taipei City 112, Taiwan, Republic of China. [3]Department of Psychiatry, Ministry of Health and Welfare, Yuli Hospital, 448 Chung-Hua Road, Yuli Township, Hualien County 981, Taiwan, Republic of China. [4]Department of Geriatrics, Mennonite Christian Hospital, 44, Minquan Rd., Hualien City, Hualien County 970, Taiwan, Republic of China. [5]Department of Psychiatry, Mennonite Christian Hospital, 44, Minquan Rd., Hualien City, Hualien County 970, Taiwan, Republic of China.

References
1. Ekramzadeh S, Javadpour A, Draper B, Mani A, Withall A, Sahraian A. Prevalence and correlates of suicidal thought and self-destructive behavior among an elderly hospital population in Iran. Int Psychogeriatr. 2012;24(9):1402–8.
2. De Leo D, Padoani W, Lonnqvist J, Kerkhof AJ, Bille-Brahe U, Michel K, Salander-Renberg E, Schmidtke A, Wasserman D, Caon F, et al. Repetition of

suicidal behaviour in elderly Europeans: a prospective longitudinal study. J Affect Disord. 2002;72(3):291–5.

3. Stillion JM, McDowell EE. Examining suicide from a life span perspective. Death Stud. 1991;15:327–54.

4. Callahan CM, Hendrie HC, Nienaber NA, Tierney WM. Suicidal ideation among older primary care patients. J Am Geriatr Soc. 1996;44(10):1205–9.

5. Shah A, Hoxey K, Mayadunne V. Suicidal ideation in acutely medically ill elderly inpatients: prevalence, correlates and longitudinal stability. Int J Geriatr Psychiatry. 2000;15(2):162–9.

6. Ponte C, Almeida V, Fernandes L. Suicidal ideation, depression and quality of life in the elderly: study in a gerontopsychiatric consultation. Span J Psychol. 2014;17:E14.

7. Kim JH, Kwon JW. The impact of health-related quality of life on suicidal ideation and suicide attempts among Korean older adults. J Gerontol Nurs. 2012;38(11):48–59.

8. Palacio-Acosta C, Garcia-Valencia J, Diago-Garcia J, Zapata C, Ortiz-Tobon J, Lopez-Calle G, Lopez-Tobon M. Characteristics of people committing suicide in Medellin, Colombia. Rev Salud Publica (Bogota). 2005;7(3):243–53.

9. Raue PJ, Morales KH, Post EP, Bogner HR, Have TT, Bruce ML. The wish to die and 5-year mortality in elderly primary care patients. Am J Geriatr Psychiatry. 2010;18(4):341–50.

10. Liu IC, Chiu CH. Case-control study of suicide attempts in the elderly. Int Psychogeriatr. 2009;21(5):896–902.

11. Chen CS, Yang MS, Yang MJ, Chang SJ, Chueh KH, Su YC, Yu CY, Cheng TC. Suicidal thoughts among elderly Taiwanese aboriginal women. Int J Geriatr Psychiatry. 2008;23(10):1001–6.

12. Yen YC, Yang MJ, Yang MS, Lung FW, Shih CH, Hahn CY, Lo HY. Suicidal ideation and associated factors among community-dwelling elders in Taiwan. Psychiatry Clin Neurosci. 2005;59(4):365–71.

13. Awata S, Seki T, Koizumi Y, Sato S, Hozawa A, Omori K, Kuriyama S, Arai H, Nagatomi R, Matsuoka H, et al. Factors associated with suicidal ideation in an elderly urban Japanese population: a community-based, cross-sectional study. Psychiatry Clin Neurosci. 2005;59(3):327–36.

14. Yip PS, Chi I, Chiu H, Chi Wai K, Conwell Y, Caine E. A prevalence study of suicide ideation among older adults in Hong Kong SAR. Int J Geriatr Psychiatry. 2003;18(11):1056–62.

15. Cheung YB, Law CK, Chan B, Liu KY, Yip PS. Suicidal ideation and suicidal attempts in a population-based study of Chinese people: risk attributable to hopelessness, depression, and social factors. J Affect Disord. 2006;90(2–3):193–9.

16. Draper BM. Suicidal behaviour and suicide prevention in later life. Maturitas. 2014;79(2):179–83.

17. Goodwin RD, Marusic A. Perception of health, suicidal ideation, and suicide attempt among adults in the community. Crisis. 2011;32(6):346–51.

18. De Leo D, Padoani W, Scocco P, Lie D, Bille-Brahe U, Arensman E, Hjelmeland H, Crepet P, Haring C, Hawton K, et al. Attempted and completed suicide in older subjects: results from the WHO/EURO multicentre study of suicidal behaviour. Int J Geriatr Psychiatry. 2001;16(3):300–10.

19. Dombrovski AY, Butters MA, Reynolds CF 3rd, Houck PR, Clark L, Mazumdar S, Szanto K. Cognitive performance in suicidal depressed elderly: preliminary report. Am J Geriatr Psychiatry. 2008;16(2):109–15.

20. Marzuk PM, Hartwell N, Leon AC, Portera L. Executive functioning in depressed patients with suicidal ideation. Acta Psychiatr Scand. 2005;112(4):294–301.

21. Juurlink DN, Herrmann N, Szalai JP, Kopp A, Redelmeier DA. Medical illness and the risk of suicide in the elderly. Arch Intern Med. 2004;164(11):1179–84.

22. Shah A, Hoxey K, Mayadunne V. Some predictors of mortality in acutely medically ill elderly inpatients. Int J Geriatr Psychiatry. 2000;15(6):493–9.

23. Lee MB, Liao SC, Lee YJ, Wu CH, Tseng MC, Gau SF, Rau CL. Development and verification of validity and reliability of a short screening instrument to identify psychiatric morbidity. J Formos Med Assoc. 2003;102(10):687–94.

24. Lung FW, Lee MB. The five-item Brief-symptom rating scale as a suicide ideation screening instrument for psychiatric inpatients and community residents. BMC Psychiatry. 2008;8:53.

25. Chen HC, Wu CH, Lee YJ, Liao SC, Lee MB. Validity of the five-item Brief symptom rating scale among subjects admitted for general health screening. J Formos Med Assoc. 2005;104(11):824–9.

26. Chen WJ, Chen CC, Ho CK, Lee MB, Chung YT, Wang YC, Lin GG, Lu RY, Sun FC, Chou FH. The suitability of the BSRS-5 for assessing elderly who have attempted suicide and need to be referred for professional mental health

27. Wu CY, Lee JI, Lee MB, Liao SC, Chang CM, Chen HC, Lung FW. Predictive validity of a five-item symptom checklist to screen psychiatric morbidity and suicide ideation in general population and psychiatric settings. J Formos Med Assoc. 2016;115(6):395–403.

28. Shaffer D, Scott M, Wilcox H, Maslow C, Hicks R, Lucas CP, Garfinkel R, Greenwald S. The Columbia suicide screen: validity and reliability of a screen for youth suicide and depression. J Am Acad Child Adolesc Psychiatry. 2004;43(1):71–9.

29. Beck AT, Kovacs M, Weissman A. Assessment of suicidal intention: the scale for suicide ideation. J Consult Clin Psychol. 1979;47(2):343–52.

30. Yao G, Chung CW, Yu CF, Wang JD. Development and verification of validity and reliability of the WHOQOL-BREF Taiwan version. J Formos Med Assoc. 2002;101(5):342–51.

31. Yao G, Wang JD, Chung CW. Cultural adaptation of the WHOQOL questionnaire for Taiwan. J Formos Med Assoc. 2007;106(7):592–7.

32. Starcevic V, Bogojevic G, Marinkovic J. The SCL-90-R as a screening instrument for severe personality disturbance among outpatients with mood and anxiety disorders. J Personal Disord. 2000;14(3):199–207.

33. Guo NW, Liu HC, Wong PF, Liao KK, Yan SH, Lin KP, Chang CY, Hsu TC. Chinese version and norms of the mini-mental state examination. J Rehabil Med. 1988;16:52–9.

34. Folstein MF, Folstein SE, McHugh PR. "Mini-mental state". A practical method for grading the cognitive state of patients for the clinician. J Psychiatr Res. 1975;12(3):189–98.

35. Williamson EJ, Forbes A. Introduction to propensity scores. Respirology. 2014;19(5):625–35.

36. Hanley JA, McNeil BJ. A method of comparing the areas under receiver operating characteristic curves derived from the same cases. Radiology. 1983;148(3):839–43.

37. Richardson JD, Thompson A, King L, Corbett B, Shnaider P, St Cyr K, Nelson C, Sareen J, Elhai J, Zamorski M. Insomnia, psychiatric disorders and suicidal ideation in a National Representative Sample of active Canadian forces members. BMC Psychiatry. 2017;17(1):211.

38. Michaels MS, Balthrop T, Nadorff MR, Joiner TE. Total sleep time as a predictor of suicidal behaviour. J Sleep Res. 2017;26(6):732–8.

39. Zuromski KL, Cero I, Witte TK. Insomnia symptoms drive changes in suicide ideation: a latent difference score model of community adults over a Brief interval. J Abnorm Psychol. 2017;126(6):739–49.

40. Escobar-Cordoba F, Quijano-Serrano M, Calvo-Gonzalez JM. Evaluation of insomnia as a risk factor for suicide. Rev Fac Cien Med Univ Nac Cordoba. 2017;74(1):37–45.

41. Moritz S, Werner R, von Collani G. The inferiority complex in paranoia readdressed: a study with the implicit association test. Cogn Neuropsychiatry. 2006;11(4):402–15.

42. Perrot C, Vera L, Gorwood P. Poor self-esteem is correlated with suicide intent, independently from the severity of depression. Encephale. 2018;44(2):122–7.

43. Bagalkot TR, Park JI, Kim HT, Kim HM, Kim MS, Yoon MS, Ko SH, Cho HC, Chung YC. Lifetime prevalence of and risk factors for suicidal ideation and suicide attempts in a Korean community sample. Psychiatry. 2014;77(4):360–73.

44. Dieserud G, Roysamb E, Ekeberg O, Kraft P. Toward an integrative model of suicide attempt: a cognitive psychological approach. Suicide Life Threat Behav. 2001;31(2):153–68.

45. Kim SH. Suicidal ideation and suicide attempts in older adults: influences of chronic illness, functional limitations, and pain. Geriatr Nnurs. 2016;37(1):9–12.

46. Fassberg MM, Cheung G, Canetto SS, Erlangsen A, Lapierre S, Lindner R, Draper B, Gallo JJ, Wong C, Wu J, et al. A systematic review of physical illness, functional disability, and suicidal behaviour among older adults. Aging Ment Health. 2016;20(2):166–94.

47. Kim YA, Bogner HR, Brown GK, Gallo JJ. Chronic medical conditions and wishes to die among older primary care patients. Int J Psychiatry Med. 2006;36(2):183–98.

48. Unni KE, Rotti SB, Chandrasekaran R. An exploratory study of the motivation in suicide attempters. Indian J Psychiatry. 1995;37(4):169–75.

49. Harrison KE, Dombrovski AY, Morse JQ, Houck P, Schlernitzauer M, Reynolds CF 3rd, Szanto K. Alone? Perceived social support and chronic interpersonal difficulties in suicidal elders. Int Psychogeriatr. 2010;22(3):445–54.

50. Barnow S, Linden M. Psychosocial risk factors of the wish to be dead in the elderly. Fortschr Neurol Psychiatr. 2002;70(4):185–91.
51. Cukrowicz KC, Jahn DR, Graham RD, Poindexter EK, Williams RB. Suicide risk in older adults: evaluating models of risk and predicting excess zeros in a primary care sample. J Abnorm Psychol. 2013;122(4):1021–30.
52. Bonnewyn A, Shah A, Bruffaerts R, Demyttenaere K. Factors determining the balance between the wish to die and the wish to live in older adults. Int J Geriatr Psychiatry. 2017;32(6):685–91.
53. Ohnsorge K, Gudat H, Rehmann-Sutter C. What a wish to die can mean: reasons, meanings and functions of wishes to die, reported from 30 qualitative case studies of terminally ill cancer patients in palliative care. BMC Palliat Care. 2014;13:38.
54. The Database for predicting suicidal ideation. 2017. https://www.dropbox.com/s/mywp9hxohxqp1k4/ROC%20computer%20-bsrs1-5.xls?dl=0.

Effectiveness of brief psychological interventions for suicidal presentations

Rose McCabe[1], Ruth Garside[2], Amy Backhouse[1] and Penny Xanthopoulou[1]* (ID)

Abstract

Background: Every year, more than 800,000 people worldwide die by suicide. The aim of this study was to conduct a systematic review of the effectiveness of brief psychological interventions in addressing suicidal thoughts and behaviour in healthcare settings.

Methods: Following PRISMA guidelines, systematic searches were conducted in MEDLINE, CINAHL, EMBASE, the Cochrane Central Register of Controlled Trials and PsycINFO databases. A predefined search strategy was used. Two independent reviewers screened titles and abstracts followed by full texts against predefined inclusion criteria. Backward and forward citation tracking of included papers was conducted. Quality appraisal was conducted using the Cochrane Risk of Bias Tool for Randomized Controlled Trials and the CASP tool for randomised controlled trials. The small number and heterogeneity of studies did not allow for meta-analysis to be conducted. A narrative synthesis was conducted.

Results: Four controlled studies of brief psychological interventions were included, conducted in Switzerland, the U.S. and across low and middle-income countries. Three studies were conducted with adults and one with adolescents. All studies were judged to be at low risk of bias. All of the interventions were implemented with patients after attending emergency departments and involved 3412 participants. The main outcomes were suicide, suicide attempts, suicidal ideation, depression and hospitalization. The components of the interventions were early therapeutic engagement, information provision, safety planning and follow-up contact for at least 12 months. The interventions drew to, different degrees, on psychological theory and techniques. Two trials that measured suicidal ideation found no impact. Two studies showed fewer suicide attempts, one showed fewer suicides and one found an effect on depression.

Conclusions: Although the evidence base is small, brief psychological interventions appear to be effective in reducing suicide and suicide attempts. All studies to date have been conducted with people who had attended the ED but the interventions could potentially be adopted for inpatient and other outpatient settings. Early engagement and therapeutic intervention based on psychological theories of suicidal behaviour, sustained in follow-up contacts, may be particularly beneficial.

Keywords: Suicide, Suicidal ideation, Systematic review, Controlled studies, Effective communication

* Correspondence: p.d.xanthopoulou@exeter.ac.uk
[1]University of Exeter Medical School, Heavitree Road, Exeter EX1 2LU, UK
Full list of author information is available at the end of the article

Background

Suicide is a serious public health concern with more than 800,000 deaths from suicide every year worldwide [1]. This is one suicide every 40 seconds [2]. Suicide prevention is a global public health priority.

Certain groups have a higher risk of suicide. The majority of deaths by suicide (78%) occur in low and middle-income countries. There are also significant gender differences with men more likely to die by suicide (male-to-female ratio 1.7 in 2015) [1]. Younger people are also more likely to die by suicide: 55% of deaths by suicide are among the 15–44 age group with suicide ranked as the second leading cause of death among 15–29 year-olds [1].

Many people who take their own life have been in contact with healthcare professionals in acute hospitals and/or primary or secondary care before they die. In the U.K., 40% of people attended the general emergency department in the year before death, having attempted suicide [3]. Around one in four people who take their own life have been in contact with mental health services the year before death in the U.K. and around one in three in the U.S. [4]. Meanwhile, 45% of people who take their life were seen in primary care the month before death in the U.K. with a similar figure of 47% in the U.S. [4].

Collectively, this is a very high number of face-to-face contacts between healthcare professionals and people who go on to take their own life. Referring patients to specialist services is often not a realistic option because they are not available or where they are available, there is not enough capacity in these services. Specialist treatment is very costly and many patients do not attend or drop out of treatment prematurely [5]. Hence, in routine contacts with people at risk of suicide, there is potential for brief therapeutic interventions. There are longer term psychological interventions (e.g. dialectical behaviour therapy, cognitive behaviour therapy) to address suicide [6, 7] and self-harm [8]. However, it is not clear if limited brief interventions that can be administered in routine frontline encounters where healthcare professionals encounter people at risk of suicide can be effective [9, 10].

Studies in healthcare and other settings (e.g. educational) [11, 12] generally report brief interventions as lasting 1–3 sessions [13, 14]. We focused on brief interventions as they are more likely to be integrated into routine clinical practice without the need for significant additional resources or extensive reconfiguration of existing services. Brief interventions that could be deployed in routine care, rather than referring people to another service, are of particular interest as they could be deployed at scale to improve patient outcome.

Objectives

The aim of this review was to evaluate the effectiveness of brief psychological interventions to address suicidal thoughts and plans, focusing on two objectives:

1. To identify controlled studies of brief psychological interventions to address suicidal thoughts and plans in healthcare settings.
2. To describe the interventions used by professionals/ paraprofessionals that are effective in addressing suicidal thoughts and plans.

Methods
Protocol and registration

Approaches to searching, methods of analysis and inclusion criteria were specified in advance and documented in a protocol [15], with some changes made in the course of the study (recorded on PROSPERO: CRD42015025867), relating mainly to the eligibility criteria. The PRISMA standards of quality for reporting meta-analyses [16] were used to plan, conduct and report this review.

Eligibility criteria

The review included published controlled studies that reported on brief psychological interventions to address suicidal thoughts and plans in healthcare settings.

Inclusion criteria

Participants Participants of any age and gender at risk of suicide.

Interventions Brief interventions delivered in any healthcare setting to the specified population:

- Interactions between professionals/paraprofessionals (e.g. lay mental health workers, nursing assistants, educators, volunteers) and patients
- Addressing suicidal thoughts and plans
- Two-way communication (i.e. not one-way communication in the form of letters/postcards/text messages or exclusively self-guided questionnaires/ instruments) between at least one professional/paraprofessional and one patient; other people can be present
- Focus on suicidal thoughts and plans rather than diagnostic conditions, e.g. depression, anxiety, borderline personality disorder
- Focus on routine clinical encounters
- Brief interventions, defined as up to three sessions delivered in/soon after presenting episode, which can be supplemented by further follow-up contact

Comparator Any comparison or no comparator/usual care.

Outcome measures Primary outcome was suicidal ideation, using any measure. Other outcomes included: Identification of suicide risk, suicide attempts, suicide, hope, patient distress and depression. Suicidal ideation is defined according to Beck's 'Scale for Suicide Ideation' [17] as the intensity of current conscious suicidal intent, examining various dimensions of self-destructive thoughts or wishes.

Types of studies No restrictions were placed on study location or publication date of included studies. We included cluster randomised controlled trials, randomised controlled trials, controlled before-and-after studies and controlled pre-test/post-test designs. We excluded non-controlled studies.

Exclusion criteria Assisted suicide; Self-harm without intent to die, i.e., direct, deliberate destruction of one's own body tissue in the absence of intent to die, which differs from suicide attempts with respect to intent, lethality, chronicity, methods, cognitions, reactions, aftermath, demographics and prevalence [18].

Search and information sources

Database searches were conducted from date of inception to June 2015, and updated in August 2016 and in April 2017. The following databases were searched: MEDLINE in Process (Ovid), PsycINFO (Ovid), EMBASE (Ovid), The Cochrane Central Register of Controlled Trials (CENTRAL) (Wiley Online Library) and CINHAL (EBSCO). Trial registers (ISRCTN registry, ClinicalTrials.gov) were searched for published and ongoing trials, references of previous systematic reviews were searched and experts in the field were contacted in order to identify any new studies.

The search strategy is presented in Additional file 1. Suicide, study design and communication/interaction terms were combined using Boolean logic (AND, OR) and specific tested filters were used for study design (The InterTASC Information Specialists' Sub-Group filters). Medical Subject Heading (MeSH) terms were also used. EndNote X7.0.2 software was used to manage searches and references.

Study selection

Search results were exported to EndNote and duplicates were automatically identified and removed. Records that were not removed automatically we identified and removed by hand. Two independent reviewers (PX, RM/AB) were involved in screening all titles and abstracts, full paper screening, quality appraisal and assessment of risk of bias of included studies. Disagreements or uncertainties were discussed in meetings and email correspondence between all authors.

Data extraction

We developed a data extraction form based on the Cochrane Risk of Bias Tool for Randomized Controlled Trials, which we modified to reflect the diversity of included studies. The extraction form was piloted (RM, AB, PX) before being finalised. Data was extracted by one author (RM/PX) and checked by another (RM, AB, PX). The authors of three included studies were contacted to obtain additional data, trial protocols and further detail on the relevant intervention. Additional information was also obtained from other publications reporting on the study [19].

Risk of bias

Risk of bias was assessed using the Cochrane Risk of Bias Tool for Randomized Controlled Trials on 6 criteria. Each criterion was rated as low, medium or high. Using these ratings, we generated an overall risk of bias score by scoring the ratings on the first 5 criteria: sequence generation, allocation concealment, blinding, incomplete outcome data and selection bias. A score of 3 was allocated to a 'low' risk, a score of 2 was allocated to 'medium' risk and a score of 1 was allocated to 'high' risk. The total score could range from 5 to 15, with a higher score indicating lower risk of bias.

Study quality was also assessed using the CASP (Critical Appraisal Skills Programme) for randomised controlled trials checklist [20]. Two raters independently assessed the risk of bias for each study (PX and RM/AB). The individual items on the score sheets were then checked by three authors (RM, AB, PX) in an inter-reviewer discussion where disagreements were resolved.

Analysis

The studies were too heterogeneous to combine in a meta-analysis, in terms of the outcomes they measured. Hence, a narrative synthesis [21] was conducted. This involved developing a preliminary synthesis, focusing on the outcomes, interventions and heterogeneity across the studies, followed by iteratively exploring relationships in the data, contexts of the interventions and mechanisms for change, using visual representations (tables) [21]. Where not available, relative risk was calculated using the MEDCALC relative risk statistical calculator (https://www.medcalc.org/calc/relative_risk.php).

Results
Study selection

After removing duplicates, a total of 17,201 titles and abstracts were identified and screened (Fig. 1). Of these, 44

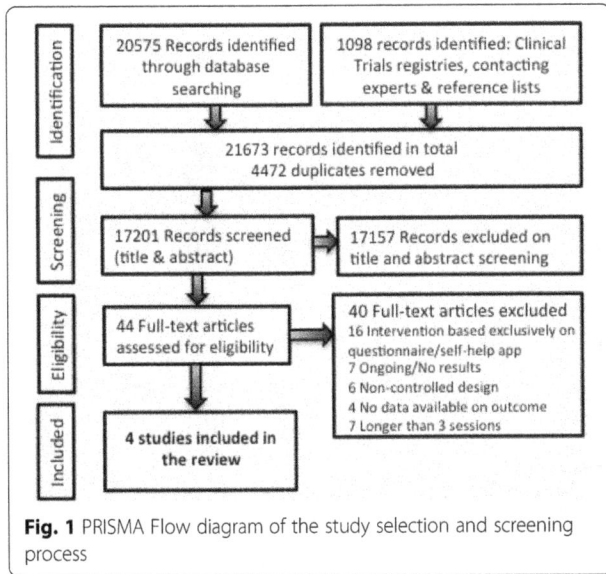

Fig. 1 PRISMA Flow diagram of the study selection and screening process

full-text articles were assessed for eligibility. Forty full-text articles were excluded studies due to a lack of control in the study design, no data available on treatment outcome, interventions were exclusively based on questionnaires or longer than three sessions. Four studies met the inclusion criteria and were included in the review.

The included studies encompassed two RCTs, one pilot RCT and a quasi-experimental study. All reported on interventions in the emergency department setting. The non-randomised controlled study used an interrupted time series design [22] and the three RCTs involved individual patient randomization [23–25]. The interventions were compared to treatment as usual (TAU) [23] and enhanced TAU [22, 24, 25].

Risk of bias

The risk of bias assessment, using Cochrane Risk of Bias Tool for Randomized Controlled Trials, is presented in Fig. 2. The overall score for each study (see Methods section for scoring) was: Fleischmann [23] 14 out 15, Gysin-Maillart [24] 13 out of 15, King [25] 13 out 15, and Miller [22] 10 out 15.

Three studies were of high quality. High/medium risk of bias was reported for blinding professionals across all studies, however, it would not have been possible to blind professionals as they were delivering the interventions. One study [22] presented medium risk of bias, where lower scores related to not using randomization to allocate interventions to participants (the study employed an interrupted time series design [26]).

Studies rated high in the CASP for randomised controlled trials checklist (results are presented in Additional file 2).

Characteristics of participants and outcomes

In total, the studies included 3412 participants (range 49–1867). Three studies included adult suicide attempters [22–24] and one [25] focused on adolescents with suicide risk factors (e.g. depression and alcohol misuse). Study characteristics are presented in Table 1.

As there were only four studies that differed in what outcomes they assessed and when these outcomes were assessed (2, 12, 18 and 24 months), a meta-analysis was not appropriate. One study was conducted across 5 countries and the included paper reports results across all 5 sites. Separate results for one of the sites (Iran) are reported elsewhere [27], however we did not include this study due to overlapping data.

Characteristics of interventions

The interventions focused on engagement, safety planning, information and follow-up contact after discharge from the emergency department. The duration of the interventions ranged from 12 to 24 months.

The four interventions in the included studies were:

a) brief intervention and contact (BIC) [23]
b) the attempted suicide short intervention program (ASSIP) [24]
c) teen options for change (TOC) [25]
d) Safety Assessment and Follow-up Telephone Intervention (SAFTI) [22]

	Sequence generation	Allocation concealment	Blinding of participants, personnel and outcome assessors	Incomplete outcome data	Selective outcome reporting	Other sources of bias
Fleischmann et al.	Low	Low	Medium	Low	Low	Unclear
Gysin-Maillart et al.	Low	Medium	Medium	Low	Low	Low
King et al.	low	Low	High	Low	Low	Unclear
Miller et al.	High	High	Medium	Low	Low	High

Fig. 2 Risk of bias assessment (Cochrane Risk of Bias Tool for Randomized Controlled Trials)

Table 1 Summary characteristics of included studies

	Participants	Nature of suicide risk	Study Design	Setting	Intervention	Control	Pre-intervention patient measures	Post-intervention patient measures	Outcomes	Follow up period
Fleischmann et al 2008 [23] 5 sites (Brazil; India; Sri Lanka; Iran; and China)	1867 Adults 57% female, median age 23 years	Patients who have attempted suicide	RCT Individual randomization	Emergency care settings	One-hour individual information session & periodic follow-up contacts after discharge for 18 months	TAU (as per norms in the respective EDs)	Questionnaire based on the European Parasuicide Study Interview Schedule (EPSIS) and adapted to each site	One-page questionnaire: if patient still alive; if not cause of death; if yes any further suicide attempts; how the patient felt; needs for support	Primary: Completed suicide	18 months
Gysin-Maillart et al 2016 [24] Switzerland	120 Adults 55% female, Mean age 37.8 years	Patients admitted to the ED who attempted suicide	RCT Individual randomization	Emergency department	3 face-to-face therapy sessions supplemented by regular, personalized letters to the participants for 24 months	Enhanced TAU: TAU (inpatient, day patient, and individual outpatient care as considered necessary by the clinicians in charge) and one clinical interview	Suicide Status Form (SSF-III) and 33-item questionnaire to collect sociodemographic, health and suicidal behaviour data	Penn Helping Alliance Questionnaire; Beck Depression Inventory; Beck Scale for Suicide Ideation	Primary: Repeat suicide attempts Secondary: Suicidal ideation, Depression, Health-care utilisation.	2 years
King et al 2015 [25] United States	49 Adolescents 65% female 14–19 years,	Patients with suicide risk factors	Pilot RCT Individual randomization	Emergency department	Personalized feedback, adapted motivational interview and follow-up note	Enhanced TAU (basic mental health resources: crisis card, written information about depression, suicide risk, firearm safety and local mental health services)	2 questions based on the Columbia-Suicide Severity Rating Scale; 15-item Suicidal Ideation Questionnaire – Junior (SIQ-JR); Reynolds Adolescent Depression Scale; Alcohol Use Disorders Identification Test; Beck Hopelessness Scale	Two questions adapted from the Columbia-Suicide Severity Rating Scale; Reynolds Adolescent Depression Scale; The Beck Hopelessness Scale; The Alcohol Use Disorders Identification Test; Motivational interviewing	Depression, hopelessness, suicidal ideation and alcohol use.	2 months
Miller et al 2017 [22] United States	1376 Adults 55.9% female median age 37	Patients attending ED with suicide attempt or ideation in previous week	Interrupted time series design	Emergency department	1. Secondary suicide risk screening 2. Self-administered safety plan & information provided by nurses 3. Telephone follow-up to patients and a significant other	TAU (usual care at each site) and contacts for 1 year	None	1. Telephone interviews using the Columbia Suicide Severity Rating Scale 2. Medical records	Suicide attempts, Suicide composite: occurrence of suicide, suicide attempt, interrupted/aborted attempts & suicide preparatory acts	1 year

A summary of the interventions is presented in Table 2. The three larger studies [22–24] used 1–3 individual sessions soon after discharge from the ED and follow-up contacts over 18, 24 and 12 months respectively. The interventions varied according to when the intervention starts, whether patients are seen soon after discharge from the ED and then how often they are contacted during the follow-up period.

Gysin-Maillart [24] implemented a therapeutic intervention focused on engaging the person in a narrative interview about the suicidal crisis in a first session soon after the ED attendance. This then progressed to case conceptualization and individualized safety planning in another 2 sessions. Then, patients were contacted via letter for 24 months, every 3 months in the first year and every 6 months in the second year. Fleischmann [23] implemented a single information session to understand and manage suicidal behaviour followed by up to 9 phone calls or visits over 18 months. In the trial by Miller et al. [22], the intervention consisted of secondary suicide screening, information provided by nurses, a self-administered safety plan and up to 7 brief (10–20 min) calls to the patient and up to 4 calls to a significant other.

Theoretical rationale and aims of the interventions

The interventions, to varying degrees, focus on informing people about suicidal behaviour, helping people to become aware of problems/vulnerability/events linked to the behaviour, exploring ambivalence and motivating people to engage in safety planning and help-seeking, problem solving and developing practical strategies to manage future suicidal crises along with signposting to helplines/professionals.

Two interventions (BIC, ASSIP) foreground the role of the relationship: BIC follow-up contacts aim to give patients a feeling of being seen and heard by someone. ASSIP aims to establish an early therapeutic alliance to maximise engagement in treatment, with the follow-up contact reinforcing the relationship.

While all of the interventions comprise information, safety planning and follow-up contact, they varied in the extent to which they used psychological theories and techniques. Gysin-Maillart's and King's interventions were based more on psychological theories (i.e. action theory and theory of health behaviour) and techniques than Fleischmann and Miller.

Completion of the intervention

Completion of the intervention ranged from 60.8% to 93% across studies. In the Fleischmann trial, it appears that 91% received the intervention. In the Gysin-Maillart trial, 93% completed the intervention. 85% of patients in

the King trial received the full intervention. Miller et al. reported that 60.8% received at least part of the intervention (i.e. 1 telephone call).

Completion of outcome assessments

Fleischmann reported a 9% loss to follow-up at 18 months. Gysin-Maillart reported a 14% loss to follow-up at 24 months. King reported low loses (6%), however this was for a very short follow up period of 2 months. Miller et al. reported that assessment of suicide attempts was conducted for all participants during the 52-week follow-up period, whereas 20% (1089 of 1376 enrolled participants) did not have a suicide composite outcome, which was derived from the telephone interview (self-reported) at 52 weeks.

Effectiveness of interventions

Brief psychological interventions were effective in reducing suicide, suicide attempts and depression (see Table 3). Interventions used a range of methods to measure these outcomes.

Suicidal ideation

Two studies found no effect for suicidal ideation [24, 25].

Suicide

One trial was effective in reducing suicide over 18 months, with a 90% relative risk reduction in completed suicides [23] (RR = 0.10, 95% CI 0.02 to 0.45, $p = 0.0025$).

Suicide attempts

Two studies reported an effect for repeat suicide attempts. Miller [22] reported a relative risk reduction of 20% for the intervention phase (RR 0.80, 95% CI 0.63 to 1.02). Gysin-Maillart [24] reported a mean hazard ratio of 0.17 (95% CI 0.07–0.46), indicating that the ASSIP group had an 83% reduced risk of attempting suicide during the 24-month follow-up period compared to the control group (Wald $\chi 2$ 1 = 13.1, 95% CI 12.4–13.7, $p < 0.001$). They also conducted an analysis removing those with BPD and found that when individuals with BPD were excluded, the ASSIP group had an 89% lower risk of attempting suicide (mean hazard ratio of 0.11 (95% CI 0.03–0.49)).

Miller [22] also reported an effect for a 'suicide composite' measure (RR 0.85, 95% CI 0.74 to 0.97), which measured 5 types of suicidal behavior: death by suicide, suicide attempt, interrupted or aborted attempts, and suicide preparatory acts.

Depression

Of the two studies assessing depression, one study by King [25] found a significant effect, however another by Gysin-Maillart [24] did not. King focused on adolescents

Table 2 Description of interventions

	Theoretical foundation	Characteristics of professionals delivering the intervention	Professional training in intervention	When was the intervention started	Intervention Components	No. & length of initial session/s	No, mode & frequency of follow up contacts	Who delivers contact/s in the ED	Who delivers contact/s after ED	Content of follow-up contacts	Intervention completion
Fleischmann et al 2008 [23]	Not described	Trained psychiatrists, medical doctors, psychologists or psychiatric nurses	Not described	Within 3 days after assessment in ED	1. Information session: information about suicidal behaviour as a sign of psychological and/or social distress, risk and protective factors, basic epidemiology, repetition, alternatives to suicidal behaviours, and referral options. 2. Follow up contacts over 18 months	One 1-hr individual information session	9 telephone / face-to-face contacts at 1, 2, 4, 7 and 11 week(s), and 4, 6,12 and 18 months)	Trained psychiatrists doctors, psychologists or psychiatric nurses	Doctor, nurse, psychologist	Phone calls or visits	91% received the full intervention
Gysin-Maillart et al 2015 [24]	Action Theory, Cognitive Behaviour Therapy, and Attachment Theory.	Four therapists: one psychiatrist, one psychologist experienced in clinical suicide prevention and two psychological therapists	1-week ASSIP training. Adherence: peer reviews and supervision	Soon after assessment in ED	1. Session 1: narrative interview - patients were asked to tell their personal stories about how they had reached the point of attempting suicide 2. Session 2: Watch session 1 video-recording & psychoeducative handout-homework 3. Session 3: Discussion & case conceptualization: goals, warning signs, and safety strategies. Written case conceptualization, safety strategies & leaflet 4. 6 follow-up letters	Three 60–90 min sessions on a weekly basis	6 letters over 24 months: every 3 months in the first year and every 6 months in the second year	Clinicians and therapists	Clinicians and therapists	Semi-standardized letters –to maintain the therapeutic relationship & reinforce safety strategy	93% completed the intervention at 24 months (95% at 12 months)
King et al 2015 [25]	Motivational Interviewing, Self Determination Theory, Theory of Health Behavior, and Theory of Planned Behavior	Three licensed Social Workers	Min 40 Hours - conducted by a member of the Motivational Interviewing Trainers' Network	After initial emergency room visit	1. Individual AMI: personalized feedback to the teen, to explore ambivalence, build discrepancy, enhance teen's problem importance and readiness to change 2. Family AMI: with parent/guardian to develop Personalized	One individual 30–45 min session One family 15–20 min session	Handwritten follow-up note and a telephone check-in two to five days after ED visit to support and facilitate action plan implementation	Study therapists	Study therapists	Personalized follow up note & telephone check-in: Half receive telephone follow-up only.	85% received the full intervention

Table 2 Description of interventions *(Continued)*

Theoretical foundation	Characteristics of professionals delivering the intervention	Professional training in intervention	When was the intervention started	Intervention Components	No. & length of initial session/s	No., mode & frequency of follow up contacts	Who delivers contact/s in the ED	Who delivers contact/s after ED	Content of follow-up contacts	Intervention completion
				Action Plan Form, provide supplemental resource materials 3. Follow-up letter & telephone call						
Miller et al 2017 [22] Not described	ED physicians & nurses	Detailed manual of procedures, meetings, and monthly teleconference to receive training updates, and problem solve	In the ED	1. Secondary suicide risk screening by ED physician following an initial positive screen 2. self-administered safety plan and information to patients by nursing staff 3. follow-up telephone calls	Not described	Up to 7 brief (10–20 min) telephone calls to the patient and up to 4 calls to a significant other, at 6, 12, 24, 36, and 52 weeks	ED physicians and nursing staff	10 advisors: 6 PhD psychologists, 3 psychology fellows, and 1 masters-level counselor	Case management, individual psychotherapy and significant other involvement following Coping Long Term with Active Suicide (CLASP)-ED protocol	1. Secondary suicide risk screening: 89.4% 2. Safety plan: 37.4% 3. Follow-up: 60.8% patients completed at least 1 phone call: of these median number 6 calls (range 2–7). 19.9% patients had a significant other who completed at least 1 call: of these median number of 4 calls (range 3–4)

Table 3 Primary and Secondary Outcomes

Type of outcome	Suicide	Repeat suicide attempts	Suicide composite	Suicidal ideation	Depression	Health-care utilization	Hopelessness	Alcohol Use
	Behavioural	Behavioural	Behavioural	Self-rated	Self-rated	Self-report & records	Self-rated	Self-rated
Fleischmann et al 2008 [23] n = 1867 Risk of bias score[a]: 14/15	Fewer suicides: 0.2% intervention vs. 2.2% control (x^2 = 13.83; $P < 0.001$) RR = 0.10 (0.02 to 0.45)	n/a	n/a	n/a	n/a	n/a	n/a	n/a
Gysin-Maillart et al 2016 [24] n = 120 Risk of bias score: 13/15	n/a	Fewer suicide attempts 8.3% intervention vs. 26.7% control (Wald x_1^2 = 13.1, 95% CI 12.4–13.7, $p < 0.001$) HR 0.17 (0.07–0.46)	n/a	No difference found	No difference found	72% fewer days in hospital after 1 year (ASSIP: 29 d; control group: 105 d; W = 94.5, $p = 0.038$) but not significant at 2 years	n/a	n/a
King et al 2015 [25] n = 49 Risk of bias score: 13/15	n/a	n/a	n/a	No difference found	Lower depression intervention Mean (SD) 25.4 (4.7) vs. 30.9 (4.0) control, F = 10.84, df = 1,44; $p < .01$ (Cohen's d = 1.07; large effect size)	n/a	No difference found	No difference found
Miller et al 2017 [22] n = 1376 Risk of bias score: 10/15	n/a	Fewer suicide attempts: TAU, 22.9% (114/497); INT, 18.3% (92/502) RR 0.80 (0.63 to 1.02)	Lower suicide composite: TAU: 48.9% (243/497) INT: 41.4% (208/502) RR 0.85 (0.74 to 0.97)	n/a	n/a	n/a	n/a	n/a

TAU treatment as usual, *INT* intervention

[a]Higher score indicates lower risk of bias

over a shorter follow-up period of 2 months while Gysin-Maillart focused on adults (with longer-standing difficulties) over a longer follow-up of 2 years.

Healthcare use

Gysin-Maillart [24] found a significant reduction in hospitalization, with 72% fewer days in hospital over 1 year, which was no longer significant after 2 years ($p = 0.08$).

Alcohol use and hopelessness

Where assessed [25], no effect was found for alcohol use and hopelessness.

Analysis Miller [22] and Gysin-Maillart [24] used intention to treat analysis. However, Fleischmann [23] did not: they analysed the participants who were not lost to follow-up which corresponded to 91% of the sample. King's [25] analysis of intervention effect used per protocol, rather than intention to treat, analysis. We cannot tell the direction or magnitude of impact of this, but there was little loss to follow-up (< 10% LTFU).

Discussion

Four controlled studies of brief psychological interventions to reduce suicidal behaviour and suicide were identified, three with adults and one with adolescents. All of the interventions were implemented with patients who had attended the ED and involved a total of 3412 participants. The interventions had three common components, namely information about/understanding of the suicidal crisis, safety planning and follow-up contact along with different degrees of psychological input. One (out of one study assessing suicide) found fewer suicides [23]. One (out of one study) assessed a 'suicide composite' score [22] and found a lower suicide composite score. Two (out of two studies assessing suicide attempts) found fewer suicide attempts [22, 24]: Miller found a small but meaningful difference with a number needed to treat of 22 and Gysin found an 83% reduced risk of attempting suicide during the 24-month follow-up period. Two (out of two) studies measuring suicidal ideation did not show an effect [24, 25]. One (out of two studies measuring depression) found an improvement in depression [25]. One (out of one study measuring hopelessness) found no improvement in hopelessness [25]. One (of one study assessing hospitalisation) found 72% fewer days in hospital after 1 year but no significant difference after 2 years [24]. Hence, there appear to be greater changes in behavioural outcomes than in symptom outcomes, suggesting that patients may still be experiencing suicidal ideation but make fewer suicide attempts and are less likely to die by suicide.

One trial [23] found an effect on suicide, which was conducted across 5 low and middle-income countries. The authors concluded that a brief intervention was likely to have reduced suicide by providing a social support network for people with limited social support in countries with modest infrastructure and financial/human resources. Two trials found an effect on suicide attempts. One was a large trial in the U.S. with 1376 participants [22] and one a small trial in Switzerland with 120 participants [24]: the large trial found a 20% relative risk reduction and the smaller trial with a 83% relative risk reduction. The large trial focused on information provided by nurses and a self-administered safety plan in the ED, followed by 7 telephone calls to the patient and 4 calls to a significant other over one year. Meanwhile, the smaller trial demonstrating the larger effect, focused on 3 face-to-face therapeutic sessions soon after discharge from the ED and follow-up letters over 24 months.

Given the low prevalence of suicide as an outcome, studies in this area use various proxy and composite measures. One study reported on completed suicide, two studies reported on suicide re-attempts and only one study reported healthcare utilisation (i.e. hospitalisation). Suicide attempts were measured using hospital records, however Miller also used telephone interviews to collect information on this outcome, which could address some of the issues of reliability and accuracy of hospital records. This area would benefit from more RCTs with larger populations, that report on completed suicide [6].

What might explain the large effect in the smaller trial? The two trials recruited participants with a similar age range (mean = 37.8 in Gysin's smaller trial, and median = 37 in Miller's larger trial) and male-to-female ratio (Gysin 55% female, Miller 56% female). However, the smaller trial [24] was conducted in one ED while the larger trial [22] was conducted across 8 EDs so local championing and fidelity to the intervention may have been stronger in the single site smaller trial. In addition, the smaller trial involved more intensive psychological input with an emphasis on an early therapeutic alliance in face-to-face sessions along with follow-up contact by the same rather than different professionals. A better therapeutic alliance was associated with a lower rate of suicide attempts [28], suggesting that early engagement and therapeutic intervention soon after the ED attendance may be particularly beneficial.

The interventions varied on some important factors, most notably the psychological theories underpinning the intervention, the intensity of and the proposed mechanisms and wider socioeconomic context of the intervention. These were to some extent reflected in when, how and by whom the initial and follow-up contacts were made and what happened in these contacts. The BIC intervention leading to fewer deaths by suicide in low/middle-income countries focused on information, practical advice and signposting and was delivered by doctors, psychologists or nurses. Interventions leading to fewer suicide attempts in countries where better mental health services exist were based more on psychological theories underpinning suicidal behaviour [24, 25] and psychological techniques to explore motivation for change and safety strategies delivered by trained clinicians or therapists [24, 25]. These differences are consistent with realist evaluation [29] pointing to what works in which circumstances and for whom. In three studies, follow-up contact was over the telephone. This makes interventions more viable and cost-effective when resources are scarce while also allowing for flexibility and improved access to treatment when, for example it might be geographically unavailable [30].

Similar to a previous review of suicide interventions [7], the contribution of the individual components of the interventions is unclear as the interventions were evaluated as a whole. Moreover, it is not clear what the contribution of more frequent contacts is and up until which point these contacts are optimally effective.

One of the four studies was conducted in low and middle-income countries, which has implications for the generalizability of the results to countries with stronger health and social care systems. Treatment as Usual is described in the studies as usual care in clinical practice. This is likely to have varied considerably as the studies were conducted in different countries with different healthcare systems. For example, this consisted of inpatient, day patient and outpatient care in the study by Gysin in Switzerland. However, this is likely to have been considerably less ("as per the norms in the respective EDs") in the Fleischmann study which was conducted across 5 different low and middle-income countries. This introduces considerable heterogeneity in interpreting the findings.

All of the studies evaluated interventions that were implemented with people after attending the ED, with two interventions explicitly also involving family or significant others [22, 25] Two studies focus on high risk populations, i.e., people in low and middle-income countries [23] and young people [25]. The ED setting is particularly important as a large number of at-risk individuals use emergency services [31]. People who attend the emergency department are at high risk of a further suicide attempt, with studies showing that around 20% re-present within one year [31]. It is estimated that hospitals in England manage over 200,000 episodes of self-harm each year. Many people who attend the ED in a crisis do not attend specialist mental health services for follow-up. Hence, brief ED interventions to reduce suicide risk may be especially useful [32]. Although the identified studies were conducted in the ED, the interventions – as a whole or components of the interventions - could be tested in other treatment settings such as inpatient or outpatient community treatment settings.

Strengths and limitations This review used a systematic approach to identify controlled studies of brief psychological interventions for suicidal thoughts and behaviour. It identified the usefulness of brief interventions to address suicidality in the ED. However, and as previously found [11], the evidence base is small. As is commonly found in systematic reviews with a limited evidence base, the included studies were disparate in their design, outcome measurement tools, measurement intervals and types of interventions offered. As they assessed different outcomes at differing time points, a meta-analysis was not appropriate. In addition, one of the four studies was conducted in low and middle-income countries, which has implications for the generalizability of the results. The findings from this study may not be generalizable to higher income countries with stronger health and social care systems. However, the narrative synthesis allowed us to summarise the state of the art across somewhat heterogeneous studies. Detailed information was lacking on specific aspects of the intervention (e.g. length of components and randomisation procedure) in some studies, which restricted the interpretation of the methodological quality. Risk of bias may be reduced if those assessing outcomes are blinded to treatment allocation. However, as some of the outcomes are objective, such as suicide [23], these are not subject to bias. With suicide attempts, there is some element of judgment but, if assessors are blinded, there is less chance of bias. Assessors were blinded in Miller and King but not in Gysin. Suicidal ideation is self-rated and so cannot be blinded. Finally, as they are receiving a psychological intervention, it is not possible to blind participants to treatment allocation.

The review focused on brief interventions that aimed to enhance treatment. While, these interventions often included considerable follow-up contact, we did not include studies solely focusing on follow-up contact. For example, a study in France consisting of a single telephone contact one month after attending the ED was categorized as a follow-up intervention rather than enhancing the index treatment episode/s [33].

Conclusions

Although there are relatively few studies to date, brief psychological interventions appear to be effective in reducing suicide and suicide attempts. However, it is unclear to what extent the effect is due to specific psychological techniques/components or to more frequent contacts, which should be investigated in future studies. All studies to date have been conducted in the ED. The interventions tested do not appear to reduce suicidal ideation, suggesting that although patients may still be in considerable distress, the interventions affect change in behaviour, i.e., fewer suicide attempts and suicides, by targeting information and understanding about the suicidal crisis, safety planning for future crises and follow-up contact to monitor and support patients. Early engagement and therapeutic intervention based on psychological theories of suicidal behaviour, sustained in follow-up contacts, may be particularly beneficial.

Abbreviations
ASSIP: Attempted suicide short intervention program; BIC: Brief intervention and contact; CASP: Critical appraisal skills programme; ED: Emergency department; RCT: Randomised controlled trial; SAFTI: Safety assessment and follow-up telephone intervention; TAU: Treatment as usual; TOC: Teen options for change

Acknowledgements
We thank the PenCLAHRC Evidence Synthesis Team and Mr Chris Cooper for their support.

Funding
National Institute for Health Research (NIHR) Collaboration for Leadership in Applied Health Research and Care South West Peninsula (McCabe).

Authors' contributions
RM, PX and RG designed the systematic review. RM, PX, AB screened all records. All authors contributed to the design of the methods and extraction form. RM and PX wrote the initial draft of the paper, which was then revised by AB and RG. The final manuscript was read and approved by all authors.

Consent for publication
Not applicable.

Competing interests
The funder had no role in the design or conduct of the study, collection, analysis, interpretation and management of data, preparation and review of the manuscript, or decision to submit for publication.

Author details
[1]University of Exeter Medical School, Heavitree Road, Exeter EX1 2LU, UK. [2]European Centre for Environment and Human Health, Knowledge Spa, Royal Cornwall Hospital, Truro TR1 3HD, UK.

References
1. World health organisation. Suicide: fact sheet. Updated 2017. http://www. who.int/mediacentre/factsheets/fs398/en/. Accessed 24 Apr 2017.
2. Office for National Statistics: Suicides in the UK : 2015 registrations. https:// www.ons.gov.uk/peoplepopulationandcommunity/ birthsdeathsandmarriages/deaths/bulletins/suicidesintheunitedkingdom/ 2015registrations. Accessed 30 May 2017.
3. Gairin I, House A, Owens D. Attendance at the accident and emergency department in the year before suicide: retrospective study. Br J Psychiatry. 2003;183(1):28–33.
4. Appleby L, Kapur N, Shaw J, Windfuhr K, Hunt IM, Flynn D, While D, Roscoe A, Rodway C, Ibrahim S et al. The National Confidential Inquiry into Suicide and homicide by people with mental illness annual report 2015: England, Northern Ireland, Scotland and Wales. University of Manchester.
5. Monti K, Cedereke M, Öjehagen A. Treatment attendance and suicidal behavior 1 month and 3 months after a suicide attempt: a comparison between two samples. Archives of Suicide Research. 2003;7(2):167–74.
6. Inagaki M, Kawashima Y, Kawanishi C, Yonemoto N, Sugimoto T, Furuno T, Ikeshita K, Eto N, Tachikawa H, Shiraishi Y, Yamada M. Interventions to prevent repeat suicidal behavior in patients admitted to an emergency department for a suicide attempt: a meta-analysis. J Affect Disord. 2015 Apr 1;175:66–78.
7. Mann JJ, Apter A, Bertolote J, Beautrais A, Currier D, Haas A, Hegerl U, Lonnqvist J, Malone K, Marusic A, Mehlum L. Suicide prevention strategies: a systematic review. JAMA. 2005;294(16):2064–74.
8. Hawton K, Witt KG, Salisbury TL, Arensman E, Gunnell D, Hazell P, Townsend E, van Heeringen K. Psychosocial interventions following self-harm in adults: a systematic review and meta-analysis. Lancet Psychiatry. 2016;3(8):740–50.
9. Da Cruz D, Pearson A, Saini P, Miles C, While D, Swinson N, Williams A, Shaw J, Appleby L, Kapur N. Emergency department contact prior to suicide in mental health patients. Emerg Med J. 2011;28(6):467–71.
10. O'Connor RC, Ferguson E, Scott F, Smyth R, McDaid D, Park AL, Beautrais A, Armitage CJ. A brief psychological intervention to reduce repetition of self-harm in patients admitted to hospital following a suicide attempt: a randomised controlled trial. The Lancet Psychiatry. 2017;4(6):451–60.
11. Milner AJ, Carter G, Pirkis J, Robinson J, Letters SMJ. Green cards, telephone calls and postcards: systematic and meta-analytic review of brief contact interventions for reducing self-harm, suicide attempts and suicide. Br J Psychiatry. 2015;206(3):184–90.
12. Hsiao RC, Walker LR. Substance use disorders: part I, an issue of child and adole scent psychiatric clinics of North America, E-book. Elsevier Health Sci. 2016;25(3).
13. Miller WR, Rollnick S. Motivational interviewing: preparing people to change addictive behavior. New York. London: Guilford Press; 1991.
14. Kaner EF, Beyer F, Dickinson HO, Pienaar E, Campbell F, Schlesinger C, et al. Effectiveness of brief alcohol interventions in primary care populations. Cochrane Database Syst Rev. 2007;2:CD004148.
15. McCabe R, Garside R, Backhouse A, Xanthopoulou P. Effective communication in eliciting and responding to suicidal thoughts: a systematic review protocol. Systematic reviews. 2016;5(1):31.
16. Moher D, Shamseer L, Clarke M, Ghersi D, Liberati A, Petticrew M, Shekelle P, Stewart LA. Preferred reporting items for systematic review and meta-analysis protocols (PRISMA-P) 2015 statement. Systematic reviews. 2015;4(1)
17. Beck AT, Kovacs M, Weissman A. Assessment of suicidal intention: the scale for suicide ideation. J Consult Clin Psychol. 1979;47(2):343–52.
18. Butler AM, Malone K. Attempted suicide v. Non-suicidal self-injury: behaviour, syndrome or diagnosis? Br J Psychiatry. 2013;202(5):324–5.
19. Boudreaux ED, Camargo CA, Arias SA, Sullivan AF, Allen MH, Goldstein AB, Manton AP, Espinola JA, Miller IW. Improving suicide risk screening and detection in the emergency department. Am J Prev Med. 2016;50(4):445–53.
20. Critical Appraisal Skills Programme. CASP (insert name of checklist i.e. Systematic Review) Checklist [online]. Available at: http://www.casp-uk.net/ casp-tools-checklists. Accessed 20 Apr 2015.
21. Popay J, Roberts H, Sowden A, Petticrew M, Arai L, Rodgers M, Britten N, Roen K, Duffy S. Guidance on the conduct of narrative synthesis in systematic reviews. A product from the ESRC methods programme Version. 2006;1:b92.
22. Miller IW, Camargo CA, Jr., Arias SA, Sullivan AF, Allen MH, Goldstein AB, Manton AP, Espinola JA, Jones R, Hasegawa K et al: Suicide prevention in an emergency department population: the ED-SAFE study. JAMA Psychiatry 2017; 74(6):563–570.
23. Fleischmann A, Bertolote JM, Wasserman D, De Leo D, Bolhari J, Botega NJ, De Silva D, Phillips M, Vijayakumar L, Värnik A, et al. Effectiveness of brief intervention and contact for suicide attempters: a randomized controlled trial in five countries. Bull World Health Organ. 2008;86:703–9.
24. Gysin-Maillart A, Schwab S, Soravia L, Megert M, Michel KA. Novel brief therapy for patients who attempt suicide: a 24-months follow-up randomized controlled study of the attempted suicide short intervention program (ASSIP). PLoS medicine. Public Libr Sci. 2016;13(3):e1001968.
25. King CA, Gipson PY, Horwitz AG, Opperman KJ. Teen options for change: an intervention for young emergency patients who screen positive for suicide risk. Psychiatr Serv. 2015;66(1):97–100.

26. Bridge JA, Horowitz LM, Campo JV. Ed-safe—can suicide risk screening and brief intervention initiated in the emergency department save lives? JAMA Psychiatry. 2017;74(6):555–6.

27. Hassanzadeh M, Khajeddin N, Nojomi M, Fleischmann A, Eshrati T. Brief intervention and contact after deliberate self-harm: an Iranian randomized controlled trial. Iranian Journal of Psychiatry and Behavioral Sciences. 2010; 4(2):5–12.

28. Gysin-Maillart AC, Soravia LM, Gemperli A, Michel K. Suicide ideation is related to therapeutic alliance in a brief therapy for attempted suicide. Arch Suicide Res. 2017;21(1):113–26.

29. Pawson R, Tilley N. Realistic evaluation. London: Sage; 1997.

30. Mohr DC, Hart SL, Julian L, Catledge C, Honos-Webb L, Vella L, Tasch ET. Telephone-administered psychotherapy for depression. Arch Gen Psychiatry. 2005;62(9):1007–14.

31. Cooper J, Steeg S, Gunnell D, Webb R, Hawton K, Bennewith O, House A, Kapur N. Variations in the hospital management of self-harm and patient outcome: a multi-site observational study in England. J Affect Disord. 2015; 174:101–5.

32. Stanley B, Brown GK. Safety planning intervention: a brief intervention to mitigate suicide risk. Cogn Behav Pract. 2012;19(2):256–64.

33. Vaiva G, Ducrocq F, Meyer P, Mathieu D, Philippe A, Libersa C, Goudemand M. Effect of telephone contact on further suicide attempts in patients discharged from an emergency department: randomised controlled study. BMJ. 2006;332(7552):1241–5.

Association between migraine and suicidal behavior among Ethiopian adults

Hanna Y. Berhane[1*], Bethannie Jamerson-Dowlen[2], Lauren E. Friedman[2], Yemane Berhane[1], Michelle A. Williams[2] and Bizu Gelaye[2]

Abstract

Background: Despite the significant impact of migraine on patients and societies, few studies in low- and middle-income countries (LMICs) have investigated the association between migraine and suicidal behavior. The objective of our study is to examine the extent to which migraines are associated with suicidal behavior (including suicidal ideation, plans, and attempts) in a well-characterized study of urban dwelling Ethiopian adults.

Methods: We enrolled 1060 outpatient adults attending St. Paul hospital in Addis Ababa, Ethiopia. Standardized questionnaires were used to collect data on socio-demographics, and lifestyle characteristics. Migraine classification was based on the International Classification of Headache Disorders-2 diagnostic criteria. The Composite International Diagnostic Interview (CIDI) was used to assess depression and suicidal behaviors (i.e. ideation, plans and attempts). Multivariable logistic regression models were used to estimate adjusted odds ratio (AOR) and 95% confidence intervals (95% CIs).

Results: The prevalence of suicidal behavior was 15.1%, with a higher suicidal behavior among those who had migraines (61.9%). After adjusting for confounders including substance use and socio-demographic factors, migraine was associated with a 2.7-fold increased odds of suicidal behavior (AOR = 2.7; 95% CI 1.88–3.89). When stratified by their history of depression in the past year, migraine without depression was significantly associated with suicidal behavior (AOR: 2.27, 95% CI: 1.49–3.46). The odds of suicidal behavior did not reach statistical significance in migraineurs with depression (AOR: 1.64, 95% CI: 0.40–6.69).

Conclusion: Our study indicates that migraine is associated with increased odds of suicidal behavior in this population. Given the serious public health implications this has, attention should be given to the treatment and management of migraine at a community level.

Keywords: Migraine, Suicidal behavior, Ethiopia

Background

Migraine is an under diagnosed and recurrent headache that is associated with sensitivity to light, nausea, or a reduced ability to function [1]. Migraine is a highly prevalent neurological disorder, affecting 1 out of every 10 individuals globally [1–3]. In Africa, though it is estimated that 5–10% of the population suffer from migraines [4, 5]; there is a scarcity of researches focusing on migraine.Higher prevalence have been reported among urban residents [4, 6], and women [5–8]. Earlier studies have also shown that migraine is higher among young adults (18–29) years [5].

Depending on the level of intensity during each episodes, migraine often has direct and immediate impact on patients' daily activities. Its manifestations range from inability to lead a productive life due to loss of work/school days to withdrawal from social and leisure activities which ultimately affect the quality of life [9, 10]. Additionally, migraine disorders have been associated with psychiatric comorbidities including substance abuse, mood and anxiety disorders, depression, and suicidal behaviors [11–20]. Suicidal thoughts and behaviors (hereafter referred to as suicidal behaviors) which include suicidal ideation, plans, and attempts are predictors of completed suicide [21, 22].

* Correspondence: hannayaciph@gmail.com
Addis Continental Institute of Public Health, Addis Ababa, Ethiopia
Full list of author information is available at the end of the article

Annually more than half a million people die due to suicide; while three-fourth of this deaths are in low and middle income countries (LAMICs) [23].Despite the profound personal, societal, and economic consequences both these problems have; knowledge pertaining to their association remain limited, particularly in LAMICs. Though previous research have shown the association between migraine and suicidal behaviors [16, 19, 20, 24]; no studies in sub-Saharan Africa have investigated this association. Due to the high burden of migraine in sub-Saharan Africa and the existing knowledge gap, we sought to evaluate the extent to which migraine headaches are associated with suicidal behaviors, including suicidal ideation, plan, and attempts, in a well-characterized study of urban dwelling Ethiopian adults.

Methods
Study design and population
This cross-sectional study enrolled 1060 participants attending the outpatient facility at the Saint Paul Hospital in Addis Ababa, Ethiopia. All patients evaluated in the internal medicine, general surgery and gynecological outpatient departments during the period of December to July 2011 were eligible to be included in the study. Those who were unable to communicate with the interviewers directly (those with diagnosed mental disabilities and hearing disabilities) were excluded. Interviewer administered structured questionnaires were used to collect data from all individuals who have consented to participate. Prior to data collection; the interviewers who were nurses by training were given an intensive training on: the contents of the questionnaire, interview techniques and ethical conduct of human subjects research. Continuous supervision and support was provided by the research coordinator throughout the period of data collection.

Major depressive disorder and suicidal behavior
Major depressive disorder (MDD) and suicidal behavior were assessed using the depression module of the Composite International Diagnostic Interview (CIDI) 3.0 [25]. The CIDI is a fully-structured interview that assesses mental disorders according to the definitions and criteria of the ICD-10 [26] and DSM-IV [27]. For this study we used the DSM-IV definition of MDD: presence of five out of nine depressive symptoms that persist for 2 weeks or longer, are present for most of the day nearly every day, and cause significant distress or impairment [27].

Suicidal behavior was classified as ideation, attempt, and plan based on participant self-report [28]. Participants answered questions relevant to the presence of ideation, plan(s) and/or attempts during their most crucial depressive episode within the past year. In particular, the following questions were included: "During that period, did you ever think that it would be better if you were dead?", "Did you make a suicide plan?" and "Did you make a suicide attempt?" if the respondent responded "Yes" to either of the three questions the individual was classified as having suicidal behaviors.

Migraine disorders
For migraine, we used a structured migraine assessment questionnaire adapted from previously validated tool [29] . Migraine was classified according to the ICHD-II criteria [30]; it was defined by at least 5 lifetime headache attacks lasting 4–72 h, with at least 2 of the four qualifying pain characteristics (unilateral location, pulsating quality, moderate or severe pain intensity, aggravation by or causing avoidance of routine physical activity) and at least one of the associated symptoms (nausea and/or vomiting, or photo and photophobia).

Other covariates
Structured questionnaires were used to collected data on socio-demographic characteristics, including sex, age (in years), and marital status (married, never married, other). Other socio-demographic covariates included: education (≤primary, secondary education, college graduate), smoking status (never, former, current), past year alcohol consumption (non-drinker, < once per month, ≥ 1 day per week), khat chewing (never, former, current), body mass index (BMI) (<18.5, 18.5–24.9, 24.9–29.9, ≥30 kg/m^2), and self-reported physical and mental health status (excellent/very good/good vs. fair/poor).

Statistical analysis
Data analyses was conducted using SPSS version 23.0 (IBM SPSS, Chicago, IL). Continuous variables were summarized as means (± standard deviation), and categorical variables as number and percentages. Multivariable logistic regression models were used to estimate odds ratios (ORs) and 95% confidence intervals (95% CI). Forward logistic regression modeling procedures combined with the change in-estimate approach were used to select the final multivariable adjusted models on the association between migraine and suicidal behaviors. Variables of a priori interest (e.g., age and sex) were included in final models. Previous studies have shown that depression is associated with suicidal behaviors and migraine. We therefore performed a sensitivity analysis stratifying our analysis by current(past year) depression status. Reported p-values are two-sided with a statistical significance set at $p < 0.05$.

Results
A total of 1060 individuals with a mean age of 35.7 ± 12.1 years took part in this study. Of those, the majority

were women (60%), married (51.3%) and had a low educational level (< grade 6) (44.7%). Current smoking and Khat use was reported by 4.1% and 20.6% of participants, respectively. When asked about their health status more than half of the participants reported having a good, very good, or excellent physical (56.2%) and mental health (65.9%). Percentage of those having depression (life time and in past year) was 24.7% while any suicidal behavior was 15.1% (Table 1).

Any suicidal behavior was reported by 160 (15.1%) study participants; which included suicidal ideation (14.5%), suicide plan (6.1%) or suicide attempt (4.2%). Characteristics of study participants by migraine status is also presented in Table 1. Migrainuers were more likely to be women, have less education and were more likely to report their physical or mental health status as fair or poor. Participants with migraine were also more likely to report depression (both past year and lifetime) and suicidal behaviors, including suicide ideation, plan, or attempt ($p \leq 0.001$).

Characteristics of the study population according to suicidal behavior are shown in Table 2. Participants with any suicidal behavior were more likely to be women, married, and more likely to have self-reported fair/poor physical and mental health status. Participants with any suicidal behaviors were also more likely to have past year or lifetime depression ($p < 0.01$).

The presence of migraine was associated with a 2.91-fold increased odds of suicidal behavior (OR: 2.91, 95% CI: 2.06–4.12) as compared to participants without migraine. After adjusting for confounders including age, sex, education, and BMI, migrainuers were 2.71-times more likely to report suicidal behaviors compared to non-migrainuers (AOR:2.71, 95% CI: 1.89–3.89). The results remained similar after further adjusting for khat chewing and past year alcohol consumption (AOR: 2.70, 95% CI: 1.88–3.89). When life time history of depression was added to the model, the association between migraine and suicidal behaviors was greatly attenuated and became statistically insignificant (AOR: 1.49, 95% CI: 0.93–2.39) (Table 3).

We next explored the association between migraine and suicidal behavior after stratifying by past year depression status (Table 4). Among individuals without a history of depression (in the past year), the odds of suicidal behavior was 2-times higher among those with migraine as compared to those without migraine in a fully adjusted model (AOR: 2.27, 95% CI: 1.49–3.46). Among individuals with a history of depression (in the past year), the odds of suicidal behavior was modestly increased but did not reach statistical significance for migraineurs as compared with those without migraine (AOR: 1.64 95% CI: 0.40–6.69).

Discussion

Our results show that migraine is significantly associated with suicidal behaviors (including suicidal ideation, plan, or attempts), after adjusting for confounders including age, sex, BMI, education, khat use, and past year alcohol consumption. However, when lifetime depression was fitted in the model, a statistically significant association was not observed. Following further analysis to understand the effect of depression; it was found that migrainuers without history of depression in the past year had a 2.27-fold increased odds of suicidal behaviors as compared to non-migrainuers.

Migraine had a strong positive association with increased odds of suicidal ideation and attempts; this association has been also established from previous studies in high income countries including the US, Canada, Taiwan, Norway, Italy, and Korea [15, 20]. For example, a recent study among members of a Health Maintenance Organization in Michigan found that migraineurs had an increased risk of suicidal attempts during a 2 year follow-up [19]. The pooled analysis from a recent meta-analysis also found that migraine with aura was associated with increased odds of suicidal ideation (AOR: 1.31; 95% CI: 1.10–1.55), while no statistical association was observed for migraine without aura [31]. Similarly, suicidal attempts were found to be 3 to 7 times higher among those with migraines in a two- year follow up study [14, 16].

Chronic migraine is often comorbid with other conditions such as depression;a recent study in India found significant comorbidity between psychiatric disorders, including anxiety, depressive disorders, suicidality, and headache disorders [32]. Likewise, a study from Lima, Peru found that migrainuers without depression had an 1.8-fold increased odds of suicidal ideation while those with both migraine and depression had a 4.1 folds increased odds after adjusting for confounder [20]. This is contrary to our finding, adding history of life-time depression to the model resulted in no statically significant association between migraine and suicidal behaviors.However when we stratified individuals with their current (past year) depression status; participants with migraine and no depression has 2.27 fold increased odds of suicidal behavior (95% CI: 1.49–3.46). In line with this, Pompili et al. in their review found that the association of migraine and suicidal attempts was not necessarily due to coexting depression; but rather the chronic pain and loss of pleasure to engage in activities that is an independent risk factor for suicide [33].

Previous studies have documented the biological links between migraine and suicidal behaviors. Investigators suggest that the levels of cortisol and functioning of the hypothalamic-pituitary-adrenocortical (HPA) axis are

Table 1 Socio-demographic and reproductive characteristics of the study population according to types of migraine ($N = 1060$)

Characteristics	All participants (N = 1060)		No migraine (N = 639)		Migraine (N = 421)		P-value
	n	%	n	%	n	%	
Age (years)[a]	35.68 ± 12.08		35.95 ± 12.10		35.28 ± 12.05		0.378
Sex							
Women	637	60.1	330	51.6	307	72.9	< 0.001
Men	423	39.9	309	48.4	114	27.1	
Marital Status							
Married	542	51.3	342	53.7	200	47.6	0.011
Never married	335	31.7	204	32.0	131	31.2	
Other	180	17.0	91	14.3	89	21.2	
Education							
≤ Primary (1–6)	474	44.7	248	38.8	226	53.7	< 0.001
Secondary (7–12)	357	33.7	233	36.5	124	29.5	
College graduate	229	21.6	158	24.7	71	16.9	
Smoking status							
Never	913	86.1	534	83.6	379	90.0	0.010
Former	104	9.8	76	11.9	28	6.7	
Current	43	4.1	29	4.5	14	3.3	
Alcohol consumption past year							
Non-drinker	601	56.7	340	53.2	261	62.0	0.002
< once a month	357	33.7	223	34.9	134	31.8	
≥ 1 day a week	102	9.6	76	11.9	26	6.2	
Khat chewing							
Never	783	73.9	455	71.2	328	77.9	0.052
Former	59	5.6	39	6.1	20	4.8	
Current	218	20.6	145	22.7	73	17.3	
Body mass index (kg/m²)							
< 18.5	174	16.5	111	17.4	63	15.1	0.252
18.5–24.9	629	59.7	373	58.6	256	61.4	
24.9–29.9	184	17.5	118	18.5	66	15.8	
≥ 30	67	6.4	35	5.5	32	7.7	
Self-reported physical health							
Excellent/very good/good	596	56.2	410	64.2	186	44.2	< 0.001
Poor/fair	464	43.8	229	35.8	235	55.8	
Self-reported mental health							
Excellent/very good/good	699	65.9	478	74.8	221	52.5	< 0.001
Poor/fair	361	34.1	161	25.2	200	47.5	
Depression (past year)	70	6.6	23	3.6	47	11.2	< 0.001
Depression (lifetime)	192	18.1	73	11.4	119	28.3	< 0.001
Suicidal behavior (any type) [b]	160	15.1	61	9.5	99	23.5	< 0.001
Suicidal ideation	154	14.5	60	9.4	94	22.3	< 0.001
Suicidal plan	65	6.1	25	3.9	40	9.5	< 0.001
Suicidal attempt	44	4.2	16	2.5	28	6.7	0.001

Due to missing data, percentages may not add up to 100%
[a]Mean ± standard deviation (SD)
[b]Non-mutually exclusive subcomponents
For continuous variables, P-value was calculated using the one-way ANOVA; for categorical variables, P-value was calculated using the Chi-square test

Table 2 Socio-demographic and reproductive characteristics of the study population according to suicidal behavior (N = 1060)

Characteristics	No suicidal behavior (N = 900)		Any suicidal behavior (N = 160)		P-value
	n	%	n	%	
Age (years)[a]	35.73 ± 12.13		35.42 ± 11.83		0.766
Sex					
Women	526	58.4	111	69.4	0.011
Men	374	41.6	49	30.6	
Marital Status					
Married	474	52.8	68	42.5	0.004
Never married	284	31.7	51	31.9	
Other	139	15.5	41	25.6	
Education					
≤ Primary (1–6)	402	44.7	72	45.0	0.850
Secondary (7–12)	301	33.4	56	35.0	
College graduate	197	21.9	32	20.0	
Smoking status					
Never	778	86.4	135	84.4	0.628
Former	85	9.4	19	11.9	
Current	37	4.1	6	3.8	
Alcohol consumption past year					
Non-drinker	499	55.4	102	63.7	0.098
< once a month	309	34.3	48	30.0	
≥ 1 day a week	92	10.2	10	6.3	
Khat chewing					
None	667	74.1	116	72.5	0.569
Former	52	5.8	7	4.4	
Current	181	20.1	37	23.1	
Body mass index (kg/m^2)					
< 18.5	147	16.4	27	17.1	0.549
18.5–24.9	539	60.2	90	57.0	
24.9–29.9	157	17.5	27	17.1	
≥ 30	53	5.9	14	8.9	
Self-reported physical health					
Excellent/very good/good	537	59.7	59	36.9	< 0.001
Poor/fair	363	40.3	101	63.1	
Self-reported mental health					
Excellent/very good/good	631	70.1	68	42.5	< 0.001
Poor/fair	269	29.9	92	57.5	
Depression (past year)	21	2.3%	49	30.6	< 0.001
Depression (lifetime)	69	7.7	123	76.9	< 0.001

Due to missing data, percentages may not add up to 100%
[a]Mean ± standard deviation (SD)
For continuous variables, P-value was calculated using the one-way ANOVA; for categorical variables, P-value was calculated using the Chi-square test

affected by stressful events. Specifically, HPA activity has been found to be correlated with low grade cognitive stress in migraineurs [34]. Individuals with history of suicidal attempts were also found to have lower basal cortisol levels [35]. Furthermore in a study conducted among adolescent females, HPA-axis responses were associated

Table 3 Association between migraine and suicidal behavior (N = 1060)

	No suicidal behavior (N = 900)		Any suicidal behavior (N = 160)		Unadjusted OR (95% CI)	Adjusted OR (95% CI)[a]	Adjusted OR (95% CI)[b]	Adjusted OR (95% CI) [c]
	n	%	n	%				
No Migraine	578	64.2	61	38.1	Reference	Reference	Reference	Reference
Migraine	322	35.8	99	61.9	2.91 (2.06–4.12)	2.71 (1.89–3.89)	2.70 (1.88–3.89)	1.49 (0.93–2.39)

Abbreviations: OR odds ratio, *CI* confidence interval

[a]Adjusted for age (continuous), sex, education, and BMI categories

[b]Adjusted for age (continuous), sex, education, BMI categories, khat chewing, and past year alcohol consumption

[c]Adjusted for age (continuous), sex, education, BMI categories, khat chewing, past year alcohol consumption, and lifetime depression

Table 4 Association between migraine and suicidal behavior stratified by past year depression status (N = 1060)

Migraine	No suicidal behavior (N = 879)		Any suicidal behavior (N = 111)		Unadjusted OR (95% CI)	Adjusted OR (95% CI)[a]	Adjusted OR (95% CI)[b]
Without Depression	n	%	n	%			
No migraine	570	64.8	46	41.4	Reference	Reference	Reference
Migraine	309	35.2	65	58.6	2.61 (1.74–3.90)	2.27 (1.49–3.46)	2.27 (1.49–3.46)
Migraine	No suicidal behavior (N = 21)		Any suicidal behavior (N = 49)				
With Depression							
No migraine	8	38.1	15	30.6	Reference	Reference	Reference
Migraine	13	61.9	34	69.4	1.40 (0.48–4.07)	1.22 (0.36–4.13)	1.64 (0.40–6.69)

Abbreviations: OR odds ratio, *CI* confidence interval

[a]Adjusted for age (continuous), sex, education, and BMI categories

[b]Adjusted for age (continuous), sex, education, BMI categories, khat chewing, and past year alcohol consumption

to stress and risk of suicidal ideation [36]. Stressful events, including migraines, depression, and suicidal behaviors, may also be associated with serotonin levels. Changes in regulation and abnormalities of serotonergic mechanisms, including serotonin transporters, receptors, and metabolites have been associated with migraines and suicidal behaviors [37, 38]. Lastly chronic pain conditions, including migraine headaches, have been associated with suicidality [39–41]. Specifically, Ilgen et al. found an association between measures of head pain and suicidal ideation or attempts [40]. Chronic pain patients have an increased prevalence of suicidal ideation and attempts [42].

In the present study, there are a few limitations that should be considered. We used a cross-sectional study design which limits our inferences on the temporality between migraine and suicidal behaviors. Additionally, our hospital-based study population may limit our study findings generalizability to a broader general population. Our study used interviewer administered questionnaires in which the participants were asked questions about their physical and mental health, due to the social desirability bias participants may under-report their history of suicidal thought and behaviors and substance use. Migraine status could also be under reported as it could be affected by recall bias.

Conclusion

Migraine is associated with increased odds of suicidal behaviors, including suicidal ideation, plans, and attempts, among urban Ethiopian adults. Studies should further investigate this comorbidity and possible risk factors for these disorders. Efforts should also be made to raise awareness about the burdens posed by migraine among the public as well as health professionals. In addition, health professionals should be aware of the comorbidity between migraine, depression, and suicidal thought and behaviors to implement effective screening and treatment of these comorbid disorders.

Abbreviations
AOR: Adjust Odds Ratio; CI: Confidence Interval; CIDI: Composite International Diagnostic Interview; DSM-IV: Diagnostic and Statistical Manual of Mental Disorders, 4th Edition; ICD-10: International Classification of Diseases, 10th revision; ICHD-II: International Classification of Headache Disorders-2; LMICs: Low- and Middle-Income Countries; MMD: Major Depressive Disorder; OR: Odds Ratio

Acknowledgments
The authors wish to thank the staff of Addis Continental Institute of Public Health for their expert technical assistance. The authors would also like to thank the Saint Paul Hospital for granting access to conduct the study.

Funding
This research was supported by an award from the National Institutes of Health (NIH), the National Institute for Minority Health and Health Disparities (T37-MD0001449). The sponsor had no role in the design of the study, nor in the data collection, analysis and write up of this research article.

Authors' contributions
HB and BJD analyzed, interpreted the data and drafted the manuscript. BG assisted the analysis process as well as the drafting the results section. LF, YB, MW, and BG were responsible for the conceptualization of the research project, data collection and management and have contributed in the interpretation of the results. All authors have read and approved the final manuscript.

Consent for publication
Not applicable.

Competing interests
The authors declare that they have no competing interests.

Author details
[1]Addis Continental Institute of Public Health, Addis Ababa, Ethiopia.
[2]Department of Epidemiology, Harvard T.H. Chan School of Public Health, Boston, MA, USA.

References
1. Charles A. Migraine. N Engl J Med. 2017;377(6):553–61.
2. Leonardi M, Raggi A. Burden of migraine: international perspectives. Neurol Sci. 2013;34(Suppl 1):S117–8.
3. Woldeamanuel YW, Cowan RP. Migraine affects 1 in 10 people worldwide featuring recent rise: a systematic review and meta-analysis of community-based studies involving 6 million participants. J Neurol Sci. 2017;372:307–15.
4. Woldeamanuel YW, Andreou AP, Cowan RP. Prevalence of migraine headache and its weight on neurological burden in Africa: a 43-year systematic review and meta-analysis of community-based studies. J Neurol Sci. 2014;342(1–2):1–15.
5. Gelaye B, Peterlin BL, Lemma S, Tesfaye M, Berhane Y, Williams MA. Migraine and psychiatric comorbidities among sub-saharan african adults. Headache. 2013;53(2):310–21.
6. Domingues R, Aquino C, Santos J, Silva A, Kuster G. Prevalence and impact of headache and migraine among Pomeranians in Espirito Santo, Brazil. Arq Neuropsiquiatr. 2006;64(4):954–7.
7. Smitherman TA, Burch R, Sheikh H, Loder E. The prevalence, impact, and treatment of migraine and severe headaches in the United States: a review of statistics from national surveillance studies. Headache. 2013;53(3):427–36.
8. Breslau N, Rasmussen BK. The impact of migraine: epidemiology, risk factors, and co-morbidities. Neurology. 2001;56(suppl 1):S4–S12.
9. Risal A, Manandhar K, Holen A, Steiner TJ, Linde M. Comorbidities of psychiatric and headache disorders in Nepal: implications from a nationwide population-based study. J Headache Pain. 2016;17:45.
10. Mannix S, Skalicky A, Buse DC, Desai P, Sapra S, Ortmeier B, et al. Measuring the impact of migraine for evaluating outcomes of preventive treatments for migraine headaches. Health Qual Life Outcomes. 2016;14(1):143.
11. Buse D, Silberstein S, Manack A, Papapetropoulos S, RB L. Psychiatric comorbidities of episodic and chronic migraine. J Neurol. 2013;260(8):1960–9.
12. Bruti G, Magnotti MC, Iannetti G. Migraine and depression: bidirectional co-morbidities? Neurol Sci. 2012;33(Suppl 1):S107–9.
13. Breslau N, Schultz L, Stewart W, Lipton R, Welch K. Headache types and panic disorder: directionality and specificity. Neurology. 2001;56(3):350–4.
14. Breslau NDG, Andreski P. Migraine, psychiatric disorders, and suicide attempts: an epidemiologic study of young adults. Psychiatry Res. 1991;37(1):11–23.
15. Novic A, Kolves K, O'Dwyer S, De Leo D. Migraine and suicidal behaviors: a systematic literature review. Clin J Pain. 2016;32(4):351–64.
16. Breslau N. Migraine, suicidal ideation, and suicide attempts. Neurology. 1992;42(2):392–5.
17. Breslau NDG, Schultz LR, Peterson EL. Joint 1994 Wolff award presentation. Migraine and major depression: a longitudinal study. Headache. 1994;34(7):387–93.
18. Breslau N, Lipton R, Stewart W, Schultz L, Welch K. Comorbidity of migraine and depression: investigating potential etiology and prognosis. Neurology. 2003;60(8):1308–12.

19. Breslau N, Schultz L, Lipton R, Peterson E, Welch K. Migraine headaches and suicide attempt. Headache. 2012;52(5):723–31.

20. Friedman LE, Gelaye B, Rondon MB, Sanchez SE, Peterlin BL, Williams MA. Association of Migraine Headaches with Suicidal Ideation among Pregnant Women in lima. Peru Headache. 2016;56(4):741–9.

21. Nock MK, Borges G, Bromet EJ, Cha CB, Kessler RC, Lee S. Suicide and suicidal behavior. Epidemiol Rev. 2008;30:133–54.

22. Whittier AB, Gelaye B, Deyessa N, Bahretibeb Y, Kelkile TS, Berhane Y, et al. Major depressive disorder and suicidal behavior among urban dwelling Ethiopian adult outpatients at a general hospital. J Affect Disord. 2016;197:58–65.

23. Saxena S, Krug EG, Chestnov O and World Health Organization, eds. Preventing Suicide: A Global Imperative. Geneva: World Health Organization; 2014.

24. Wang S, Fuh J, Juang K, Lu S. Migraine and suicidal ideation in adolescents aged 13 to 15 years. Neurology. 2009;72(13):1146–52.

25. (WHO) WHO. Composite international diagnostic interview (CIDI). 1990.

26. (WHO) WHO. International statistical classification of diseases and health related problems: (the) ICD-10. 2004.

27. American Psychiatric Association, American Psychiatric Association. Task Force on DSM-IV. Diagnostic and statistical manual of mental disorders: DSM-IV-TR. 4.th ed. Washington, DC: American Psychiatric Association; 2000.

28. Nock MK, Hwang I, Sampson NA, Kessler RC. Mental disorders, comorbidity and suicidal behavior: results from the National Comorbidity Survey Replication. Mol Psychiatry. 2010;15(8):868–76.

29. Samaan Z, Macgregor EA, Andrew D, McGuffin P, Farmer A. Diagnosing migraine in research and clinical settings: the validation of the structured migraine interview (SMI). BMC Neurol. 2010;10:7.

30. Society HCCotIH. The international classification of headache disorders, 3rd edition (beta version). Cephalalgia. 2013;33(9):629–808.

31. Friedman LE, Gelaye B, Bain PA, Williams MA. A systematic review and meta-analysis of migraine and suicidal ideation. Clin J Pain. 2016;33(7):659-65.

32. Desai SD, Pandya RH. Study of psychiatric comorbidity in patients with headache using a short structured clinical interview in a rural neurology clinic in western India. J Neurosci Rural Pract. 2014;5(Suppl 1):S39–42.

33. Pompili M, Di Cosimo D, Innamorati M, Lester D, Tatarelli R, Martelletti P. Psychiatric comorbidity in patients with chronic daily headache and migraine: a selective overview including personality traits and suicide risk. J Headache Pain. 2009;10(4):283–90.

34. Leistad RB, Stovner LJ, White LR, Nilsen KB, Westgaard RH, Sand T. Noradrenaline and cortisol changes in response to low-grade cognitive stress differ in migraine and tension-type headache. J Headache Pain. 2007;8(3):157–66.

35. Keilp JG, Stanley BH, Beers SR, Melhem NM, Burke AK, Cooper TB, et al. Further evidence of low baseline cortisol levels in suicide attempters. J Affect Disord. 2016;190:187–92.

36. Giletta M, Calhoun C, Hastings P, Rudolph K, Nock M, Prinstein M. Multi-level risk factors for suicidal ideation among at-risk adolescent females: the role of hypothalamic-pituitary-adrenal Axis responses to stress. J Abnorm Child Psychol. 2015;43(5):807–20.

37. Pandey G. Biological basis of suicide and suicidal behavior. Bipolar Disord. 2013;15(5):524–41.

38. Gupta S, Nahas SJ, Peterlin BL. Chemical mediators of migraine: preclinical and clinical observations. Headache. 2011;51(6):1029–45.

39. Ilgen M, Kleinberg F, Ignacio R, Bohnert A, Valenstein M, McCarthy J, et al. Noncancer pain conditions and risk of suicide. JAMA Psychiatry. 2013; 70(7):692–7.

40. Ilgen MA, Zivin K, McCammon RJ, Valenstein M. Pain and suicidal thoughts, plans and attempts in the United States. Gen Hosp Psychiatry. 2008;30(6):521–7.

41. Ratcliffe G, Enns M, Belik S, Sareen J. Chronic pain conditions and suicidal ideation and suicide attempts: an epidemiologic perspective. Clin J Pain. 2008;24(3):204–10.

42. Tang NK, Crane C. Suicidality in chronic pain: a review of the prevalence, risk factors and psychological links. Psychol Med. 2006;36(5):575–86.

9

Binge eating disorder and depressive symptoms among females of child-bearing age: the Korea Nurses' Health Study

O. Kim[1,2], M. S. Kim[3], J. Kim[4], J. E. Lee[5] and H. Jung[6*] (iD)

Abstract

Background: Most studies regarding the relationship between binge eating disorder (BED) and depression have targeted obese populations. However, nurses, particularly female nurses, are one of the vocations that face these issues due to various reasons including high stress and shift work. This study investigated the prevalence of BED and the correlation between BED and severity of self-reported depressive symptoms among female nurses in South Korea.

Methods: Participants were 7,267 female nurses, of which 502 had symptoms of BED. Using the propensity score matching (PSM) technique, 502 nurses with BED and 502 without BED were included in the analyses. Data were analyzed using descriptive statistics, Spearman's correlation, and multivariable ordinal logistic regression analysis.

Results: The proportion of binge eating disorder was 6.90% among the nurses, and 81.3% of nurses displayed some levels of depressive symptoms. Multivariable ordinal logistic regression analysis revealed that age (40 years old and older), alcohol consumption (frequent drinkers), self-rated health, sleep problems, and stress were associated with self-reported depression symptoms. Overall, after adjusting for confounders, nurses with BED had 1.80 times the risk (95% CI = [1.41–2.30]; p-value < 0.001) of experiencing a greater severity of self-reported depression symptoms.

Conclusions: Korean female nurse showed a higher prevalence of both binge eating disorder and depressive symptoms, and the association between the two factors was proven in the study. Therefore, hospital management and health policy makers should be alarmed and agreed on both examining nurses on such problems and providing organized and systematic assistance.

Keywords: Binge eating disorder, Depression, DSM, Korea nurses' health study, Nursing, Public health, South Korea

Background

Binge eating disorder (BED) is characterized by recurring eating behaviors wherein a significantly large amount of food is consumed when an individual experiences a lack of control [1]. BED has the highest prevalence rate among all of the eating disorders [2], and this differs according to the characteristics of the subjects and the diagnostic standards. For instance, the lifetime prevalence of BED by the age of 20 years was reported as 3.0% in a study targeting a community sample of 496 female adolescents [3]. In another study, the lifetime prevalence in non-clinical samples was 2.0% for men and 3.5% for women [4]. The clinical samples

consisting of obese patients seeking treatment for weight loss had a lifetime prevalence ranging from 5% to 30% [5].

BED has mostly been related to obesity or depression, and recent studies have shown comorbidity with gender (female), age (young), and high level of anxiety and stress [2]. Depression is both a risk factor of BED as well as a potential cause [5]; it is a disorder that has a high prevalence rate and is a significant health issue [6]. Women in particular have a high prevalence of depression; the prevalence rate of Koreans in 2014 was 6.7% (9.1% for women and 4.2% for men) according to the research by Korea Centers for Disease Control and Prevention [7]. According to a systematic literature review, 10 out of 14 studies showed a significant relationship between BED and depression [5]. Female BED patients showed a higher rate of loss of control than male patients [8] and reported

---
* Correspondence: jhj1215@konyang.ac.kr; jhjice@gmail.com
[6]College of Nursing, Konyang University, Daejeon, Republic of Korea
Full list of author information is available at the end of the article

higher levels of depression when compared to the general population [9]. Until now, however, most studies regarding the relationship between BED and depression have targeted obese populations. Therefore, it is necessary to study the nature of that association within different groups and occupations.

Among various occupational groups, nurses' shift-works and high work stress were proven to be associated with binge eating and other abnormal eating behaviors [10]. In addition, nurses can be assumed as a high-risk group of depression as they undergo a high level of stress [11]. However, there has been a lack of research proving the association between BED and depression among nurses. Although depression has recently arisen as a major mental health problem for nurses [11], limited research was done confirming the influence of eating disorders such as binge eating on depression. This research aims to establish the association between BED and depressive symptoms among nurses by analyzing the data collected from the Korean Nurses' Health Study, which is a large-scale prospective cohort research targeting female nurses.

Methods
Study design and participants
The target population was 7,267 female Registered Nurses (RNs) aged 20 to 45 years, who were in their childbearing years. Nurses with either psychiatric comorbidities or history of using psychiatric drugs were excluded. These nurses have either been medically diagnosed with depression or have taken any psychiatric drugs including Selective Serotonin Reuptake Inhibitator (SSIR) type antidepressants, other antidepressants, or Minor tranquilizers. The data was collected from July of 2013 to September of 2015 via online survey through voluntary participation. Participants had completed the first and second surveys as part of the Korea Nurses' Health Study [12]. The Korea Nurses' Health Study is a grand-scale research that the Korean Nurses Association and Korea Centers of Disease Control and Prevention jointly conducted using a similar survey protocol and format of the Nurses' Health Study 3 (NHS 3) [13] of the United States. The first baseline study was conducted for 3 years, from March 2013 to December 2015. The KNHS consisted of six modules including two special modules asking about one's early stages of pregnancy and postpartum experiences with consent in case the participants got pregnant or gave birth. This study utilized the data from the first phase of the KNHS. The second phase of the KNHS has been underway since 2016 and is scheduled to be completed in 2018. The first survey, which served as baseline data, was closed while the other surveys are still open.

Measures
All the survey questionnaires used in this study were translated and back-translated into Korean, modified, and redeemed to suit the Korean context after discussions with an advisory committee of multidisciplinary experts. In this research, we measured whether one has binge eating disorder with 10 questions of self-report measures using the diagnostic criteria (definition of binge eating episode) of Diagnostic and Statistical Manual of Mental Disorders, fifth edition (DSM-5) [1]. The last question was a negative-form question related to inappropriate compensatory behaviors and was converted into positive-form for this research. For each question, participants could answer with either "yes" or "no," and the BED criteria of DSM-5 was met if she answered "yes" for both of the questions: 1) did you eat an amount of food that is definitely larger than most people would eat in a similar period of time under similar circumstances in a discrete period of time? and 2) did you feel a sense of lack of control over eating? Once a participant responded "yes" to both of these questions, then five additional questionnaires were asked. These questions were: a) did you eat much more rapidly than normal? b) did you eat until feeling uncomfortably full?, c) did you eat large amounts of food when not feeling physically hungry?, d) did you eat alone because of feeling embarrassed by how much you eat?, and e) did you feel disgusted with yourself, depressed, or very guilty after overeating? Participants who answered "yes" to at least 3 of the above 5 questions and "yes" to 'did you feel often upset both during and after the binge eating?' and 'did you experience binge eating episodes at least once a week over the past 3 months?' were categorized as experiencing binge eating disorder. Additionally, we excluded participants who answered "yes" to a question regarding inappropriate compensatory behaviors like laxatives, diuretics, and self-induced vomiting.

We measured the degree of self-reported depressive symptoms using the Patient Health Questionnaire (PHQ-9), which is a self-report instrument with 9 questions. The possible score range is 0–27, divided into 0–4, 5–9, 10–14, 15–19, and above 20, representing minimal, mild, moderate, moderately severe, and severe depressive symptoms respectively. The higher the score, the severer one's depressive symptom [14]. The Cronbach's alpha value in our study was 0.90, and that of the original research by Arroll et al. was 0.87 [15].

In order to find the association between BED and depressive symptoms, this research considered potential confounders through literature reviews. Confounders included a) age [11], level of education [16], annual income [11], and marital status [16] as socio-demographic factors, b) alcohol consumption [17], body mass index (BMI) [11], self-rated health [18], sleep [19], stress [20] as health-behavior factors and c) shift work as a work-related factor [11].

Stress, a control variable in this study, was measured using the Perceived Stress Scale-4 (PSS-4) [21], which consists of 4 questions regarding the frequency of emotions and thoughts during the last 30 days. The possible score range is 0–16; the higher the score, the greater the degree of stress. For sleep, another control variable, we used the Jenkins Sleep Questionnaire [22], which consists of 4 questions about the amount of sleep during the last 30 days, with possible score range of 0–20; a high score implies a sleep disorder. We measured self-rated health using one question asking if a participant think of herself as healthy in three categories, which are good, fair, and poor.

Statistical analysis

We analyzed the data using the Statistical Package for Social Sciences (SPSS) Version 23 (SPSS Inc., Chicago, IL, USA). We calculated frequency and percentage as parts of descriptive statistics and the Spearman's correlation to identify the associations between variables. Since the data were extremely skewed with 6.9% of nurses having symptoms of binge eating, we used propensity score matching (PSM) to match the BED group and the non-BED group. This was done through estimating an average treatment effect from observational data using the following selected potential predictive variables based on prior studies: age, marital status, BMI, self-rated health, alcohol consumption, stress, sleep, and shift work. Smoking was considered as a potential predictive variable; however, almost all of the study participants were non-smokers, and we excluded it as a confounder from the analyses. After matching using the PSM, the sample size was reduced from 7,267 to 1,004 with an evenly distributed sample size of 502. The PSM technique helps to reduce the bias due to distorted samples between the group with BED and the group without it. Finally, we performed multivariable ordinal logistic regression analysis to see the relationship between BED and depressive symptoms and showed the result using odds ratios (OR) and 95% confidence intervals (CIs). The threshold for statistical significance for this study was $p < 0.05$.

Results

Participant characteristics

Out of the 7,267 nurses, 6.9% ($n = 502$) nurses had symptoms for BED. Distributions of key variables with and without BED as well as the differences between the two groups by key variables are presented in Table 1. According to the descriptive analysis, 81.3% of nurses displayed some levels of depressive symptoms (from mild to severe), and majority of them were younger than

30 years old (42.9%) or in the ages between 30 and 39 (45.5%). Majority of the study participants had completed either a 3-year college (51.7%) or 4-year university (42.9%), had earned either annual income in ranges of $30,000–39,999 (42.0%) or $40,000–49.999 (37.8%), and were single (76.1%). With regard to health related characteristics and shift work, majority of the nurses consumed alcohol occasionally (70.2%), had a normal BMI (61.8%), rated their health as fair (50.7%), expressed some levels of sleep problems (14.9% with the least sleep problems) and stress (26.1% with the lowest level of stress), and worked shifts (77.9%).

BED and severity of self-reported depressive symptoms

Multicollinearity was examined with no variance inflation factor (VIF) values over 10 [23]. Spearman's correlation analyses showed that all variables showed moderate correlation below 0.6 (Table 2), which justified proceeding to conduct multivariable ordinal logistic regression [24]. Table 3 shows the results of the multivariable ordinal logistic regression analysis. In model 2, socio-demographic characteristics, such as age, level of education, annual income, and marital status, were controlled; health behaviors including alcohol consumption, BMI, self-rated health, sleep, and stress were included as control variables in Model 3. In the final model (Model 4), shift work was also included. Out of the control variables, age (40 years old and older), alcohol consumption (frequent drinkers), self-rated health, sleep problems, and stress were associated with depressive symptoms in the final model. Overall, after adjusting for confounders, nurses with binge eating disorders had 1.80 times the risk of experiencing a greater severity of self-reported depressive symptoms when compared to those without BED. Table 3 shows that as we add more confounders, both the Nagelkerke R-square values and the risk of nurses with binge eating disorders to experience a greater severity of depressive symptoms increase.

Discussion

First, we confirmed high prevalence rates in both BED and self-reported depressive symptoms among Korean female nurses. While the BED prevalence rate in a prior research targeting a community sample by using the same DSM-5 criteria was 3.0% [3], 6.9% of our research targets met the BED criteria. Besides this, we found that the prevalence rate in our research targeting female nurses was higher even when compared to the BED prevalence rate of 3.53% from a study done on female college students in Wuhan, China [25]. Similarly, the prevalence rate of BED from a phone interviewed study of Canadian women was 3.8% [26], and the rate from an Australian adolescent cohort study was 5.6% [27]. In the current research, the high BED prevalence rate supports

Table 1 Descriptive characteristics according to BED after matching groups using the PSM

	All (N = 1,004)		No (N = 502)		Yes (N = 502)		
	n	%	n	%	n	%	P
Depressive symptom							
Normal	188	18.7	95	18.9	93	18.5	0.882
Mild	386	38.4	194	38.6	192	38.2	
Moderate	23.1	23.1	116	23.1	115	22.9	
Moderately severe	140	13.9	65	12.9	75	14.9	
Severe	59	5.9	32	6.5	27	5.5	
Age (in years)							
≤ 29	431	42.9	219	43.6	212	42.2	0.895
30–39	457	45.5	225	44.8	232	46.2	
≥ 40	116	11.6	58	11.6	58	11.6	
Level of education							
Masters or higher	54	5.4	26	5.2	28	5.6	0.562
3-year college	519	51.7	268	53.4	251	50.0	
4-year university	431	42.9	208	41.4	223	44.4	
Annual income							
< $20,000	50	5.1	26	5.2	24	4.8	0.640
$20,000–$29,999	130	12.9	58	11.6	72	14.3	
$30,000–$39,999	422	42.0	208	41.4	214	42.6	
$40,000–$49,999	380	37.8	198	39.4	182	36.3	
≥ $50,000	22	2.2	12	2.4	10	2.0	
Marital status							
Single	764	76.1	394	78.5	370	73.7	0.076
Married	240	23.9	108	21.5	132	26.3	
Alcohol consumption							
Never	161	16.1	71	14.2	90	17.9	0.211
Occasionally	705	70.2	364	72.5	341	67.9	
Frequently	138	13.7	67	13.3	71	14.2	
BMI (in kg/m^2)*							
Normal (18.5–22.9)	621	61.8	308	61.4	313	62.3	0.000
Underweight (< 18.5)	114	11.4	81	16.1	33	6.6	
Overweight (≥23)	269	26.8	113	22.5	156	31.1	
Self-rated health							
Poor	188	18.7	94	18.7	94	18.7	0.937
Fair	509	50.7	257	51.2	252	50.2	
Good	307	30.6	151	30.1	156	31.1	
Sleep (quartile)							
1 (least sleep problem)	150	14.9	74	14.7	76	15.1	0.946
2	263	26.2	128	25.5	135	26.9	
3	252	25.1	127	25.3	125	24.9	
4	339	33.8	173	34.5	166	33.1	
Stress (quartile)							
1 (least stressed)	262	26.1	139	27.7	123	24.5	0.584

Table 1 Descriptive characteristics according to BED after matching groups using the PSM *(Continued)*

	All (N = 1,004)		No (N = 502)		Yes (N = 502)		
	n	%	n	%	n	%	P
2	301	30.0	146	29.1	155	30.9	
3	256	25.5	122	24.3	134	26.7	
4	185	18.4	95	18.9	90	17.9	
Shift work							
No	222	22.1	106	21.1	116	23.1	0.447
Yes	782	77.9	396	78.9	386	76.9	

Note: Occasionally: sometimes in a month; Frequently: sometimes in a week; BMI: body mass index
*BMI categories are according to the World Health Organization Asia Pacific Region and the Korean Society for the Study of Obesity

that the female nurses are a BED high-risk group, corroborated by a previous research [10].

The prevalence of depressive symptoms among Korean nurses in the current research was 81.2% (38.4% with mild, 23.1% with moderate, 13.9% with moderately severe and 5.9% with severe); we could confirm that the level of depressive symptoms among Korean nurses was considerably high. Prior studies showed lower prevalence rates [28, 29]. A cross-sectional research conducted on 441 Korean nurses using the South Korean version of the Center for Epidemiologic Studies rating scale for Depression (CESD) showed a prevalence rate of 38% [28]. Another prior study done on 1,592 nurses of hospitals in Liaoning, China, using the PHQ-P measurement, showed a prevalence rate 61.7% [29].

Using the BED criteria of the DSM-5 and PHQ-9, this study confirmed the association between BED and self-reported depressive symptoms among female nurses. In our research, the results from the multivariable ordinal logistic regression showed that the nurses with BED were 1.80 times more likely to have self-reported depressive symptoms compared with the nurses without BED

controlling the potential confounders. Previous researches have also shown that BED was significantly related to depression including a study by Borges [30] targeting Brazilian women who participated in a weight loss program and Celic et al. [31] showing the connection between BED and the level of depression within a type 2 diabetes mellitus (T2DM) patient group. Other studies also confirmed the association between the two variables including a study revealing the high correlation between BED and depression in general adult population [32] and another study on young women in the United States [33]. Overall, we can say that the result of this research was a reconfirmation of the fact that BED is a major influential factor of depressive symptoms.

Although female nurses are rationally a group to be studied on the association between BED and depression, limited studies have examined the association among female nurses. We have seen from our own data of Korea Nurses' Health Study that Korean female nurses show high prevalence of self-reported depressive symptoms, but majority of them do not seek medical help [11]. This alarmed us and made us to further investigate the associations between

Table 2 Correlation coefficients for variables

		1	2	3	4	5	6	7	8	9	10	11	12
1	Depressive symptoms	1											
2	BED	.008	1										
3	Age	.012	−.177**	1									
4	Level of education	.025	.014	.131**	1								
5	Annual income	.040	−.050	.430**	.112**	1							
6	Marital status	.056	−.209**	.542**	.078*	−.241**	1						
7	Alcohol consumption	−.028	.001	−.050	−.051	.005	−.033	1					
8	BMI	.026	.001	.157**	−.037	.004	.174**	.005	1				
9	Self-rated health	.008	−.403**	.006	.020	−.015	.069*	.015	−.051	1			
10	Sleep	−.017	.513**	−.113**	.000	.053	−.182**	.035	.021	−.332**	1		
11	Stress	.019	.392**	−.118**	−.001	.108**	−.113**	−.004	−.056	−.253**	.189**	1	
12	Shift work	−.024	.171**	−.269**	−.066*	.026	−.303**	.083**	−.019	−.099**	.227**	.079*	1

Note: BMI: body mass index
*p < .05, **p < .01, ***p < .001

Binge eating disorder and depressive symptoms among females of child-bearing...

85

Table 3 Result of the multivariate ordinal logistic regression analysis

Variables	Model 1 OR	Model 1 95% CI	Model 2 OR	Model 2 95% CI	Model 3 OR	Model 3 95% CI	Model 4 OR	Model 4 95% CI
BED								
No	Ref.		Ref.		Ref.		Ref.	
Yes	1.456**	1.163–1.823	1.537**	1.223–1.931	1.795**	1.410–2.286	1.800**	1.414–2.292
Age (in years)								
≤ 29			Ref.		Ref.		Ref.	
30–39			0.904	.685–1.193	0.780	0.581–1.047	0.785	0.585–1.055
≥ 40			0.308**	0.176–0.536	0.359**	0.195–0.659	0.372**	0.200–0.690
Level of education								
3-year college			Ref.		Ref.		Ref.	
4-year college			1.096	0.857–1.401	1.122	0.866–1.454	1.130	0.872–1.464
Master or higher			1.251	0.686–2.279	1.321	0.700–2.496	1.320	0.699–2.494
Annual income								
< $20,000			Ref.		Ref.		Ref.	
$20,000–29,999			1.140	0.618–2.103	0.798	0.412–1.544	0.800	0.413–1.549
$30,000–39,999			1.378	0.775–2.448	0.913	0.491–1.699	0.916	0.492–1.706
$40,000–49,999			1.332	0.733–2.419	0.860	0.451–1.639	0.873	0.457–1.666
≥ $50,000			0.965	0.361–2.577	0.546	0.194–1.538	0.556	0.197–1.569
Marital status								
Single			Ref.		Ref.		Ref.	
Married			1.691**	1.217–2.351	1.393	0.983–1.974	1.371	0.964–1.951
Alcohol consumption								
Never					Ref.		Ref.	
Occasionally					0.759	0.543–1.062	0.759	0.543–1.062
Frequently					0.572*	0.365–0.897	0.565*	0.360–0.887
BMI, kg/m^2								
Normal (18.5–22.9)					Ref.		Ref.	
Underweight (< 18.5)					1.356	0.910–2.019	1.354	0.909–2.018
Overweight(≥ 23)					1.087	0.821–1.440	1.084	0.818–1.435
Self-rated health								
Poor					Ref.		Ref.	
Fair					0.457**	0.327–0.639	0.454**	0.325–0.635
Good					0.317**	0.215–0.468	0.317**	0.214–0.467
Sleep (quartile)								
1 (least problem)					Ref.		Ref.	
2					2.821**	1.852–4.295	2.783**	1.823–4.246
3					5.439**	3.511–8.425	5.341**	3.438–8.299
4					12.494**	7.991–19.535	12.272**	7.823–19.253
Stress (quartile)								
1 (least stress)					Ref.		Ref.	
2					2.094**	1.493–2.937	2.092**	1.492–2.934
3					3.671**	2.583–5.217	3.650**	2.568–5.190
4					7.346**	4.907–10.998	7.310**	4.882–10.945

Table 3 Result of the multivariate ordinal logistic regression analysis *(Continued)*

Variables	Model 1		Model 2		Model 3		Model 4	
	OR	95% CI	OR	95% CI	OR	95% CI	OR	95% CI
Shift work								
No							Ref.	
Yes							0.903	0.656–1.243
Nagelkerke R^2	0.011**		0.092***		0.421***		0.421***	
x^2/df	10.758/1		91.507/10		507.345/22		507.717/23	

Note: OR: odds ratio; *95% CI*: 95% confidence interval; *Ref*: reference group; Occasionally: sometimes in a month; Frequently: sometimes in a week; BMI: body mass index

*$p < .05$, **$p < .01$, ***$p < .001$

depressive symptoms and other health issues among the population. Our findings might not bring any brilliantly new clinical findings to the current understanding of binge eating and depression. However, we strongly believe that it is meaningful to investigate the association between the two factors among female nurses since they show high prevalence in both BED and depressive symptoms and are not investigated enough compare to other groups.

This research has both strengths and limitations. Our research outcome is as unique as a pioneer research that found a relationship between BED and depressive symptoms among a specific occupation group. It is also quite significant that we confirmed the BED prevalence rate, while excluding the comorbidity of night eating syndrome; we also saw a meaningful association between self-reported BED symptoms and depressive symptoms, especially on a non-clinical population. Despite these significant advantages, there are some limitations in this research. First, while we controlled certain related variables to find the association between BED and depressive symptoms, we failed to control other potential confounders, such as a dissatisfaction about one's body image and other work or family related factors, which should be considered in future researches. Second, we used only the DSM-5 criteria to diagnose BED. Using a broader measurement, such as the DSM-5 criteria could have influenced the high prevalence rate of BED in our study. For further studies, we suggest more conservative measurement of BED by combining self-report measures to identify BED symptoms with a 2-stage screening processes either including expert interviews or additional surveys. Lastly, our research only included Korean female RNs aged 20 to 45. Findings may not be generalized beyond this specific population. Therefore more research in this area needs to be conducted on different study subjects including various occupations and ethnicities.

Conclusions

This research aimed to find the relationship between BED and depressive symptoms among Korean female nurses, and we were able to confirm a high correlation between the two variables as a pioneer study. Currently, depression is a major mental and psychological health problem in the Korean society, and eating disorders including BED are not gaining enough attention in Korea. Based on the findings of this study, hospital management and health policy makers should be alarmed and agreed on both examining nurses on such problems and providing organized and systematic assistance.

Abbreviation

BED: Binge eating disorder; DSM-5: Diagnostic and Statistical Manual of Mental Disorders, fifth edition; KNHS: Korea Nurses' Health Study; NHS: Nurses' Health Study; PHQ-9: Patient Health Questionnaire-9; PSM: Propensity Score Matching

Acknowledgements

Not applicable

Funding

The Korea Nurses' Health Study is funded (2013E6300600, 2013E6300601, 2013E6300602) by the Korea Centers for Disease Control and Prevention (KCDC) of the Korea National Institute of Health (KNIH).

Authors' contributions

OK and HJ have planned study, MSK is responsible for the design and analysis of data. OK, HJ, MSK, JK, and JEL are responsible for drafting the manuscript. All authors have read and approved of the final manuscript.

Consent for publication

Not applicable.

Competing interests

The authors declare that they have no competing interests.

Author details

[1]Korean Nurses Association, Seoul, Republic of Korea. [2]College of Nursing, Ewha Womans University, Seoul, Republic of Korea. [3]Jeju Institute of Public Health and Health Policy, Jeju, Republic of Korea. [4]Department of Nursing, Dongeui University, Busan, Republic of Korea. [5]Department of Food and Nutrition, Seoul National University, Seoul, Republic of Korea. [6]College of Nursing, Konyang University, Daejeon, Republic of Korea.

References

1. American Psychiatric Association. Diagnostic and statistical manual of mental disorders. 5th ed. Washington, D.C.: American Psychiatric Association; 2013.
2. Kessler RC, Berglund PA, Chiu WT, Deitz AC, Hudson JI, Shahly V, et al. The prevalence and correlates of binge eating disorder in the World Health Organization world mental health surveys. Biol Psychiatry. 2013;73:904–14. https://doi.org/10.1001/jama.291.21.2581.
3. Stice E, Marti CN, Rohde P. Prevalence, incidence, impairment, and course of the proposed DSM-5 eating disorder diagnoses in an 8-year prospective community study of young women. J Abnorm Psychol. 2013;122:445–57. https://doi.org/10.1037/a0030679.
4. Hudson JI, Hiripi E, HG Jr P, Kessler RC. The prevalence and correlates of eating disorders in the National Comorbidity Survey Replication. Biol Psychiatry. 2007;61:348–58. https://doi.org/10.1016/j.biopsych.2006.03.040.
5. Araujo DM, Santos GF, Nardi AE. Binge eating disorder and depression: a systematic review. World J Biol Psychiatry. 2010;11:199–207. https://doi.org/10.3109/15622970802563171.
6. Park JH, Kim KW. A review of the epidemiology of depression in Korea. J Korean Med Assoc. 2011;54:362–9. https://doi.org/10.5124/jkma.2011.54.4.362.
7. Korea Centers for Disease Control and Prevention: 2014 Korea health statistics[December 23rd, 2015]. Available from: http://www.cdc.go.kr/CDC/eng/main.jsp. Accessed 7 Aug 2017.
8. Reslan S, Saules KK. College students' definitions of an eating "binge" differ as a function of gender and binge eating disorder status. Eat Behav. 2011;12:225–7. https://doi.org/10.1016/j.eatbeh.2011.03.001.
9. Vancampfort D, De Herdt A, Vanderlinden J, Lannoo M, Soundy A, Pieters G, et al. Health related quality of life, physical fitness and physical activity participation in treatment-seeking obese persons with and without binge eating disorder. Psychiatry Res. 2014;216:97–102. https://doi.org/10.1016/j.psychres.2014.01.015.
10. Almajwal AM. Stress, shift duty, and eating behavior among nurses in Central Saudi Arabia. Saudi Med J. 2016;37:191–8. https://doi.org/10.15537/smj.2016.2.13060.
11. Lee HY, Kim MS, Kim O, Lee IH, Kim HK. Association between shift work and severity of depressive symptoms among female nurses: the Korea Nurses' health study. J Nurs Manag. 2015;24:192–200. https://doi.org/10.1111/jonm.12298.
12. Kim O, Ahn Y, Jang HJ, Kim S, Lee JE, Jung H, et al. The Korea Nurses' health study: a prospective cohort study. J Women's Health. https://doi.org/10.1089/jwh.2016.6048.
13. Gaskins AJ, Rich-Edwards JW, Lawson CC, Schernhammer ES, Missmer SA, Chavarro JE. Work schedule and physical factors in relation to fecundity in nurses. Occup Environ Med. 2015;72:777–83. https://doi.org/10.1136/oemed-2015-103026.
14. Kroenke K, Spitzer RL, Williams JB. The PHQ-9: validity of a brief depression severity measure. J Gen Intern Med. 2001;16:606–13.
15. Arroll B, Goodyear-Smith F, Crengle S, Gunn J, Kerse N, Fishman T, et al. Validation of PHQ-2 and PHQ-9 to screen for major depression in the primary care population. Ann Fam Med. 2010;8:348–35. https://doi.org/10.1370/afm.1139.
16. Jang SN, Kawachi I, Chang J, Boo K, Shin HG, Lee H, et al. Marital status, gender, and depression: analysis of the baseline survey of the Korean longitudinal study of ageing (KLoSA). Soc Sci Med. 2009;69:1608–15. https://doi.org/10.1016/j.socscimed.2009.09.007.
17. Fergusson DM, Boden JM, Horwood LJ. Tests of causal links between alcohol abuse or dependence and major depression. Arch Gen Psychiatry. 2009;66:260–6. https://doi.org/10.1001/archgenpsychiatry.2008.543.
18. Badawi G, Pagé V, Smith KJ, Gariépy G, Malla A, Wang J, et al. Self-rated health: a predictor for the three year incidence of major depression in individuals with type II diabetes. J Affect Disord. 2013;145:100–5. https://doi.org/10.1016/j.jad.2012.07.018.
19. Sivertsen B, Harvey AG, Lundervold AJ, Hysing M. Sleep problems and depression in adolescence: results from a large population-based study of Norwegian adolescents aged 16–18 years. Eur Child Adolesc Psychiatry. 2013;23:681–9. https://doi.org/10.1007/s00787-013-0502-y.
20. Yusoff MS, Abdul Rahim AF, Baba AA, Ismail SB, Pa MN, Esa AR. Prevalence and associated factors of stress, anxiety and depression among prospective medical students. Asian J Psychiatry. 2013;6:128–33. https://doi.org/10.1016/j.ajme.2016.01.005.
21. Cohen S, Kamarch T, Mermelstein RA. Global measure of perceived stress. J Health Soc Behav. 1983;24:385–96.
22. Jenkins CD, Stanton BA, Niemcryk SJ, Rose RM. A scale for the estimation of sleep problems in clinical research. J Clin Epidemiol. 1988;41:313–21. https://doi.org/10.1016/0895-4356(88)90138-2.
23. Mansfield ER, Helms BP. Detecting multicollinearity. Am Stat. 1982;36:158–60.
24. Bottles K, Cohen MB, Holly EA, Chiu S, Abele JS, Cello JP, et al. A step-wise logistic regression analysis of hepatocellular carcinoma an aspiration biopsy study. Cancer. 1988;62:558–63.
25. Tong J, Miao S, Wang J, Yang F, Lai H, Zhang C, et al. A two-stage epidemiologic study on prevalence of eating disorders in female university students in Wuhan, China. Soc Psychiatry Psychiatr Epidemiol. 2014;49:499–505. https://doi.org/10.1007/s00127-013-0694-y.
26. Gauvin L, Steiger H, Brodeur JM. Eating disorder symptoms and syndromes in a sample of urban-dwelling Canadian women: contributions toward a population health perspective. Int J Eat Disord. 2009;42:158–65. https://doi.org/10.1002/eat.20590.
27. Hay P, Girosi F, Mond J. Prevalence and sociodemographic correlates of DSM-4 eating disorders in the Australian population. J Eat Disord. 2015;3:2–7. https://doi.org/10.1186/s40337-015-0056-0.
28. Yoon SL, Kim JH. Job-related stress, emotional labor, and depressive symptoms among Korean nurses. J Nurs Scholarsh. 2013;45:169–76. https://doi.org/10.1111/jnu.12018.
29. Gao YQ, Pan BC, Sun W, Wu H, Wang JN, Wang L. Depressive symptoms among Chinese nurses: prevalence and the associated factors. J Adv Nurs. 2011;68:1166–75. https://doi.org/10.1111/j.1365-2648.2011.05832.x.
30. Borges MB, Jorge MR, Morgan CM, Silveira DX, Custodio O. Binge eating disorder in Brazilian women on a weight loss program. Obes Res. 2002;10:1127–34. https://doi.org/10.1038/oby.2002.153.
31. Çelik S, Kayar Y, Önem Akçakaya R, Türkyılmaz Uyar E, Kalkan K, Yazısız V, et al. Correlation of binge eating disorder with level of depression and glycemic control in type II diabetics mellitus patients. Gen Hosp Psychiatry. 2015;37:116–9. https://doi.org/10.1016/j.genhosppsych.2014.11.012.
32. Brownley KA, Berkman ND, Peat CM, Lohr KN, Cullen KE, Bann CM, et al. Binge-eating disorder in adults: a systematic review and meta-analysis. Ann Intern Med. 2016;165:409–20. https://doi.org/10.7326/M15-2455.
33. Skinner HH, Haines J, Austin SB, Field AE. A prospective study of overeating, binge eating, and depressive symptoms among adolescent and young adult women. J Adolesc Health. 2012;50:478–83. https://doi.org/10.1016/j.jadohealth.2011.10.002.

10

Entrapment as a mediator of suicide crises

Shuang Li[†], Zimri S. Yaseen[†], Hae-Joon Kim, Jessica Briggs, Molly Duffy, Anna Frechette-Hagan, Lisa J. Cohen and Igor I. Galynker[*]

Abstract

Background: Prior research has validated the construct of a suicide crisis syndrome (SCS), a specific psychological state that precedes and may precipitate suicidal behavior. The feeling of entrapment is a central concept of the SCS as well as of several other recent models of suicide. However, its exact relationship with suicidality is not fully understood. In efforts to clarify the exact role of entrapment in the suicidal process, we have examined if entrapment mediates the relationship of other components of the SCS, including ruminative flooding, panic-dissociation, fear of dying and emotional pain, with suicidal ideation (SI) in recently hospitalized psychiatric inpatients.

Methods: The Suicide Crisis Inventory (SCI) and Beck Scale for Suicidal Ideation (BSS) were administered to 200 high-risk adult psychiatric inpatients hospitalized following SI or suicide attempt, assessing SCS and SI levels at admission, respectively. The possible mediation effects of entrapment on the relationship between the other components of the SCS and SI at admission were evaluated.

Results: Entrapment significantly and fully mediated the relationship of ruminative flooding, panic-dissociation, and fear of dying with SI, with no direct relationships between these variables and SI reaching statistical significance. Further, no reverse mediation relationships between these variables and SI were found, indicating that the mediation effects of entrapment were unidirectional. While entrapment did mediate the association between emotional pain and SI, the direct relationship between emotional pain and SI was also significant. Moreover, in reverse mediational analysis, emotional pain was a partial mediator of the relationship between entrapment and SI.

Conclusion: Entrapment and emotional pain may have a more direct association with SI than the other components of the SCS, including ruminative flooding, panic-dissociation, and fear of dying, the effects of which are mediated by the former. This suggests entrapment and emotional pain may represent key symptomatic targets for intervention in acutely suicidal individuals. Further research is needed to determine the relationship of these constructs to suicidal behavior.

Keywords: Suicide, Suicidal ideation, Entrapment, Emotional pain, Suicide crisis

Background

Suicide is a major public health concern, ranking as the 10th leading cause of death in the United States, and accounts for over 42,773 deaths in the US each year [1]. Suicide is a complex behavior reflecting a multi-level interplay of biological, psychological, social, and material factors such as access to means. Although the predictive value of long-term risk factors including biomarkers (e.g., serotonin levels), demographic factors (sex, age), and clinical factors (diagnosis of mental illness, prior

* Correspondence: Igor.Galynker@mountsinai.org
[†]Equal contributors
Department of Psychiatry, Beth Israel Medical Center NY, 1st Avenue and 15th Street, New York, NY 10003, USA

suicide attempt) has been well established [2, 3], a recent meta-analysis of 50 years of research on risk factors for suicidal thoughts and behaviors (STB) highlights the consistently small effect sizes of such risk factors and that no risk factor category or subcategory is substantially stronger than any other [4]. Likewise, reliable predictors of acute suicide risk have also remained elusive. Recently, however, a small but growing body of evidence suggests the existence of an acute suicide crisis syndrome (SCS) [5, 6], characterized by the experience of entrapment accompanied by intense negative affect, loss of cognitive control, hyper-arousal, and social withdrawal, which may precipitate the transition from chronic suicidal ideation (SI) to acute suicide attempt (SA) [7–12]. Our previous work on a series of instruments aiming to define the SCS has shown several clinical factors, proposed as criterion symptoms of a clinical syndrome that characterizes the suicidal crisis, are indeed related to each other and short-term risk for suicidal behavior. These include the constructs of entrapment, ruminative flooding (a cognitive control symptom), panic-dissociation and fear of dying (hyper-arousal symptoms), and emotional pain (an intense negative affect symptom) [10–13] and encompass the affective, cognitive, and somatic aspects of the hypothesized SCS. Notably, the Suicide Crisis Inventory (SCI) has demonstrated strong internal consistency, and significant predictive as well as incremental predictive validity over standard suicide predictors (SI, depression, state and trait anxiety) for short-term post-discharge suicidal behavior [12].

The first construct, entrapment, has recently been proposed as a key psychological element of several models of suicidal behavior, notably the Arrested Flight/Cry of Pain model by Williams and Pollock [14] and O'Connor's Integrated Motivational-Volitional Theory (IMV) [15]. According to these models, entrapment, defined as a felt urgency to escape from an unbearable situation from which there is no perceived escape [16], could be a core psychological mechanism in causal pathways to suicide. In agreement with this hypothesis, a strong positive association was found between perceptions of entrapment and suicidality in a range of subacute outpatient populations [17–23]. O'Connor's group also demonstrated that entrapment added incremental predictive validity for suicidal behaviors over depression, hopelessness, SI, and the frequency of previous suicide attempts [24]. Similar to their findings, in our group's latest study of the SCS, entrapment was the strongest individual predictor of suicidal behavior within the 2 months following discharge from an inpatient unit [12].

Surprisingly, although entrapment is a core concept of many models of suicide and of the hypothesized SCS, its role as a possible mediator of the relationship between other acute risk factors and SI/suicidal behavior has never been examined in *acutely suicidal patients.* The IMV model [15] posits that ruminations increase the likelihood of stressful experiences leading to perceptions of entrapment, which in turn may trigger SI. Alternatively, entrapment may lead to a cognitive search for escape routes resulting in rumination, thus triggering SI. Uncovering these relationships may not only help clarify theoretical models of suicidal behavior, but also establish important targets for therapeutic interventions in acutely suicidal individuals.

The second hypothesized component of the SCS, ruminative flooding, is characterized by uncontrollable perseverative thinking involving continual thoughts about the causes, meaning, and consequences of one's negative mood. Ruminative flooding differs from simple ruminations in that it is experienced as an uncontrollable and overwhelming profusion of negative thoughts, often associated with somatic symptoms inside the head, such as headaches or head pressure [10]. Similar constructs have been associated with elevated suicide risk by other research teams [25, 26]. The third construct, panic-dissociation, describes somatic symptoms commonly associated with a panic-like dissociative state, and involves somatic experiences of unfamiliar sensations felt all over the body, and derealization [11, 13]. Similar constructs have also been described by other suicide researchers [27, 28]. The fourth construct, fear of dying, describes morbid cognitions during panic, which may mediate the transition from latent SI to active SI and suicide attempt in some depressed subjects [29–34].

Finally, the fifth hypothesized component of the SCS is emotional pain, a mixture of intense and painfully felt negative emotions such as guilt, shame, hopelessness, disgrace, rage, and defeat, which arises when the essential needs to love, to have control, to protect one's self image, to avoid shame, guilt, and humiliation, or to feel secure are frustrated [35]. Emotional pain is similar to entrapment in that it is strongly correlated with but distinct from anxiety and depression, and can be so intense that the individual seeks to escape by – suicide [35–39]. However, those in emotional pain may lack the desperation caused by the perception that all escape routes are blocked, whereas this desperation and subsequent escape motivation are intrinsic components of entrapment.

Severe or pervasive SI is consistently found to be a significant predictor of subsequent suicidal behaviors [40]. Even passive ideation, such as a wish to die, has been identified as a risk factor for death by suicide [41]. Although the relationship between SI, suicidal behavior, and suicide is not straightforward, and several other symptom dimensions may synergistically influence suicide risk [20, 42], SI has a much higher base rate than suicides or suicide attempts and thus represents a scientifically useful and clinically meaningful modifiable element of suicide risk.

Given the evidence of the central role of entrapment in the suicidal process, the goal of the present report was to establish whether entrapment mediates the relationship between the other clinical factors of the SCS and SI in psychiatric inpatients recently hospitalized for suicide risk. As, the SCS is conceptualized as a clinical syndrome that activates SI, motivating the transition from SI to SA, in the context of the current study, severity of SI serves as a proxy for nearness to suicidal action. We therefore reanalyze the data from our published validation study of the SCI [12] to examine the interrelationships among the SCI subscales and sever- ity of suicidal ideation. We hypothesized that entrap- ment will mediate the relationships between SI and ruminative flooding, panic-dissociation, fear of dying, and emotional pain.

Methods

Study subjects

Participants between the ages of 18–65 hospitalized for SI or SA were recruited from the inpatient psychiatric units at Mount Sinai Beth Israel (MSBI) in New York City between April 2013 and July 2015. Potential partici- pants were identified and referred to the study by a clin- ician. Within 72 h of observation and admission to the psychiatric inpatient unit, a trained research assistant approached each eligible patient to explain the study, its aims, and the risks and benefits of participation. To avoid reporting bias that might be associated with pre- senting the study as explicitly focused on suicidality, the study was titled "Predicting Emotional Dysregulation: In- ternal Consistency and Predictive Validity of the Emo- tional Dysregulation Scale" and the phrases "SI" and "suicide attempt" were replaced with the term "emo- tional dysregulation" in the consent form. Following an explanation of what the study entailed, he or she was then presented with a consent form to review and sign, and study measures were completed concurrently.

Participants were excluded if they had cognitive or lin- guistic limitations precluding their understanding the consent or research questions, significant medical or neurological disease, or possible delirium that might interfere with study participation or informed consent. The study was approved by the MSBI Institutional Re- view Board, project #223–14.

Measures

The suicide crisis inventory (SCI)

The 49-item SCI, comprises 5 subscales: entrapment (13 items), panic-dissociation (9 items), ruminative flooding (7 items), emotional pain (4 items), and fear of dying (3 items). The remaining items contribute to the total SCI score but are not assigned to a subscale. Items are rated by self- report on a five-point scale ranging from 'not at all = 0' to 'extremely = 4'. Each subscale, as previously reported, demonstrates good to excellent internal consistency in the study sample (entrapment: $\alpha = 0.946$; panic-dissociation: $\alpha = 0.882$; ruminative flooding: $\alpha = 0.892$; emotional pain: $\alpha = 0.878$ and fear of dying: $\alpha = 0.796$) [12].

Suicidal ideation (SI)

Severity of SI was assessed with the Part 1 total score of the Beck Scale for Suicidal Ideation (BSS) [43], a 21-item self-report measure of SI. Scores on each item range from 0 to 2, with higher scores indicating greater severity of SI. Part 1 of the BSS was used because Part 2 is completed only if items 4 and 5 in Part 1 are scored >0, and thus total scores were not calculated for the entire sample.

Depression severity

Severity of depression (exclusive of suicidal ideation) at admission was assessed with the Beck Depression Inven- tory II (BDI) [44, 45], a 21-item self-report measure of depression with item 9 (suicidal ideation) excluded. Scores on each item range from 0 to 3, with higher scores indicating greater severity of SI.

Statistical analysis

To investigate the hypothesis that the relationship be- tween each construct and SI was fully mediated by the perception of entrapment, a simple mediation model was applied, with severity of SI as the dependent variable.

Table 1 Demographic characteristic of study participants

Age (years)	Mean = 35.3	SD = 13.4
Education (years)	Mean = 13.7	SD = 2.9
Variable	N	Percent
Gender		
Male	91	46.3
Transgender	2	1.0
Female	107	53.7
Race		
Asian	20	10.0
Black	43	21.5
White	76	38.0
Other	61	30.5
Ethnicity (Latino)	68	34.0
Marital status		
Never married	136	68.0
Married	25	12.5
Divorced/widowed/separated	39	19.5
Diagnosis		
Psychotic spectrum disorders	20	10
Bipolar spectrum disorders	26	13
Unipolar depressive disorders	84	42
Other disorders[a]	70	35
Substance use		
EtOH use disorder	75	37.5
Illicit substance use disorder	97	48.5
Any substance use disorder	120	60

[a]Mood disorder not otherwise specified, adjustment disorder, substance-induced disorders, personality disorder only, anxiety disorders

Table 2 Inter-correlations among study variables ($N = 200$)

	Entrapment	Panic /Dissociation	Ruminative Flooding	Fear of dying	Emotional Pain	SI
Entrapment	1					
Panic/Dissociation	.510***	1				
Ruminative Flooding	.671***	.609***	1			
Fear of dying	.519***	.572***	.496***	1		
Emotional Pain	.708***	.500***	.619***	.454***	1	
SI	.422***	.228**	.316***	.145*	.417***	1

SI suicidal ideation
*$p < 0.05$ (2-tailed), **$p < 0.01$ (2-tailed), ***$p < 0.001$ (2-tailed)

Direct, indirect and total effects together with their bias-corrected 95% confidence intervals were calculated based on 5000 bootstraps. The mediation effect was assessed by (a) Preacher & Kelley's [46] Kappa-squared test, where κ^2 = the proportion (ranging from 0 to 1) of the maximum possible indirect effect observed and (b) the completely standardized effect size (CS) interpreted relative to zero with larger values indicating larger effect size. In those tests, a bootstrapped 95% confidence interval (CI) excluding zero indicates statistical significance. The Sobel test was chosen as a conservative confirmation of significance of the mediation effect, with a threshold alpha value of 0.05 for significance. To test the unidirectionality of the mediation effects, 'reversed' mediation models were calculated with entrapment as the independent variable and each of the other SCS constructs as the mediator. If no mediation is found in these reversed models, a unidirectional mediation effect of entrapment is supported. In other words, if a mediation effect is significant but the reversed mediation is not, we can say with more confidence that (for example) entrapment accounts for the effect of ruminative flooding on SI and not the other way around.

Finally, in supplementary analyses we examined whether a) SI severity as assessed by the BSS and mediation effects differed between patients admitted in the context of recent suicide attempt and patients admitted with SI only, and b) mediation effects were retained when age and concurrent depression severity were controlled for.

All statistical tests were performed using the Statistical Package for the Social Sciences (SPSS), version 21. Mediation analyses were performed using Hayes [47] PROCESS module model 4 for SPSS.

Results

Demographics

Two hundred and one patients met inclusion criteria and provided informed consent. Data from one participant were excluded because the patient did not complete the BSS. Among these, 142 were hospitalized after presenting with SI, while 58 made attempts leading to their hospitalization. Table 1, summarized below, presents the demographic characteristics of the study participants as previously described [12]. The remaining sample of 200 participants was roughly 50% female and had a racial composition approximately equivalent to that of the general New York City population. Among the participants, nearly half had a unipolar mood disorder, and approximately one quarter had a psychotic or bipolar mood disorder, while roughly a third were diagnosed with other disorders such as an unspecified adjustment disorder. Over half also were diagnosed with a comorbid substance use disorder.

Table 3 Regression coefficients of entrapment and ruminative flooding predicting suicidal ideation

Predicted variable								
M(entrapment)					Y (suicidal ideation)			
Predictor variable		Coeff.	SE	P		Coeff.	SE	P
X (Ruminative Flooding)	a	1.192	0.094	<0.001	c'	0.023	0.033	0.494
M (Entrapment)		–	–	–	b	0.082	0.019	<0.001
Constant	i_1	13.187	1.684	<0.001	i_2	0.387	0.504	0.443
$R^2 = 0.450$					$R^2 = 0.180$			
$F(1,198) = 162.000, p = <0.001$					$F(2,197) = 21.649, p < 0.001$			

"a" is the regression coefficient predicting entrapment by ruminative flooding
"b" is the coefficient predicting suicidal ideation by entrapment
"c'" is the coefficient predicting suicidal ideation from ruminative flooding independent of entrapment

Table 4 Total, direct and indirect effects and effects sizes for indirect effects of ruminative flooding on suicidal ideation mediated by entrapment

	Raw effect	SE	lower	upper	p	CS	SE	κ^2	SE	Z Score
Indirect effect	0.097	0.023	0.054	0.142	<0.001	0.256	0.061	0.202	0.047	4.140
Direct effect	0.023	0.033	−0.043	0.088	0.494					
Total effect	0.120	0.026	0.070	0.171	<0.001					

SE standard error, *lower* lower bound of 95% confidence interval, *upper* upper bound of 95% confidence interval, *CS* completely standardized effect size, κ^2 Kappa-squared test, Z score by Sobel test

Inter-correlations among each component of the suicidal crisis syndrome

Current SI and each of the subscales of the SCI had significant positive correlations with each other with r values ranging from 0.15 to 0.71. See Table 2.

Mediation analyses

Ruminative flooding

As indicated in Tables 3 and 4, the total effect of ruminative flooding on SI was significant at $p < 0.001$ with a standardized regression coefficient of 0.120. The direct effect of ruminative flooding on SI was not significant (95% CI including 0). In contrast, the indirect effect of ruminative flooding on SI was significant (95% CI did not include 0 and Sobel test: z = 4.140, $p < 0.001$), suggesting that entrapment fully mediates the relationship between ruminative flooding and SI with small to mediate effect size (CS = 0.256, $\kappa^2 = 0.202$). As indicated in Table 11, the reversed mediation analysis with entrapment as the independent variable and ruminative flooding as the mediator showed no significant indirect effect (Sobel test: $p = 0.494$). Both the direct effect and the total effect of entrapment on SI were significant. These results show that entrapment fully mediates the relationship between ruminative flooding and SI, and conversely, that ruminative flooding is not a mediator of the relationship between entrapment and SI.

Panic-dissociation

As shown in Tables 5 and 6, the total effect of panic-dissociation on SI was significant at $p = 0.001$ with a standardized regression coefficient of 0.077. The direct effect of panic-dissociation on SI was not significant ($p = 0.821$). In contrast, the indirect effect of panic-dissociation on SI was significant (95% CI did not include 0 and Sobel test: z = 4.573, $p < 0.001$). This suggests that the effect of panic-dissociation on SI was fully mediated by entrapment.

As indicated in Table 11, the reversed mediation analysis with entrapment as the independent variable and panic-dissociation as the mediator showed no indirect effect (Sobel test: $p = 0.822$) while both the direct effect and the total effect of entrapment on SI were significant. This confirms that entrapment fully mediates the relationship between panic-dissociation and SI, and this relationship is unidirectional.

Fear of dying

As indicated in Tables 7 and 8, the total effect of fear of dying on SI was significant at $p = 0.041$ with a standardized regression coefficient effect of 0.117. The direct effect of fear of dying on SI was not significant as the corresponding confidence interval includes zero. In contrast, the indirect effect of fear of dying on SI was significant (95% CI did not include 0 and Sobel test: z = 5.058, $p < 0.001$).

As indicated in Table 11, the reversed mediation analysis with entrapment as the independent variable and fear of dying as the mediator showed no significant indirect effect (Sobel test: $p = 0.185$). Both the direct effect and the total effect of entrapment on SI were significant. This indicates that entrapment fully mediates the

Table 5 Regression coefficients of entrapment and panic-dissociation predicting suicidal ideation

Predicted variable								
M (entrapment)					Y (suicidal ideation)			
Predictor variable		Coeff.	SE	P		Coeff.	SE	P
X (Panic dissociation)	a	0.810	0.097	<0.001	c'	0.006	0.026	0.821
M (Entrapment)		–	–	–	b	0.088	0.016	<0.001
Constant	i_1	23.164	1.408	<0.001	i_2	0.469	0.489	0.339
$R^2 = 0.260$					$R^2 = 0.174$			
$F(1,198) = 69.432, P = <0.001$					$F(2,197) = 21.394, P < 0.001$			

"*a*" is the regression coefficient predicting entrapment by panic-dissociation
"*b*" is the coefficient predicting suicidal ideation by entrapment
"*c'*" is the coefficient predicting suicidal ideation from panic-dissociation independent of entrapment

Table 6 Total, direct and indirect effects and effects sizes for indirect effects of panic-dissociation on suicidal ideation mediated by entrapment

	Raw effect	SE	lower	upper	p	CS	SE	κ^2	SE	Z Score
Indirect effect	0.072	0.015	0.044	0.105	<0.001	0.211	0.0451	0.190	0.039	4.573
Direct effect	0.006	0.026	−0.045	0.056	0.821					
Total effect	0.077	0.024	0.031	0.124	0.001					

SE standard error, *lower* lower bound of 95% confidence interval, *upper* upper bound of 95% confidence interval, CS completely standardized effect size, κ^2 Kappa-squared test, Z score by Sobel test

relationship between fear of dying and SI, and fear of dying is not a mediator of the relationship between entrapment and SI.

Emotional pain
As indicated in Tables 9 and 10, the total effect of emotional pain on SI was significant at $p < 0.001$ with a standardized regression coefficient effect of 0.250. In contrast to the other SCS constructs, the direct effect of emotional pain on SI was significant with a standardized regression coefficient effect of 0.141, $p = 0.009$. Nevertheless, the indirect effect was also significant (95% CI did not include 0 and Sobel test: z = 2.774, $p = 0.006$), indicating that entrapment is a *partial* mediator of the relationship between emotional pain and SI.

Partial mediation by entrapment was further confirmed by the reversed mediation analyses with entrapment entered as the independent variable and emotional pain as the mediator. As shown in Table 11, while the total effect of entrapment on SI was significant ($p < 0.001$), both the direct effect ($p = 0.005$) and the indirect effect (Sobel test: $p = 0.010$) were also significant, which suggests that the mediation is not unidirectional. Thus, the mediating relationships of emotional pain and entrapment with SI appear to be reciprocal.

Supplementary analyses
In supplementary analyses, no differences were found in SI between patients admitted with SA and patients admitted with SI, nor were there substantive differences in the strength of mediation effects.

When age and depression severity were added as covariates to the mediation models the mediation effects of entrapment remained significant for each SCI subscale except emotional pain. (See Additional file 1.) Both entrapment and emotional pain, however, were independent predictors of SI (in separate models controlling for depression), and partially mediated the relation between depression severity and SI severity. (See Additional file 2.)

Discussion
The primary aim of the present study was to test the hypothesis that entrapment mediates the relationships between other constructs of the SCS (ruminative flooding, panic-dissociation, fear of dying, and emotional pain) and SI. To our knowledge, this is the first study to show that entrapment plays a central role in the relationship between the symptoms of the SCS and SI in acutely suicidal individuals. Further, ruminative flooding, panic-dissociation, and fear of dying did not significantly mediate the effect of entrapment on SI, indicating that entrapment fully mediated the relationships between each of these constructs and SI. However, entrapment was only a partial mediator of the relationship between emotional pain and SI, and emotional pain was a significant partial mediator of the effect of entrapment on SI. This suggests both common and independent effects of entrapment and emotional pain on SI.

These results are consistent with our previous work, which has documented the prominence of entrapment in several populations of acutely suicidal patients both in the psychiatric emergency department and among

Table 7 Regression coefficients of entrapment and fear of dying predicting suicidal ideation

Predicted variable								
M(entrapment)					Y (suicidal ideation)			
Predictor variable		Coeff.	SE	P		Coeff.	SE	P
X (Fear of dying)	a	1.959	0.229	<0.001	c′	−0.082	0.061	0.177
M (Entrapment)		–	–	–	b	0.102	0.016	<0.001
Constant	i_1	22.413	1.452	<0.001	i_2	0.524	0.488	0.284
$R^2 = 0.270$					$R^2 = 0.186$			
$F(1,198) = 73.161, P = <0.001$					$F(2,197) = 22.476, P < 0.001$			

"a" is the regression coefficient predicting entrapment by fear of dying
"b" is the coefficient predicting suicidal ideation by entrapment
"c′" is the coefficient predicting suicidal ideation from fear of dying independent of entrapment

Table 8 Total, direct and indirect effects and effects sizes for indirect effects of fear of dying on suicidal ideation mediated by entrapment

	Raw effect	SE	lower	upper	p	CS	SE	κ^2	SE	Z Score
Indirect effect	0.199	0.040	0.129	0.286	<0.001	0.247	0.049	0.222	0.042	5.058
Direct effect	−0.082	0.061	−0.202	0.038	0.178					
Total effect	0.117	0.057	0.005	0.229	0.041					

SE standard error, *lower* lower bound of 95% confidence interval, *upper* upper bound of 95% confidence interval, *CS* completely standardized effect size, κ^2 Kappa-squared test, Z score by Sobel test

psychiatrically hospitalized patients [11, 13]. Our data also support the central role of entrapment in the SCS, as assessed by the Suicide Crisis Inventory [12].

Ruminations have been previously linked to SI and suicidal behavior [25, 48, 49] although prior research has also pointed to an indirect rather than direct effect. Smith, Alloy [50] demonstrated that hopelessness partially mediated the relationship between ruminations and SI, and fully mediated the association between ruminations and duration of suicidality. Notably, Teismann and Forkmann [51] reported no direct relationship between ruminations and SI in two outpatient populations, as the link between the two was fully mediated by entrapment. Our results also show that the relationship between the ruminative flooding subscale of the SCI and SI is fully mediated by entrapment. This finding complements that by Teismann and Forkmann [51], and suggests that as ruminations during a suicidal crisis become uncontrollable and overwhelming, the perception of being trapped may precipitate SI.

Similarly, although numerous studies have shown that the experience of somatic symptoms, [11, 13, 27, 28, 52] and fear of dying [29–34], particularly in the context of anxiety and panic, predict SI or suicidal behavior, our current study indicates that in the acute suicidal state there are no direct linkages between either somatic symptoms or fear of dying and SI. Our results indicate instead that the somatic symptoms of panic, dissociation, and fear of dying are indirectly linked with SI via a pathway of entrapment. Thus, as with ruminative flooding, experiencing a fear of dying and dissociative symptoms

may increase or simply be correlated with the intensity of stressful experiences that result in a sense of entrapment, which in turn might trigger SI.

Our results show that the relationship between emotional pain and SI was only partially mediated by entrapment, indicating a direct link between emotional pain and SI. Furthermore, the finding that the association between entrapment and SI was partially mediated by emotional pain suggests that these two constructs have both a direct and mutually mediatory relationship to SI. It may be that both of these constructs substantially entail the other. Namely, emotional pain may reliably produce the escape motivation that is necessary for entrapment, and the perception of entrapment may necessarily induce emotional pain. This understanding of the findings is consistent with Baumeister's Escape Theory of Suicide [53] which conceptualizes suicide as an escape from otherwise seemingly inescapable painful self-states. Likewise, Shneidman [35] defines emotional pain or mental pain as a compilation of negative emotions (e.g., anxiety, helplessness, and despair) that reflects frustration with one's inability to fulfill basic psychological needs. In Orbach and Mikulincer's formulation, emotional pain includes loss of self-esteem, as well as feelings of failure, abandonment, emotional flooding, and emptiness and, notably, irreversibility [36–39]. Thus, emotional pain as assessed in studies using the Orbach Mikulincer Mental Pain scale, appears to be substantially convergent with the entrapment subscale of the SCI. The emotional pain subscale of the SCI, on the other hand, comprises only items directly descriptive of an

Table 9 Regression coefficients of entrapment and emotional pain predicting suicidal ideation

Predicted variable								
M (entrapment)					Y (suicidal ideation)			
Predictor variable		Coeff.	SE	P		Coeff.	SE	P
X (Emotional pain)	a	1.986	0.141	<0.001	c'	0.141	0.054	0.009
M (Entrapment)		–	–	–	b	0.055	0.019	0.005
Constant	i_1	13.358	1.525	<0.001	i_2	0.279	0.486	0.566
$R^2 = 0.502$					$R^2 = 0.206$			
$F(1,198) = 199.332, P = <0.001$					$F(2,197) = 25.549, P < 0.001$			

"a" is the regression coefficient predicting entrapment by emotional pain
"b" is the coefficient predicting suicidal ideation by entrapment
"c'" is the coefficient predicting suicidal ideation from emotional pain independent of entrapment

Table 10 Total, direct and indirect effects and effects sizes for indirect effects of emotional pain on suicidal ideation mediated by entrapment

	Raw effect	SE	lower	upper	p	CS	SE	κ^2	SE	Z Score
Indirect effect	0.108	0.042	0.027	0.193	0.006	0.181	0.070	0.140	0.052	2.774
Direct effect	0.141	0.054	0.035	0.248	0.009					
Total effect	0.250	0.039	0.173	0.326	<0.001					

SE standard error, *lower* lower bound of 95% confidence interval, *upper* upper bound of 95% confidence interval, *CS* completely standardized effect size, κ^2 Kappa-squared test, Z score by Sobel test

emotional experience described in terms of pain. Past research has indicated that emotional pain mediates the relationship between perfectionism and suicidality [54], between hopelessness and SI [55], and between non-suicidal self-injury and suicide risk [56]. Shneidman [35], and later Orbach [36] further suggested that unbearable psychological pain may mediate the relationships between other relevant psychological factors and suicide. Similarly, in Klonsky & May's recent Three Step Theory of suicide, the combination of pain and hopelessness drives the development of suicidal ideation; our findings for entrapment, which may be understood as a product of emotional pain and hopelessness, are thus also broadly consistent with the three-step theory [57]. Orbach's studies and the strong correlation we found between entrapment and emotional pain suggest that entrapment is an emotionally painful experience. At the same time, however, the aversive experience of emotional pain may drive an urgency for escape which itself is requisite for the experience of entrapment. Our finding in supplementary analyses that controlling for severity of depression in mediation models of entrapment and emotional pain reduced mediation effects to non-significance points to the variance common to all three constructs. Nonetheless, entrapment and emotional pain each show incremental prediction of SI with respect to depression severity, highlighting the pertinence of each of these constructs.

Thus, taken altogether, our data indicate that in the SCS, entrapment acts as a conduit between most of the associated symptoms and SI. This finding is highly consistent with recent theoretical models of suicide including the Cry of Pain Model [14, 58] and the IMV Model of suicide [15], as well as Baumeister's Escape Theory of Suicide [53] and Gilbert's phenomenon of 'arrested flight' [16] and Galynker's Narrative Crisis model [6]. Williams and Pollock [14] posit that suicide results from a feeling of defeat in response to humiliation or rejection, which in turn leads to a perception of entrapment. When the latter is combined with a failure to find alternative ways to solve a problem, i.e. cognitive rigidity [59], a suicidal person may see no exit out of his or her perceived entrapment other than suicide. One interpretation of the mediating role of entrapment is that perceptions of entrapment may constitute a final common pathway to SI. Therefore, therapeutic interventions aimed at reducing the perception of entrapment and creating actionable alternatives may eventually reduce suicide risk. In addition, clinical evaluation of entrapment, as illustrated in our previous reports [11, 13] by explicitly asking whether a patient felt "trapped," or that "there was no way out," or that he or she "had no good options," would be essential for a suicide risk assessment. Further, our data suggest that in addition to explicitly asking whether patients feel trapped in their current life situation, relationship, or within themselves, it is important to assess whether they have experienced fear of dying, felt unusual sensations in their bodies or pressure inside their heads, and lost the ability to control and stop their ruminative thoughts, as such experiences were robustly correlated with entrapment and may provide a path of approach to assessment of suicidal thoughts that the patient might not otherwise disclose.

Based on our current results, and our findings from the complementary study of prediction of suicidal behavior [12], it can be hypothesized that while either unbearable emotional pain or entrapment may mediate the relationship between other symptoms of the SCS and SI, it is entrapment that may be the final mediator of the relationship of

Table 11 Regression models for mediation of entrapment effects on SI by SCS components (reversed analysis)

Mediating variable	Total effect of Entrapment on SI: coefficient effect; (T score)	Direct effect of Entrapment on SI: coefficient effect; (T score)	Indirect effect of Entrapment on SI by Normal theory test: coefficient effect; (Z score)
Ruminative flooding	0.090; (6.553)***	0.082; (4.393)***	0.009; (0.683)
Panic-dissociation	0.090; (6.550)***	0.088; (5.509)***	0.002; (0.225)
Fear of dying	0.090; (6.550)***	0.102; (6.314)***	−0.011; (−1.327)
Emotional pain	0.090; (6.553)***	0.055; (2.836)**	0.036; (2.573)*

SI severity of suicidal ideation, *SCS* suicide crisis syndrome
*p < 0.05, **p < 0.01, ***p < 0.001

multiple psychological factors and suicidal action. A mediation analysis of prospective suicidal behavior using a larger sample size may provide support for this testable hypothesis. As the SCS is proposed to be a syndrome, the strong inter-correlations among the SCI subscales are certainly supportive of the SCS concept. Nonetheless, further study is needed to determine whether such a syndrome is more predictive of STB than simple severity of entrapment.

The results of this study need to be considered in the context of its limitations. This study represents a novel analysis of our previously published scale-validation data and thus all conclusions are tempered by the need for replication. Further, the study examines the relationship between the SCS constructs and SI rather than suicidal behavior or actual suicide, making the results less relevant to the urgent clinical task of suicide prevention. However, both active and passive SI have been shown to predict death by suicide marking it as a significant modifiable element of suicide risk [40, 41]; thus, understanding the mediation effects of the relationships of psychiatric symptoms in acutely suicidal individuals with SI can improve our understanding of the suicidal process in general. Second, the cross-sectional design of the study limits any causal interpretation of our findings. Third, the current study utilized only a self-report measure of SI, and the data may be confounded if some participants were not forthcoming in revealing their suicidality. Finally, the study was conducted at a single site, and study findings need to be replicated at other locations.

Conclusion

Within its limitations, the current study highlights the central links between SI and entrapment and emotional pain in high-risk patients. The results suggest that psychiatric symptoms of a suicide crisis, such as ruminative flooding, panic-dissociation, and fear of dying may result in SI when they are experienced as painful states lacking routes for escape. The study further suggests that for individuals in a state of suicide crisis, the psychological processes tying entrapment and emotional pain to SI are highly similar, and generally consistent with models conceptualizing suicide as an escape behavior. Further research is warranted to establish the respective mediatory roles of entrapment and emotional pain with regard to future suicidal behavior.

Abbreviations

BSS: Beck Scale for Suicide Ideation; IMV: Integrated Motivational-Volitional Model; MSBI: Mount Sinai Beth Israel; SCI: Suicide Crisis Inventory; SCS: Suicide Crisis Syndrome; SI: Suicidal Ideation; STB: Suicidal Thoughts and Behaviors

Funding

This work was supported by the focus grant # RFA-1-015-14 from the American Foundation for Suicide Prevention. The content is solely the responsibility of the authors and does not necessarily represent the official views of the American Foundation for Suicide Prevention. The funders had no role in study design, data collection and analysis, decision to publish, or preparation of the manuscript.

Authors' contributions

SL, ZY, and IG contributed to the concept and design of the study. JB, MD, and AFH collected the data. SL and ZY analyzed the data. SL, ZY, IG, HK, JB, MD, AFH, and LC wrote and revised the manuscript. All authors read and approved the final manuscript.

Consent for publication

Not applicable.

Competing interests

The authors declare that they have no competing interests.

References

1. Control, C.f.D. and Prevention, WISQARS™(web-based injury statistics query and reporting system). 2014.
2. Pandey GN, Dwivedi Y. Peripheral biomarkers for suicide. In: Dwivedi Y, editor. The neurobiological basis of suicide. London: CRC Press; 2012. p. 407-24.
3. Suokas J, et al. Long-term risk factors for suicide mortality after attempted suicide-findings of a 14-year follow-up study. Acta Psychiatr Scand. 2001; 104(2):117–21.
4. Franklin JC, et al. Risk factors for suicidal thoughts and behaviors: a meta-analysis of 50 years of research. Psychol Bull. 2017;143(2):187–232.
5. Rogers ML, et al. An overview and comparison of two proposed suicide-specific diagnoses: acute suicidal affective disturbance and suicide crisis syndrome. Psychiatr Ann. 2017;47(8):416–20.
6. Galynker I. The suicidal crisis: clinical guide to the assessment of imminent suicide risk. New York: Oxford University Press; 2017.
7. Fawcett J, et al. Time-related predictors of suicide in major affective disorder. Am J Psychiatry. 1990;147(9):1189.
8. Hendin H, et al. Role of intense affects in predicting short-term risk for suicidal behavior: a prospective study. J Nerv Ment Dis. 2010;198(3):220–5.
9. Hendin H, Maltsberger JT, Szanto K. The role of intense affective states in signaling a suicide crisis. J Nerv Ment Dis. 2007;195(5):363–8.
10. Yaseen Z, et al. Construct development: the suicide trigger scale (STS-2), a measure of a hypothesized suicide trigger state. BMC Psychiatry. 2010;10(1):110.
11. Yaseen ZS, et al. Predictive validity of the suicide trigger scale (STS-3) for post-discharge suicide attempt in high-risk psychiatric inpatients. PLoS One. 2014;9(1):e86768.
12. Galynker I, et al. Prediction of suicidal behavior in high risk psychiatric patients using an assessment of acute suicidal state: the suicide crisis inventory. Depress Anxiety. 2017;34(2):147–58.
13. Yaseen ZS, et al. Emergency room validation of the revised suicide trigger scale (STS-3): a measure of a hypothesized suicide trigger state. PLoS One. 2012;7(9):e45157.
14. Williams JMG, Pollock LR. Psychological aspects of the suicidal process. Underst Suicidal Behav. 2001:76–93.
15. O'Connor RC, Cleare S, Eschle S, Wetherall K, Kirtley OJ. The integrated motivational-volitional model of suicidal behavior. In: O'Connor RC, Pirkis J, editors. The international handbook of suicide prevention. Chichester: John Wiley & Sons, Ltd; 2016. p. 220–40.
16. Gilbert P, Allan S. The role of defeat and entrapment (arrested flight) in depression: an exploration of an evolutionary view. Psychol Med. 1998; 28(3):585–98.
17. Maria P, et al. Negative self-appraisals and suicidal behavior among trauma victims experiencing Ptsd symptoms: the mediating role of defeat and entrapment. Depress Anxiety. 2012;29(3):187–94.
18. Panagioti M, et al. A model of suicidal behavior in posttraumatic stress disorder (PTSD): the mediating role of defeat and entrapment. Psychiatry Res. 2013;209(1):55–9.
19. Panagioti M, Gooding PA, Tarrier N. Hopelessness, defeat, and entrapment in posttraumatic stress disorder: their association with suicidal behavior and severity of depression. J Nerv Ment Dis. 2012;200(8):676–83.

20. Rasmussen SA, et al. Elaborating the cry of pain model of suicidality: testing a psychological model in a sample of first-time and repeat self-harm patients. Br J Clin Psychol. 2010;49(1):15–30.

21. Siddaway AP, et al. A meta-analysis of perceptions of defeat and entrapment in depression, anxiety problems, posttraumatic stress disorder, and suicidality. J Affect Disord. 2015;184:149–59.

22. Taylor PJ, et al. Defeat and entrapment in schizophrenia: the relationship with suicidal ideation and positive psychotic symptoms. Psychiatry Res. 2010;178(2):244–8.

23. Taylor PJ, et al. Appraisals and suicidality: the mediating role of defeat and entrapment. Arch Suicide Res. 2010;14(3):236–47.

24. O'connor RC, et al. Psychological processes and repeat suicidal behavior: a four-year prospective study. J Consult Clin Psychol. 2013;81(6):1137.

25. Miranda R, Nolen-Hoeksema S. Brooding and reflection: rumination predicts suicidal ideation at 1-year follow-up in a community sample. Behav Res Ther. 2007;45(12):3088–95.

26. Tucker RP, et al. Rumination and suicidal ideation: the moderating roles of hope and optimism. Personal Individ Differ. 2013;55(5):606–11.

27. Garcia-Campayo J, et al. The reason for medical consultations in patients with psychiatric diseases: somatization phenomena and suicide attempts. Medicina Clinica. 1997;108(9):321–4.

28. Öztürk E, Sar V. Somatization as a predictor of suicidal ideation in dissociative disorders. Psychiatry Clin Neurosci. 2008;62(6):662–8.

29. Bolton JM, et al. Anxiety disorders and risk for suicide attempts: findings from the Baltimore epidemiologic catchment area follow-up study. Depress Anxiety. 2008;25(6):477–81.

30. Capron DW, Lamis DA, Schmidt NB. Test of the depression distress amplification model in young adults with elevated risk of current suicidality. Psychiatry Res. 2014;219(3):531–5.

31. Capron DW, et al. Distress tolerance and anxiety sensitivity cognitive concerns: testing the incremental contributions of affect dysregulation constructs on suicidal ideation and suicide attempt. Behav Ther. 2013;44(3):349–58.

32. Tucker RP, et al. Maladaptive five factor model personality traits associated with borderline personality disorder indirectly affect susceptibility to suicide ideation through increased anxiety sensitivity cognitive concerns. Psychiatry Res. 2016;246:432–7.

33. Yaseen ZS, et al. Fear of dying in panic attacks predicts suicide attempt in comorbid depressive illness: prospective evidence from the national epidemiological survey on alcohol and related conditions. Depress Anxiety. 2013;30(10):930–9.

34. Yaseen ZS, et al. Panic as an independent risk factor for suicide attempt in depressive illness: findings from the National Epidemiological Survey on alcohol and related conditions (NESARC). J Clin Psychiatry. 2011;72(12):1628–35.

35. Shneidman ES. Suicide as psychache: a clinical approach to self-destructive behavior. Northfield: Jason Aronson; 1993.

36. Orbach I. Mental pain and suicide. Isr J Psychiatry Relat Sci. 2003;40(3):191.

37. Orbach I, et al. Mental pain and its relationship to suicidality and life meaning. Suicide Life Threat Behav. 2003;33(3):231–41.

38. Orbach I, et al. Mental pain: a multidimensional operationalization and definition. Suicide Life Threat Behav. 2003;33(3):219–30.

39. Troister T, Holden RR. Factorial differentiation among depression, hopelessness, and psychache in statistically predicting suicidality. Meas Eval Couns Dev. 2013;46(1):50–63.

40. Brown GK, et al. Risk factors for suicide in psychiatric outpatients: a 20-year prospective study. J Consult Clin Psychol. 2000;68(3):371.

41. Brown GK, et al. The internal struggle between the wish to die and the wish to live: a risk factor for suicide. Am J Psychiatr. 2005;162(10):1977–9.

42. Yaseen ZS, et al. Functional domains as correlates of suicidality among psychiatric inpatients. J Affect Disord. 2016;203:77–83.

43. Beck AT, Steer RA. BSI, Beck scale for suicide ideation: manual. San Antonio: Psychological Corporation; 1991.

44. Beck AT, Steer RA, Brown GK. Beck depression inventory-II. San Antonio. 1996;78(2):490–8.

45. Steer RA, et al. Mean Beck depression inventory-II scores by severity of major depressive episode. Psychol Rep. 2001;88(3_suppl):1075–6.

46. Preacher KJ, Kelley K. Effect size measures for mediation models: quantitative strategies for communicating indirect effects. Psychol Methods. 2011;16(2):93.

47. Hayes AF. Introduction to mediation, moderation, and conditional process analysis: a regression-based approach. New York: Guilford Press; 2013.

48. Levi-Belz Y, et al. Mental pain, communication difficulties, and medically serious suicide attempts: a case-control study. Arch Suicide Res. 2014;18(1):74–87.

49. Miranda R, et al. Cognitive inflexibility and suicidal ideation: mediating role of brooding and hopelessness. Psychiatry Res. 2013;210(1):174–81.

50. Smith JM, Alloy LB, Abramson LY. Cognitive vulnerability to depression, rumination, hopelessness, and suicidal ideation: multiple pathways to self-injurious thinking. Suicide Life Threat Behav. 2006;36(4):443–54.

51. Teismann T, Forkmann T. Rumination, entrapment and suicide ideation: a mediational model. Clin Psychol Psychother. 2017;24(1):226–34.

52. Rappaport LM, et al. Panic symptom clusters differentially predict suicide ideation and attempt. Compr Psychiatry. 2014;55(4):762–9.

53. Baumeister RF. Suicide as escape from self. Psychol Rev. 1990;97(1):90.

54. Flamenbaum R, Holden RR. Psychache as a mediator in the relationship between perfectionism and suicidality. J Couns Psychol. 2007;54(1):51.

55. Flamenbaum, R., Testing Shneidman's theory of suicide: Psychache as a prospective predictor of suicidality and comparison with hopelessness. 2009.

56. Nahaliel S, et al. Mental pain as a mediator of suicidal tendency: a path analysis. Compr Psychiatry. 2014;55(4):944–51.

57. Klonsky ED, May AM. The three-step theory (3ST): a new theory of suicide rooted in the "ideation-to-action" framework. Int J Cogn Ther. 2015;8(2):114–29.

58. Williams M. Cry of pain: understanding suicide and the suicidal mind. London: Little, Brown Book Group; 2014.

59. Schotte DE, Clum GA. Problem-solving skills in suicidal psychiatric patients. J Consult Clin Psychol. 1987;55(1):49.

11

Accuracy of risk scales for predicting repeat self-harm and suicide

Sarah Steeg[1]*[iD], Leah Quinlivan[1], Rebecca Nowland[1], Robert Carroll[4], Deborah Casey[2], Caroline Clements[1], Jayne Cooper[1], Linda Davies[5], Duleeka Knipe[4], Jennifer Ness[3], Rory C. O'Connor[6], Keith Hawton[2], David Gunnell[4] and Nav Kapur[1,7]

Abstract

Background: Risk scales are used widely in the management of patients presenting to hospital following self-harm. However, there is evidence that their diagnostic accuracy in predicting repeat self-harm is limited. Their predictive accuracy in population settings, and in identifying those at highest risk of suicide is not known.

Method: We compared the predictive accuracy of the Manchester Self-Harm Rule (MSHR), ReACT Self-Harm Rule (ReACT), SAD PERSONS Scale (SPS) and Modified SAD PERSONS Scale (MSPS) in an unselected sample of patients attending hospital following self-harm. Data on 4000 episodes of self-harm presenting to Emergency Departments (ED) between 2010 and 2012 were obtained from four established monitoring systems in England. Episodes were assigned a risk category for each scale and followed up for 6 months.

Results: The episode-based repeat rate was 28% (1133/4000) and the incidence of suicide was 0.5% (18/3962). The MSHR and ReACT performed with high sensitivity (98% and 94% respectively) and low specificity (15% and 23%). The SPS and the MSPS performed with relatively low sensitivity (24–29% and 9–12% respectively) and high specificity (76–77% and 90%). The area under the curve was 71% for both MSHR and ReACT, 51% for SPS and 49% for MSPS. Differences in predictive accuracy by subgroup were small. The scales were less accurate at predicting suicide than repeat self-harm.

Conclusions: The scales failed to accurately predict repeat self-harm and suicide. The findings support existing clinical guidance not to use risk classification scales alone to determine treatment or predict future risk.

Keywords: Self-harm, Suicide, Risk factors, Classification, Outcome

Background

Emergency Departments (EDs) in England treat over 200,000 presentations for self-harm (intentional self-poisoning or self-injury) each year [1], and the appropriate management of these individuals is important. Clinicians are required to manage a number of risks when treating this population. People who have self-harmed are at greater risk of suicide [2], other causes of premature mortality [3] and comorbid conditions such as alcohol misuse [4] compared to the general population. In efforts to help mental health and non-specialist clinicians manage patients, many hospitals use risk scales, which aim to score or classify patients according to their risk of future self-harm or suicide based on the presence or absence of a specified set of characteristics.

Psychosocial assessment by a mental health clinician is a central component of clinical care and is recommended for each episode of self-harm [5]. These in-depth assessments help clinicians to formulate decisions about follow-

* Correspondence: sarah.steeg@manchester.ac.uk
[1]Centre for Mental Health and Safety, Manchester Academic Health Science Centre, University of Manchester, Manchester, England
Full list of author information is available at the end of the article

up care and reach an informed decision about the risk of further self-harm. There is also evidence that psychosocial assessment may reduce the risk of a further self-harm episode [6, 7]. Formal risk scales are used often by ED and psychiatric clinicians. One study of 32 hospitals across England found that over 20 different risk scales were being used with people who presented after self-harm [8]. This suggests they are in widespread use, with little consensus about which should be used or how well they predict future risk.

A recent systematic review compared the diagnostic accuracy of predicting repeat self-harm of a number of scales [9]. There were no scales that performed well enough to be recommended for use in clinical practice. Another recent meta-analysis pooled positive predictive values from 52 studies of psychological scales predicting repeat self-harm and suicide [10]. The results suggested high-risk classification approaches were unlikely to be clinically useful but also reported high between-study heterogeneity. Another study measured the accuracy of the SAD PERSONS Scale (SPS) for predicting suicide following an emergency department presentation, using administrative data to identify suicide deaths [11]. The study found that the predictive accuracy of the SPS was inadequate to support the use of this risk scale. However, there have been few head-to-head comparisons of risk scales within the same cohort. A comparatively small study ($n = 483$) found that the levels of diagnostic accuracy reached by the five scales investigated meant they had limited clinical utility [12]. The risk scales also performed worse at predicting repeat self-harm than simply asking the clinician or patient to rate their risk. However, the study only recruited individuals receiving a psychosocial assessment from mental health clinician (typically only around 55% of all self-harm patients who present to the ED receive a psychosocial assessment) [6, 13]. This study was too small to consider the outcome of most concern to clinicians – suicide, or to examine diagnostic accuracy of the scales in different subgroups. In the current study we therefore aimed to test four of the risk scales tested in previous research, using data from a large unselected cohort of people presenting to the ED after self-harm.

Aims of the study

Our specific objectives were:

- To estimate predictive accuracy of the risk scales, using established cut-off points, for identifying a) repeat self-harm and b) suicide
- To test for differences in the predictive accuracy of the scales by groups (age, sex, method of self-harm,

professional background of the assessor and self-harm history)

Our hypothesis was that the poor predictive ability of risk scales found in previous smaller studies would hold for this larger unselected hospital cohort and would be replicated for suicide as an outcome.

Methods
Data sources

Data were obtained from self-harm cohorts in four separate centres in England. Each centre has an established system to collect data relating to episodes of self-harm presenting to the study EDs. Two of the centres (Bristol and Oxford) are based in the South of England, one in the Midlands (Derby) one in the North (Manchester). The centres collected data from one hospital each with the exception of Manchester, which included three hospitals. The EDs in the study hospitals each had access to psychiatric liaison teams alongside emergency out-of-hours cover from crisis teams or junior psychiatrists.

For all self-harm episodes, basic data were available on method of self-harm (including drugs taken in self-poisoning), time of presentation, age, gender and initial hospital management (for example, admission to a medical bed, referral for a psychiatric assessment). For individuals who were subsequently referred to liaison psychiatry services for a psychosocial assessment, additional data were available including factors precipitating the self-harm, circumstances of the act (such as planning and suicidal intent), social circumstances (such as living arrangements and marital status) and symptoms of depression. For the present study, 1000 consecutive episodes of self-harm, including any repeat episodes by the same individuals, were extracted from each centre's cohort. The presentations took place over different time periods in each centre but all were between 2010 and 2012. Repeat episodes of self-harm by individuals were included to reflect the real-world ED environment and to be in line with clinical guidance that each episode of self-harm should be assessed comprehensively [5]. In order to preserve the observational nature of the data, no selection/exclusion criteria were applied.

In addition to information from the study hospitals, individuals in three of the centres were matched to Office for National Statistics (ONS) records held by the National Health Service [https://digital.nhs.uk]. For individuals who died, information about the cause of death, verdict and date of death were available. In one of the centres, suicide deaths were identified from the local coroner's office.

Scales

We compared the predictive accuracy of the following risk scales: the Manchester Self-Harm Rule (MSHR) [14], the ReACT Self-Harm Rule (ReACT) [15], the SAD PERSONS Scale (SPS) [16] and the Modified SAD PERSONS Scale (MSPS) [17]. The MSHR and ReACT both consist of four items, with a 'yes' to at least one of the items resulting in a high risk categorisation and 'no' to all items corresponding to low risk. The SPS and the MSPS both include ten items and classify episodes into three risk categories (low, moderate and high). The MSPS also weights four of the items, resulting in maximum score of 14. The items included in each of these scales and the cut-off points for the risk categories are shown in Additional file 1: Table S1. Scales were selected based on an existing systematic review of the diagnostic accuracy of risk scales for predicting self-harm [9]. We included scales that could be re-constructed from routinely recorded information following a self-harm hospital presentation. The scales were also included in a previous study that compared their predictive accuracy when administered by a mental health clinician as part of the psychosocial assessment [12].

Due to the observational nature of the study, some of the individual items for the risk scales were derived from variables related to the core items of interest. For example, the item 'Stated future intent' from the two SAD PERSONS Scales was derived in three centres from the Suicide Intent Scale [18] and in another from a binary 'yes/no' question about current suicidal plans. In another example, the SPS item 'Depression or hopelessness' was available for two of the four sites: in one site it was derived from the presence of either one or two of the items 'depression' and 'hopelessness' within a list of eight symptoms of depression and in another it was derived from the presence of a diagnosis of affective disorder at the time of presentation.

Outcome measures

Repeat attendance to the study hospitals with an episode of self-harm within 6 months was our first outcome measure. This was selected because it is a marker for continued distress and need for ongoing clinical care, and has been an outcome in many previous studies [19]. We chose 6 months as the follow-up period as the majority of repeat episodes occur within this time-frame [20]. Our second outcome measure was suicide within 6 months of the self-harm episode. Many studies are insufficiently powered to examine suicide as an outcome, due to low event numbers, but large observational datasets are well suited to this purpose. Individuals who could not be matched to ONS records ($n = 38/3157$) were excluded from the analyses of suicide. Finally, we were interested to see if there were differences in the

predictive accuracy of the scales by demographic and clinical sub-groups (age, sex, method of self-harm, self-harm history and according to the professional background of the assessor). These have been identified as factors which may influence the assessment of risk [21].

Missing data

Data were relatively complete (median levels of completeness for variables 69% (IQR 45% to 92%, range 34% to 100%) with lower completeness for certain variables (e.g. future suicidal intent and depression). Data were more likely to be missing for variables where the individual did not have a psychosocial assessment. For episodes where no assessment took place, there was evidence of bias towards clinicians recording the variable if it was 'present' and not if it was 'absent'. In these instances, variables were imputed as absent, prior to multiple imputation. The potential effect of this would be to underestimate sensitivity and overestimate specificity (defined in Table 1). This included the following items from the SPS/MSPS: depression or hopelessness, organised or serious attempt and rational thinking loss. This approach has been taken in a previous study with similar data [7]. The remaining missing data were largely missing at random, with potential predictors of missingness included in the imputation model. Imputation was conducted using the 'chained equations' approach [22] in Stata to generate 50 imputations. Analyses were either conducted on all imputed datasets to generate pooled results, or, where multiple imputation was not compatible with the analytic method, estimates were pooled from $m = 1-5$ using Rubin's rules [23].

In a sensitivity analysis, repeat self-harm outcomes were also examined using a dataset with missing data for scale items coded as not present. This analysis did not include one of the centres due to the unavailability of a scale item used in three of the four scales (living circumstances) in this centre. We also conducted a 'complete case' analysis of the MSHR and ReACT by excluding scale items with missing data. Due to the larger number of items in the SPS and the MSPS, too many cases would have been excluded for this approach to be feasible for these scales. For example, while 52% of cases had complete data for at least seven out of ten items on the SPS, only 2% had complete data for all ten scale items. Therefore, excluding all cases with missing data for any one scale item would result in 98% of cases excluded from the analyses.

Statistical analyses

The predictive accuracy of the scales was examined using the following measures: sensitivity (the proportion of people who repeated self-harm and were correctly identified by the scale as high risk), specificity (the

Table 1 Diagnostic accuracy definitions

Sensitivity	The proportion of episodes that were followed by a repeat self-harm episode and were correctly identified by the scale as high risk
Specificity	The proportion of episodes that were not followed by a repeat self-harm episode and were correctly identified by the scale as low risk
Positive predictive value	The probability that the episode identified as high risk by the scale was followed by repeat self-harm
Negative predictive value	The probability that the episode identified as low risk by the scale was not followed by repeat self-harm
Positive likelihood ratio	The increased likelihood of a high-risk scale result in an episode that is followed by repeat self-harm versus one that is not
Negative likelihood ratio	The decreased likelihood of a low-risk scale result in an episode that is followed by repeat self-harm versus one that is not
Diagnostic odds ratio	The odds of a high-risk result in an episode that is followed by repeat self-harm versus one that is not (interpreted the same as an odds ratio)
Receiver operating characteristic (ROC) curve	Graphically shows the overall discrimination ability of a scale to identify episodes that were followed by a repeat self-harm episode compared with those that did not at various cut-off points (plotted as sensitivity versus 1-specifcity). The performance of the scale is indicated by the calculation of the area under the curve (AUC). Higher AUC indicate greater discriminatory power.

proportion of people who did not repeat self-harm and were correctly identified by the scale as low risk), positive predictive value (the probability that the person identified as high risk went on to repeat self-harm), negative predictive value (the probability that the person identified as low risk did not repeat self-harm), positive likelihood ratio (the increased likelihood of a high risk scale result in a person who repeated self-harm vs. one who did not), negative likelihood ratio (the decreased likelihood of a low risk scale result in a person who repeated self-harm vs. one who did not) and diagnostic odds ratio (the odds of a high risk scale result in a person who repeated self-harm vs. one who did not). Receiver operator characteristic (ROC) curves, which show sensitivity on the y-axis and 1 minus specificity on the x-axis for all possible scale thresholds were plotted [24]. The area under the curve (AUC), based on the published cut-off points for each scale, was also calculated. The AUC represents the overall proportion of cases correctly predicted by the test; an AUC of 0.5 would suggest the test does not perform any better than chance while an AUC of 1.0 indicates every case is predicted correctly. Chi-square tests were used to examine differences in the AUC between subgroups. Stata V.13.1 and OpenEpi were used for the analyses.

Results

Characteristics of the cohort
The 4000 self-harm presentations involved 3157 individuals. 60% (2411) of episodes were by females, 14% (552) by individuals aged 18 or under and 22% (892) aged 45 years or over. The majority of episodes involved self-poisoning with drugs or other substances (81%, 3241) and 19% (759) presentations were by individuals who had self-injured. 55% (2206) of episodes received a psychosocial assessment. In 2759 (69%) of the episodes,

individuals had a previous history of self-harm. 28% (1133) of episodes were followed by a repeat episode within 6 months. Amongst the 3962 episodes in which individuals could be followed up for mortality status, the incidence of suicide was 0.5% ($n = 18$).

Repeat self-harm within six months by scale cut-off points
For the MSHR and ReACT the majority of the episodes that were followed by a repeat episode in the subsequent 6 months were identified as moderate to high risk (Table 2). The MSHR and ReACT both had high sensitivity for identifying repeat self-harm (98% and 94% respectively) alongside relatively low specificity for identifying those that did not go on to repeat (15% and 23% respectively) (Table 3). The reverse pattern was seen for the SPS and the MSPS: relatively low sensitivity with high specificity resulted in the correct prediction of the majority of episodes that were not followed by repetition of self-harm as low risk. Positive predictive values were similar across the four scales. The positive likelihood ratios for a high risk result on the scales were between 1.2 (MSHR) and 1.3 (MSPS). The overall area under the curve (the proportion of episodes correctly identified by the scales) was highest for the MSHR and ReACT (both 71%) and was approximately equivalent to chance for the SPS (51%) and the MSPS (49%) (Fig. 1).

Suicide within six months by scale cut-off points
Only two people who died by suicide (11% of all suicides) were identified as low risk by the MSHR and four (22%) by ReACT (Table 2). However two thirds of the suicides (12/18) were categorised as low risk by the SPS and over 80% (15/18) by the MSPS. There were no suicide deaths identified as high risk by the MSPS (Table 2). The MSHR and ReACT had relatively high sensitivity for predicting

Table 2 Self-harm episodes and repeat self-harm or suicide within 6 months by scale cut-off points (missing data imputed)

Scale	Thresholds	Repeated self-harm (N = 1133, 28.3%)	Did not repeat self-harm (N = 2867, 71.7%)	Total (N = 4000)	Died from suicide (N = 18, 0.5%)	Did not die from suicide (N = 3944)	Total (N = 3962)[a]
Manchester Self-Harm Rule (MSHR)	Low risk (0)	23 (2.0)	435 (15.2)	458 (11.5)	2 (11.1)	450 (11.4)	452 (11.4)
	Moderate/high risk (1+)	1110 (98.0)	2432 (84.8)	3542 (88.6)	16 (88.9)	3494 (88.6)	3510 (88.6)
ReACT Self-Harm Rule (ReACT)	Low risk (0)	63 (5.6)	665 (23.2)	728 (18.2)	4 (22.2)	719 (18.2)	723 (18.2)
	Moderate/high risk (1+)	1070 (94.4)	2202 (76.8)	3272 (81.8)	14 (77.8)	3225 (81.8)	3239 (81.8)
SAD PERSONS (SPS)	Low risk (0–4)	781 (68.9)	2029 (70.1)	2810 (70.3)	12 (66.7)	2766 (70.1)	2778 (70.1)
	Moderate risk (5–6)	251 (22.2)	642 (22.4)	893 (22.3)	4 (22.2)	885 (22.4)	889 (22.4)
	High risk (7–10)	101 (8.9)	196 (6.8)	297 (7.4)	2 (11.1)	293 (7.4)	295 (7.4)
Modified SAD PERSONS (MSPS)	Low risk (0–5)	1020 (90.0)	2561 (89.3)	3581 (89.5)	15 (83.3)	3532 (89.6)	3547 (89.5)
	Moderate risk (6–8)	99 (8.7)	276 (9.6)	375 (9.4)	3 (16.7)	369 (9.4)	372 (9.4)
	High risk (> 8)	14 (1.2)	30 (1.0)	44 (1.1)	0 (0)	43 (1.1)	43 (1.1)

[a]38 individuals were lost to mortality follow-up

Table 3 Measures of diagnostic accuracy[a] for repeat self-harm with 95% confidence intervals, N = 4000, m (missing data imputation) =1–5

Scale	Thresholds	Sens %	Spec %	PPV %	NPV %	LR+	LR-	DOR
MSHR	Low risk (0) vs. moderate/high risk (1+)	98 (97, 99)	15 (14, 17)	31 (30, 33)	95 (93, 97)	1.155 (1.154, 1.156)	0.13 (0.12, 0.15)	8.6 (5.6, 13.2)
ReACT	Low risk (0) vs. moderate/high risk (1+)	94 (93, 96)	23 (22, 25)	33 (31, 34)	91 (89, 93)	1.23 (1.228, 1.231)	0.240 (0.230, 0.250)	5.1 (3.9, 6.7)
SPS	Low risk (0–4) vs. moderate risk (5–6)	24 (22, 27)	76 (74, 78)	28 (25, 31)	72 (71, 74)	1.01 (0.98, 1.04)	0.996 (0.993, 0.999)	1.0 (0.9, 1.2)
	Moderate risk (5–6) vs. high risk (7–10)	29 (24, 34)	77 (74, 79)	34 (29, 40)	72 (69, 75)	1.23 (1.16, 1.30)	0.931 (0.923, 0.939)	1.3 (1.0, 1.7)
MSPS	Low risk (0–5) vs. moderate risk (6–8)	9 (7, 11)	90 (89, 91)	26 (22, 31)	72 (70, 73)	0.9 (0.7, 1.1)	1.01 (1.008, 1.012)	0.9 (0.7, 1.1)
	Moderate risk (6–8) vs. high risk (> 8)	12 (7, 20)	90 (86, 93)	32 (19, 48)	74 (69, 78)	1.3 (0.4, 3.6)	0.97 (0.95, 0.99)	1.3 (0.7, 2.6)

[a]Sens sensitivity, Spec specificity, PPV positive predictive value, NPV negative predicctive value, LR+ positive likelihood ratio, LR- negative likelihood ratio, DOR diagnostic odds ratio

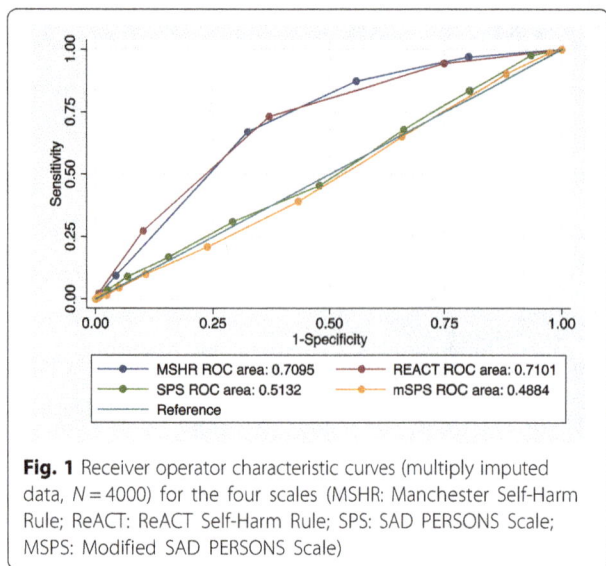

Fig. 1 Receiver operator characteristic curves (multiply imputed data, N = 4000) for the four scales (MSHR: Manchester Self-Harm Rule; ReACT: ReACT Self-Harm Rule; SPS: SAD PERSONS Scale; MSPS: Modified SAD PERSONS Scale)

suicide, while the SPS and the MSPS had higher specificity (Table 4).

Differences by subgroups

There were few differences in overall predictive accuracy (AUC) by subgroups (Table 5). There was higher AUC for episodes assessed by a psychiatrist for both the SPS (area under the curve 0.61, $p = 0.003$) and the MSPS (0.57, $p = 0.001$) than those assessed by a mental health nurse, by another profession or not assessed. The ReACT risk scale performed worse amongst episodes involving individuals with no prior episode of self-harm (0.60) compared to individuals with a history of self-harm (0.67, $p = .0.02$). However, the absolute differences between subgroups were small (Table 5).

Sensitivity analysis

In sensitivity analysis with missing items imputed as not present, the MSHR and ReACT again performed with relatively high sensitivity and low specificity, though sensitivities were lower and specificities higher, due to more individuals being rated as low risk (Additional file 1: Table S2). The measures of predictive accuracy of the SPS and MSPS were broadly similar to those in the main analyses. When we included only those cases with complete data for all scale items for the MSHR and ReACT scales, sensitivity was similar but specificity was lower. For the MSHR, 30.4% (981/3228) of episodes were followed by repetition of self-harm, sensitivity was 99.2% and specificity was 7.4%. For ReACT, the repeat rate was 27.2% (668/2459), sensitivity was 94.3% and specificity was 20.0%.

Discussion

Main findings

The MSHR and ReACT performed with high sensitivity but low specificity for prediction of repeat self-harm. This resulted in a large proportion of episodes that were not followed by repetition being placed in the higher risk category. The overall area under the curve for these scales was fair. The SPS and the MSPS had lower sensitivity and higher specificity, resulting in the majority of episodes that resulted in repetition being identified as low risk. The SPS and the MSPS were no better than chance in terms of overall predictive accuracy. The SPS and the MSPS identified the majority of suicide deaths as low risk.

Strengths and limitations

Some scale items were not available across all sites. To avoid over-estimating the prevalence of risk factors, we assumed the item was not present if data were missing. Furthermore, if there was evidence that the prevalence of a scale item was over-estimated in non-assessed episodes, missing items were imputed as absent for all non-assessed episodes before multiple imputation. The effect of this on the measures of predictive accuracy would be to underestimate sensitivity (due to fewer meeting the criteria for 'high risk') and overestimate specificity (due to more meeting the criteria for 'low risk'). When the performance of the MSHR and the ReACT scales, the two best performing scales in this study, was tested on cases with complete data for all scales items, measures of sensitivity were similar and specificities were lower. This suggests our imputation approach did not lead to over-estimation of the performance of these two scales.

The data for this study were obtained from observational self-harm cohorts with data extracted from hospital records and clinical notes. It was necessary to use proxy variables for certain scale items where an exact corresponding variable was not available, which is a limitation of this study. In addition, for some scale items, corresponding variables could be recorded differently according to the study centre. For example, suicidal intent was derived from the Suicide Intent Scale in three centres and from a binary variable in another centre. This would have had most impact on the SAD PERSONS Scales, due to the higher number of scale items. However, the measures of diagnostic accuracy are in line with a previous study which showed the area under the curve to be no better than chance for the SPS [17]. Furthermore, this novel approach resulted in a more representative, real-world sample of self-harm episodes and their management.

A potential source of bias in this study could have arisen if perceived risk influenced subsequent clinical management, which in turn may have been associated

Table 4 Measures of diagnostic accuracy[a] for suicide with 95% confidence intervals, $N = 3962$, $m = 1$–5

Scale	Thresholds	Sens %	Spec %	PPV %	NPV %	LR+	LR-	DOR
MSHR	Low risk (0) vs. moderate/high risk (1+)	89 (65, 99)	11 (10, 12)	0.5 (0.3, 0.7)	99.6 (98.4, 99.9)	1.003 (0.99, 1.02)	0.97 (0.35, 2.68)	1.03 (0.24, 4.50)
ReACT	Low risk (0) vs. moderate/high risk (1+)	78 (52, 94)	18 (17, 19)	0.4 (0.2, 0.7)	99.5 (98.6, 99.9)	0.95 (0.91, 0.99)	1.2 (0.74, 2.0)	0.8 (0.3, 2.4)
SPS	Low risk (0–4) vs. moderate risk (5–6)	25 (7, 52)	76 (74, 77)	0.5 (0.1, 1.2)	99.6 (99.3, 99.8)	1.0 (0.2, 4.5)	1.0 (0.8, 1.2)	1.0 (0.4, 3.2)
	Moderate risk (5–6) vs. high risk (7–10)	33 (4, 77)	75 (73, 78)	0.7 (0.1, 2.4)	99.6 (98.9, 99.9)	1.3 (0.2, 9.6)	0.9 (0.5, 1.5)	1.5 (0.3, 8.3)
MSPS	Low risk (0–5) vs. moderate risk (6–8)	17 (4, 41)	91 (90, 91)	0.8 (0.2, 2.3)	99.6 (99.3, 99.8)	1.8 (0.1, 4.5)	0.9 (0.8, 1.0)	1.9 (0.6, 6.6)
	Moderate risk (6–8) vs. high risk (> 8)	0 (0, 71)	90 (86, 92)	0 (0, 8)	99.2 (97.7, 99.8)	_[b]	–	–

[a]Sens sensitivity, Spec specificity, PPV positive predictive value, NPV negative predictive value, LR+ positive likelihood ratio, LR- negative likelihood ratio, DOR diagnostic odds ratio
[b]No suicides were identified as high risk by the MSPS

Table 5 Area under the curve (AUC) for repeat self-harm by subgroups, with 95% confidence intervals, $N = 4000$, m = 1–5

	MSHR	ReACT	SPS	MSPS
Overall AUC (95% CI)	0.71 (0.69, 0.73)	0.71 (0.70, 0.73)	0.51 (0.48, 0.54)	0.49 (0.47, 0.51)
Male ($n = 1589$)	0.69 (0.67, 0.72)	0.69 (0.66, 0.72)	0.54 (0.51, 0.57)	0.52 (0.49, 0.55)
Female ($n = 2411$)	0.72 (0.70, 0.74)	0.73 (0.70, 0.75)	0.51 (0.49, 0.54)	0.49 (0.46, 0.52)
Aged < 19 ($n = 552$)	0.73 (0.68, 0.78)	0.73 (0.68, 0.78)	0.47 (0.42, 0.52)	0.48 (0.42, 0.53)
Aged = > 19 to 44 ($n = 2556$)	0.71 (0.69, 0.73)	0.71 (0.69, 0.73)	0.51 (0.49, 0.54)	0.48 (0.46, 0.50)
Aged 45+ ($n = 892$)	0.71 (0.67, 0.74)	0.71 (0.68, 0.75)	0.54 (0.49, 0.58)	0.51 (0.47, 0.56)
Main method of harm				
Self-poison ($n = 3241$)	0.71 (0.69, 0.73)	0.72 (0.70, 0.74)	0.53 (0.51, 0.55)	0.50 (0.48, 0.52)
Self-injury ($n = 759$)	0.70 (0.67, 0.74)	0.67 (0.64, 0.71)	0.47 (0.43, 0.51)	0.47 (0.42, 0.51)
Assessed by:				
Psychiatrist ($n = 638$)	0.67 (0.63, 0.71)	0.64 (0.60, 0.69)	**0.61 (0.56, 0.66)**	**0.57 (0.52, 0.62)**
Mental health nurse ($n = 1273$)	0.69 (0.66, 0.72)	0.72 (0.69, 0.75)	0.51 (0.47, 0.54)	0.47 (0.44, 0.51)
Other ($n = 295$)	0.67 (0.61, 0.74)	0.71 (0.64, 0.77)	0.50 (0.42, 0.57)	0.44 (0.37, 0.51)
History of self-harm ($n = 2759$)	0.63 (0.61, 0.66)	**0.67 (0.65, 0.69)**	0.45 (0.42, 0.48)	0.44 (0.41, 0.46)
No history of self-harm ($n = 1241$)	0.64 (0.59, 0.69)	0.60 (0.53, 0.67)	0.49 (0.42, 0.55)	0.46 (0.40, 0.52)

Bold text denotes statistically significant ($p < 0.05$) difference between groups

with risks of repeat self-harm and suicide. This would have led to bias in the measures of predictive accuracy.

Comparison to previous research

A previous study used a selected sample with clinicians administering the risk scales following referral to psychiatric services [12]. The conclusion from that study was that the diagnostic accuracy of the scales was too modest for them to be of clinical use. The measures of diagnostic accuracy in the present study are comparable, suggesting that risk scales following self-harm are also unsuitable for the wider population of all those who present to hospital following self-harm, not just those seen by mental health clinicians. While the previous study recruited patients after they had been referred to liaison psychiatry for assessment, the present study also included non-referred episodes, typically just under half of all episodes [13, 25]. The present study also suggests that the risk scales are unsuitable for predicting risk of future suicide among individuals presenting with self-harm. A meta-analysis of risk scales used for predicting suicidal behaviour also found that predictive ability of risk scales was insufficient to be used to determine treatment allocation [10]. The present study addresses the high level of heterogeneity found in the meta-analysis, and reaches similar conclusions.

A comparatively small study of psychiatric inpatients recently reported a modular multi-informant approach, resulting in promising levels of accuracy for predicting further suicidal behaviour [26]. Machine learning techniques utilising medical databases are also becoming more common in the pursuit of accurate detection of

suicide risk [27]. These are potential areas for further research.

Clinical implications

This study adds to the evidence that scales, particularly the widely used SAD PERSONS Scales, are not suitable for predicting repeat episodes of self-harm or future suicide. Their overall performance as measured by the AUC did not surpass a 'fair' level of prediction, defined as between 0.7 and 0.8 [28], likelihood ratios had weak predictive ability [29] and performance did not exceed that of clinicians' ratings (measured at 0.74) found in an earlier study [12].

There is evidence that risk classification scales remain in widespread use despite growing evidence about their poor predictive abilities [8, 10]. It is possible that clinicians welcome the structure they offer or the prompts for factors to consider, such as social isolation, in their overall formulation of a follow-up plan. The use of risk scales may act as 'aide memoires' for less experienced clinicians and may help in eliciting the relevant information, provided the patient's narrative is not lost [30]. Carter and colleagues also suggest that there should be a focus on modifiable risk factors, such as hopelessness, as part of a needs-based assessment [10]. This would help focus the assessment on a person's situation and how best to help manage it [31]. There is evidence that assessment itself may be beneficial at reducing the risk of a repeat self-harm episode [6, 7], with patients valuing a positive therapeutic alliance that promotes hope and encouragement [32].

The SPS and MSPS performed slightly better for episodes assessed by a psychiatrist, though the performance was still below those of the ReACT and MSHR scales. Episodes assessed by a psychiatrist were more likely to involve individuals with a history of self-harm but not currently receiving treatment. The episodes by individuals assessed by psychiatrists were also more likely to be rated as moderate or high risk than low risk on both the SPS and the MSPS compared to episodes assessed by mental health nurses. In addition, the overall predictive accuracy of the ReACT scale was lower for episodes where individuals had no history of self-harm. These individuals were less likely to repeat self-harm, and the specificity was lower (16%), suggesting the incorrect identification of episodes that did not repeat resulted in reduced overall performance. However, the difference in predictive accuracy between these groups was small and is unlikely to be of major clinical importance.

Conclusion

The findings of this study support existing clinical guidance, which suggests scales that classify patients into risk categories should not be used alone to allocate treatment or predict future risk of further self-harm or suicide. There was no evidence to support the use of risk scales with particular subgroups of patients. While scales with high sensitivity may have some clinical use when considered alongside a comprehensive assessment [15], they are not suitable for the purpose of prediction. Given that scales continue to be widely used by clinicians, future studies could consider if they could be combined with other approaches to increase their effectiveness. For example, randomised controlled trials could combine structured risk assessment with other aspects of care, such as comprehensive follow-up planning or building therapeutic alliance. A study carried out recently in the United States found that screening in the ED combined with a brief intervention consisting of a number of components (including safety planning and follow-up telephone calls), was associated with reductions in repeat suicide attempts and overall number of repeat attempts [33]. Further studies of this kind could help to determine aspects of risk scales that might be useful in the management of self-harm.

Abbreviations
AUC: Area under the curve; ED: Emergency Department; MSHR: Manchester Self-Harm Rule; MSPS: Modified SAD PERSONS Scale; ONS: Office for National Statistics; ReACT: ReACT Self-Harm Rule; ROC: Receiver operating characteristic; SPS: SAD PERSONS Scale

Acknowledgements
The authors would like to thank Dr. Matthew Carr at the University of Manchester for statistical advice.

Funding
This paper presents independent research funded by the National Institute of Health Research (NIHR) under its Programme Grants for Applied Research Programme (Grant Reference Number RP-PG-0610-10026). The views expressed are those of the authors and not necessarily those of the NHS, the NIHR or the Department of Health. K.H. and D.G. are NIHR Senior Investigators. K.H. is also supported by the Oxford Health NHS Foundation Trust and N.K. by the Greater Manchester Mental Health NHS Foundation Trust.

Authors' contributions
NK, JC, ROC, DG and KH designed the study with input from SS and LQ. SS, LQ, DC, CC, DK, JN and RC extracted and processed the data. SS analysed the data. All authors interpreted the results and SS wrote the first draft. All the authors contributed to subsequent drafts and have approved the final version of the manuscript.

Competing interests
D.G., K.H. and N.K. are members of the Department of Health's (England) National Suicide Prevention Advisory Group. N.K. chaired the NICE guideline development group for the longer-term management of self-harm and the NICE Topic Expert Group (which developed the quality standards for self-harm services). He is currently chair of the updated NICE guideline for depression. R.O.C. was a member of the NICE guideline development group for the longer-term management of self-harm and is a member of the Scottish Government's suicide prevention implementation and monitoring group. All other authors declare no conflict of interest.

Author details
[1]Centre for Mental Health and Safety, Manchester Academic Health Science Centre, University of Manchester, Manchester, England. [2]Centre for Suicide Research, University of Oxford Department of Psychiatry, Warneford Hospital, Oxford, England. [3]Centre for Self-harm and Suicide Prevention Research, Derbyshire Healthcare NHS Foundation Trust, Derby, England. [4]Population Health Sciences, Bristol Medical School, University of Bristol, Bristol, England. [5]Institute of Population Health, University of Manchester, Manchester, England. [6]Suicidal Behaviour Research Laboratory, Institute of Health and Wellbeing, University of Glasgow, Glasgow, Scotland. [7]Greater Manchester Mental Health NHS Foundation Trust, Manchester, England.

References
1. Hawton K, Bergen H, Casey D, Simkin S, Palmer B, Cooper J, Kapur N, Horrocks J, House A, Lilley R, et al. Self-harm in England: a tale of three cities - multicentre study of self-harm. Soc Psychiatry Psychiatr Epidemiol. 2007;42(7):513–21.
2. Carroll R, Metcalfe C, Gunnell D. Hospital presenting self-harm and risk of fatal and non-fatal repetition: systematic review and meta-analysis. PLoS One. 2014;9(2):e89944.
3. Bergen H, Hawton K, Waters K, Ness J, Cooper J, Steeg S, Kapur N. Premature death after self-harm: a multicentre cohort study. Lancet. 2012; 380(9853):1568–74.
4. Ness J, Hawton K, Bergen H, Cooper J, Steeg S, Kapur N, Clarke M, Waters K. Alcohol use and misuse, self-harm and subsequent mortality: an epidemiological and longitudinal study from the multicentre study of self-harm in England. Emerg Med J. 2015;32(10):793–9.
5. NICE. The long term care and treatment of self-harm. Clinical guideline 133. London: National Institute of Health and Care Excellence; 2011.
6. Kapur N, Steeg S, Webb R, Haigh M, Bergen H, Hawton K, Ness J, Waters K, Cooper J. Does clinical management improve outcomes following self-harm? Results from the multicentre study of self-harm in England. PLoS One. 2013;8(8):e70434.
7. Steeg S, Emsley R, Carr M, Cooper J, Kapur N. Routine hospital management of self-harm and risk of further self-harm: propensity score analysis using record-based cohort data. Psychol Med. 2017;48(2):1–12.

8. Quinlivan L, Cooper J, Steeg S, Davies L, Hawton K, Gunnell D, Kapur N. Scales for predicting risk following self-harm: an observational study in 32 hospitals in England. BMJ Open. 2014;4(5):e004732.

9. Quinlivan L, Cooper J, Davies L, Hawton K, Gunnell D, Kapur N. Which are the most useful scales for predicting repeat self-harm? A systematic review evaluating risk scales using measures of diagnostic accuracy. BMJ Open. 2016;6(2):e009297.

10. Carter G, Milner A, McGill K, Pirkis J, Kapur N, Spittal MJ. Predicting suicidal behaviours using clinical instruments: systematic review and meta-analysis of positive predictive values for risk scales. Br J Psychiatry. 2017;210(6):387-+.

11. Katz C, Randall JR, Sareen J, Chateau D, Walld R, Leslie WD, Wang J, Bolton JM. Predicting suicide with the SAD PERSONS scale. Depress Anxiety. 2017; 34(9):809–16.

12. Quinlivan L, Cooper J, Meehan D, Longson D, Potokar J, Hulme T, Marsden J, Brand F, Lange K, Riseborough E, et al. Predictive accuracy of risk scales following self-harm: multicentre, prospective cohort study. Br J Psychiatry. 2017;210(6):429-+.

13. Cooper J, Steeg S, Bennewith O, Lowe M, Gunnell D, House A, Hawton K, Kapur N. Are hospital services for self-harm getting better? An observational study examining management, service provision and temporal trends in England. BMJ Open. 2013;3(11):e003444.

14. Cooper J, Kapur N, Dunning J, Guthrie E, Appleby L, Mackway-Jones K. A clinical tool for assessing risk after self-harm. Ann Emerg Med. 2006; 48(4):459–66.

15. Steeg S, Kapur N, Webb R, Applegate E, Stewart SLK, Hawton K, Bergen H, Waters K, Cooper J. The development of a population-level clinical screening tool for self-harm repetition and suicide: the ReACT Self-Harm Rule. Psychol Med. 2012;42(11):2383–94.

16. Patterson WM, Dohn HH, Bird J, Patterson GA. Evaluation of suicidal patients - the sad persons scale. Psychosomatics. 1983;24(4):343-&.

17. Bolton J, Rae Spiwak R, Sareen J. Predicting suicide attempts with the sad persons scale: a longitudinal analysis. J Clin Psychiatry. 2012;73(6):e735–41.

18. Beck RW, Morris JB, Beck AT. Cross-validation of suicidal-intent-scale. Psychol Rep. 1974;34(2):445–6.

19. Carroll R, Metcalfe C, Gunnell D. Hospital management of self-harm patients and risk of repetition: systematic review and meta-analysis. J Affect Disord. 2014;168:476–83.

20. Kapur N, Cooper J, King-Hele S, Webb R, Lawlor M, Rodway C, Appleby L. The repetition of suicidal behavior: a multicenter cohort study. J Clin Psychiatry. 2006;67(10):1599–609.

21. Hawton K, Witt KG, Taylor Salisbury TL, Arensman E, Gunnell D, Hazell P, Townsend E, van Heeringen K. Psychosocial interventions for self-harm in adults. Cochrane Database Syst Rev. 2016;5. Art. No.: CD012189. https://doi.org/10.1002/14651858.CD012189.

22. Royston P, White IR. Multiple Imputation by Chained Equations (MICE): implementation in Stata. J Stat Softw. 2011;45(4):1–20.

23. Rubin DB. Multiple imputation for non-response in surveys. New York: John Wiley & Sons; 1987.

24. Altman DG, Bland JM. Diagnostic-tests-3 - receiver operating characteristic plots .7. Br Med J. 1994;309(6948):188.

25. Kapur N, Murphy E, Cooper J, Bergen H, Hawton K, Simkin S, Casey D, Horrocks J, Lilley R, Noble R, et al. Psychosocial assessment following self-harm: results from the multi-centre monitoring of self-harm project. J Affect Disord. 2008;106(3):285–93.

26. Hawes M, Yaseen Z, Briggs J, Galynker I. The Modular Assessment of Risk for Imminent Suicide (MARIS): a proof of concept for a multi-informant tool for evaluation of short-term. Compr Psychiatry. 2017;72:88–96.

27. Walsh CG, Ribeiro JD, Franklin JC. Predicting risk of suicide attempts over time through machine learning. Clin Psychol Sci. 2017;5(3):457–69.

28. Metz CE. BASIC PRINCIPLES OF ROC ANALYSIS. Semin Nucl Med. 1978; 8(4):283–98.

29. Hancock M, Kent P. Interpretation of dichotomous outcomes: risk, odds, risk ratios, odds ratios and number needed to treat. J Physiother. 2016; 62(3):172–4.

30. Runeson B, Odeberg J, Pettersson A, Edbom T, Adamsson IJ, Waern M. Instruments for the assessment of suicide risk: a systematic review evaluating the certainty of the evidence. PLoS One. 2017;12(7):e0180292.

31. Ryan CJ, Large MM. Suicide risk assessment: where are we now? Med J Aust. 2013;198(9):462–3.

32. Hunter C, Chantler K, Kapur N, Cooper J. Service user perspectives on psychosocial assessment following self-harm and its impact on further help-seeking: a qualitative study. J Affect Disord. 2013;145(3):315–23.

33. Miller IW, Camargo CA Jr, Arias SA, Sullivan AF, Allen MH, Goldstein AB, Manton AP, Espinola JA, Jones R, Hasegawa K, et al. Suicide prevention in an emergency department population the ED-SAFE study. Jama Psychiatry. 2017;74(6):563–70.

12

Associations between health-related self-efficacy and suicidality

Vivian Isaac[1], Chia-Yi Wu[2,3], Craig S. McLachlan[4] and Ming-Been Lee[3,5,6*] ⓘ

Abstract

Background: Few studies have focused on exploring the association of self-efficacy and suicidal behaviour. In this study, we aim to investigate the association between health-related self-efficacy and suicidality outcomes, including lifetime/recent suicidal ideation, suicidal attempts and future intent of suicide.

Methods: A computer-assisted telephone interview (CATI) system was used to draw potential respondents aged over 15 in Taiwan via telephone numbers, which were selected by a stratified proportional randomization method according to the distribution of population size in different geographic areas of Taiwan. We obtained available information on suicide behaviours for the analysis of 2110 participants. Logistic regression was applied to investigate the independent effect of health-related self-efficacy on life-time suicidal thoughts and attempts.

Results: Suicidality measured as suicide ideation and attempted suicide was reported as 12.6 and 2.7% respectively in the sample. Among those with suicide ideation, 9.8% had thoughts of future suicide intent. Female gender, low education, people living alone or separated, history of psychiatric disorders, substance abuse, poor self-rated mental health and physical health were associated with suicidality factors. Low health-related self-efficacy was associated with lifetime suicide ideation, prior suicide attempt and future suicidal intent. Among those with recent suicidal ideation, low health self-efficacy was independently associated with future suicide intent after adjustment of gender, age, education, marital status, substance abuse, psychological distress, poor mental and physical health.

Conclusion: Health-related self-efficacy was associated with suicide risks across different time points from prior ideation to future intention. Evaluation of the progress of self-efficacy in health may be long-term targets of intervention in suicide prevention strategies.

Keywords: Self-efficacy, Suicidality, Computer-assisted telephone interview, Taiwan

Background

The suicide rate in Taiwan has been decreasing since 2010 from a high rate of 16.8 to 15.7 per 100,000 in 2015 according to national statistical data. Suicide poses a significant social and economic burden [1]. Developing strategies that target suicide behaviours may improve suicide rates. Suicide behaviour carries a 10–15% lifetime risk of death [2, 3]. Psychiatric morbidities such as depression and anxiety are strongly associated with suicidal ideation and suicide death in Taiwan [2, 4]. Prior suicide attempts are known to be associated with a higher level of engagement of mental health services [5]. The possible risk factors leading to suicide ideation include substance use [6], gender, aging, divorce and unemployment [7].

Suicidality is a complex multifactorial process. It is not known whether self-efficacy impacts on suicide behaviours in the cultural context of Taiwan. Health confidence and health-related self-efficacy are adaptive cognitive factors that have been shown to improve health behaviours [8]. A higher sense of self-efficacy and control has consistently shown to predict better positive health outcomes [9, 10]. Numerous studies have adopted health practices that have measured self-efficacy with respect to behavioural changes. For example, self-efficacy has been measured in chronic disease management, diet, exercise, and tobacco control [11–13].

* Correspondence: mingbeen@ntu.edu.tw
[3]Taiwan Suicide Prevention Center, Taipei, Taiwan
[5]Departments of Psychiatry, National Taiwan University College of Medicine & National Taiwan University Hospital, Taipei, Taiwan
Full list of author information is available at the end of the article

Only a few studies have globally focused on the association of self-efficacy and suicidal behaviour [14]. A community-based household survey in rural Japan showed lower general self-efficacy was associated with increased rates of suicidal ideation. Feng et al. has proposed that general self-efficacy functions as a mechanism of self-confidence to cope with challenging life stresses [15]. In this study, we aim to investigate the independent association between health-related self-efficacy and suicidal trajectories/outcomes including lifetime suicidal ideation, suicidal attempts and future intent of suicide. These aims were explored in a representative sample throughout the island of Taiwan.

Methods

Participants and procedure

Population study sampling was performed via the project administrator of Taiwan Suicide Prevention Centre (TSPC). Specifically, participants were contacted upon sampling via a telephone survey on population mental health, knowledge and behaviour of suicide prevention carried out by the Centre. The ethical approval was acquired from the general hospital the corresponding author affiliates (reference number 201204034RIC). The survey recruited a representative random sample of the general population aged over 15 in Taiwan. Data were collected between July 14th and 23th in 2015 by personnel with specific training for this survey. A computer-assisted telephone interview (CATI) system was used to draw potential respondents via telephone numbers selected by a stratified proportional randomization method according to the distribution of population size, gender and age in different geographic areas of Taiwan. In total, initially, 21,384 subjects landline phone numbers were randomly selected, and 5430 respondents aged 15 years or older were contacted, with 2110 respondents agreed to take part in the survey anonymously over the phone and accomplished the interview (with sampling error of ± 2.10% in 95% confidence interval).

Measurements

The questionnaire used in the interview included demographics (age, gender, education level, occupation and marital status) and health-related bio-behavioural measures (self-rated physical/mental health, self-efficacy), and suicide risk factors (suicide-related items, psychopathology, and substance use). Definition and assessment for these key variables are listed below.

Suicide ideation/intention to suicide: We evaluated whether the respondents had had previous suicide ideation across different time points; lifetime and in the past week. We also assessed whether they may have future suicide intent through the question, "Is it likely that you may attempt suicide in the future?"

Suicide attempts: The respondents were asked whether they had engaged in a suicide attempt and when this occurred. We determined if this attempt ever happened in their lifetime (classified as a previous attempt).

Health-related measures: A single item question was used to assess health-related self-efficacy based on standard methodology for measuring self-efficacy beliefs [16]. The participants were asked, "How much confidence, from a scale of 0 to 100, do you think you have to control over your own health conditions?" We also inquired about self-rated health conditions in both physical and mental aspects, with the ratings from 0 (very poor) to 4 (very good) [17].

Psychopathology assessment: We used the Brief Symptom Rating Scale to measure the level of psychological distress in the past week of the respondents [18]. It is a 5-item Likert scale (scores of 0 to 4) that contained the following questions [2]: (1) having trouble falling asleep (insomnia); (2) feeling tense or keyed up (anxiety); (3) feeling easily annoyed or irritated (hostility); (4) feeling low in mood (depression); and (5) feeling inferior to others (inferiority).

Substance abuse: A single question was used to assess whether a previous substance misuse leading to life impairments had occurred due to any illicit drug, prescription medication, or alcohol. Substance abuse during any period of lifetime was recorded as a binary response of yes or no based on self-report.

Data analysis

Descriptive statistics of demographic variables are presented. The following tests were used for data analyses. Univariate and bivariate tabulation was conducted as a prerequisite for multivariate analyses. Associations between independent variables and lifetime suicidal ideation, suicide attempt and future suicide intent were performed using chi-square tests and then were presented as odds ratios (ORs) with 95% confidence intervals (CIs). Self-efficacy score was significantly skewed, therefore the score was log-transformed for further analysis. In order to identify low health-related self-efficacy, a tertile spit of the self-efficacy scale was conducted. The participants in the lower tertile (represented a score of below 80) were categorised as having low health self-efficacy. Multivariate logistic regression was applied to investigate the independent effect of health-related self-efficacy on lifetime suicidal thought and attempt after separate and successive inclusion of other independent variables in the model. The independent effects of health- related self-efficacy on associations with future suicide intent were performed. The subgroup here was those with life-time suicidal ideation. The model was adjusted for age, gender, marital status, history of psychiatric disorders, substance abuse and self-rated physical & mental health. We modelled whether self-efficacy would be independently associated with different assessments of suicidality (suicide attempt, lifetime suicide ideation and future intent). All statistical analyses were performed using the SPSS v21, and statistical significance was defined as a value of $p < 0.05$.

Results

We obtained available information on suicide behaviours for the analysis of 2110 participants. Among the cohort, 53.2% were women. People who aged 15–19 years represented 20.1% of the sample; nearly half were those aged between 30 and 60 years (52.2%), and 27.7% was aged 60 years and above. About two-third (65.6%) of the participants was married and 28.2% was single. Sample characteristics were reported in Table 1. The mean (standard deviation) score of health-related self-efficacy was 78.8 (13.4). We stratified the self-efficacy subgroups based on self-efficacy score tertiles. A low tertile self-efficacy score we defined as below 80. The mean score for low self-efficacy group was 63.8 (10.8), this was significantly lower than rest of the sample 86.1 (6.9), $t = 55.8$, $p < 0.001$. Participants with psychological distress and substance abuse of drug or alcohol represented in 15 and 2.9% of the sample, respectively. One-fourth (25.4%) reported poor self-rated physical health and 14.4% had poor self-rated mental health. Suicidality measured as lifetime suicidal ideation and

Table 1 Characteristics of the sample ($N = 2110$)

	N (%)
Gender	
Female	1122 (53.2)
Male	988 (46.8)
Age	
15–29	424 (20.1)
30–59	1101 (52.2)
60 & above	585 (27.7)
Education[a]	
Elementary school and below	212 (10.0)
Junior high school	267 (12.7)
Senior/vocational high school	694 (32.9)
Technical college	274 (13.0)
College	545 (25.8)
Graduate school	113 (5.4)
Marital status[a]	
Single/Married	1979 (93.8)
Divorced/Widowed/Separated	126 (6.0)

[a]Missing = 5

prior attempted suicide were reported to be 12.6 and 2.7%, respectively. Among those with suicide ideation, 9.8% had thoughts of future intention of suicide.

Study factors associated with suicidality

Age and gender were not associated with suicidal behaviours in our sample (Table 2). However a higher education level had a protective effect with lower risk of suicidal attempt (OR = 0.4, 95% CI 0.2–0.7). People divorced or separated compared to those married or single had higher risks of suicidal thoughts (OR = 2.2, 95% CI 1.4–3.4) and attempted suicide (OR = 5.2, 95% CI 2.7–9.9). Psychological distress and substance abuse exposed a strong risk with suicidal behaviours. The risks for suicidal behaviours were about four times higher for those affected by psychopathological symptoms and six times for previous substance abuse. Specifically, the risk of suicidal thought was (OR = 4.3, 95% CI 3.2–5.7), suicidal attempt (OR = 4.6.1, 95% CI 3.5–10.4) and future suicide intent (OR = 10.9, 95% CI 5.1–22.9) for those with psychopathological symptoms. For substance abuse, the risk for suicidal thought was (OR = 6.0, 95% CI 3.5–10.1); attempted suicide (OR = 6.3, 95% CI 2.8–13.9) and future intent of suicide (OR = 6.4, 95% CI 2.4–17.3).

Poor self-rated mental health and physical health also showed associations with suicidality. The risk for suicidal ideation among those with poor self-rated mental health was (OR = 3.3, 95%CI 2.5–4.5). The risk increases for attempted suicide (OR = 5.3, 95% CI 3.1–9.1) and future suicide intent (OR = 9.7, 95% CI 4.7–19.6). For those with poor self-rated physical health the risk for suicidal ideation was (OR = 2.7, 95% CI 2.1–3.6), suicidal attempt (OR = 2.9, 95% CI 1.7–4.9) and future intent of suicide (OR = 3.9, 95% CI 1.9–7.9).

Health-related self-efficacy and suicidality

Low health self-efficacy was associated with suicidal behaviours. The risks for suicidal ideation, attempted suicide and future suicide intent were (OR = 3.2, 95% CI 2.5–4.2); (OR = 4.1, 95% CI 2.3–7.3) and (OR = 11.2, 95% CI 4.2–29.3) respectively. Tables 3 & 4 explained the stepwise logistic regression and factor adjustments. These factor adjustments were conducted individually and sequentially to investigate the independent association between low health-related self-efficacy and suicidal behaviours. Low health-related self-efficacy was associated with lifetime suicide ideation after controlling for gender, age, education, marital status, substance abuse, psychological distress, poor mental and physical health (OR = 2.0, 95% CI 1.5–2.8). Low health self-efficacy was associated with suicidal attempt after adjustment. The association weakened when sequential analysis of the factors self-rated mental and physical health were added to the models (OR = 1.9, 95% CI 1.0–3.7).

Table 2 Sample characteristics and suicidality

	Life time suicide ideation			Suicide attempt			Future suicide intent		
	No n (%)	Yes n (%)	OR (95% CI); p value	No n (%)	Yes n (%)	OR (95% CI); p value	No n (%)	Yes n (%)	OR (95% CI); p value
Gender									
Female	955 (85.1)	167 (14.9)	Ref	1086 (96.8)	36 (3.2)	Ref	1105 (98.5)	17 (1.5)	Ref
Male	889 (90.0)	99 (10.0)	0.6 (0.5–0.8); p = 0.001	968 (98.0)	20 (2)	0.6 (0.4–1.1); p = 0.10	972 (98.4)	18 (1.8)	1.0 (0.5–2.1); p = 0.86
Age									
15–29	382 (90.1)	42 (9.9)	Ref	415 (97.9)	9 (2.1)	Ref	421 (99.3)	3 (0.7)	Ref
30–59	947 (86.0)	154 (14.0)	1.5 (1.0–2.1); p = 0.03	1074 (97.5)	27 (2.5)	1.2 (0.5–2.5); p = 0.70	1080 (98.1)	21 (1.9)	2.7 (0.8–9.1); p = 0.10
60 & above	515 (88.0)	70 (12.0)	1.2 (0.8–1.8); p = 0.30	565 (96.6)	20 (3.4)	1.6 (0.7–3.6); p = 0.22	576 (98.5)	9 (1.5)	2.1 (0.6–8.1); p = 0.24
Education									
School level	1016 (86.6)	157 (13.4)	1.0	1130 (96.3)	43 (3.7)	1.0	1152 (98.2)	21 (1.8)	1.0
College & above	828 (88.4)	109 (11.6)	0.9 (0.7–1.1); p = 0.23	924 (98.6)	13 (1.4)	0.4 (0.2–0.7); p = 0.001	925 (98.7)	12 (1.3)	0.7 (0.3–1.5); p = 0.38
Marital status									
Single/Married	1742 (88.0)	237 (12.0)	1.0	1936 (97.8)	43 (2.2)	1.0	1947 (98.4)	32 (1.6)	1.0
Divorced/Widowed/ Separated	97 (77.0)	29 (23.0)	2.2 (1.4–3.4); p = 0.001	113 (89.7)	13 (10.3)	5.2 (2.7–9.9); p < 0.001	125 (99.2)	1 (0.8)	0.5 (0.06–3.5); p = 0.71
Substance abuse									
No	1810 (88.3)	239 (11.7)	1.0	2001 (97.7)	48 (2.3)	1.0	2021 (98.4)	28 (1.4)	1.0
Yes	34 (55.7)	27 (44.3)	6.0 (3.5–10.1); p < 0.001	53 (86.9)	8 (13.1)	6.3 (2.8–13.9); p < 0.001	56 (91.8)	5 (8.2)	6.4 (2.4–17.3); p = 0.002
Psychological distress									
No	1608 (90.6)	166 (9.4)	1.0	1746 (98.4)	28 (1.6)	1.0	1763 (99.4)	11 (0.6)	1.0
Yes	217 (69.1)	96 (30.9)	4.3 (3.2–5.7); p < 0.001	286 (91.1)	28 (8.9)	6.1 (3.5–10.4); p < 0.001	132 (89.2)	20 (6.4)	10.9 (5.1–22.9); p < 0.001
Poor Self-rated mental health									
No	1616 (89.9)	181 (10.1)	1.0	1767 (98.3)	30 (1.7)	1.0	1784 (99.3)	13 (0.7)	1.0
Yes	221 (72.7)	83 (27.3)	3.3 (2.5–4.5); p < 0.001	279 (91.8)	25 (8.2)	5.3 (3.1–9.1); p < 0.001	284 (93.4)	20 (6.6)	9.7 (4.7–19.6); p < 0.001
Poor self-rated physical health									
No	1421 (90.7)	145 (9.3)	1.0	1538 (98.2)	28 (1.8)	1.0	1552 (99.1)	14 (0.8)	1.0
Yes	418 (78.0)	118 (22.0)	2.7 (2.1–3.6); p < 0.001	509 (95.0)	27 (5.0)	2.9 (1.7–4.9); p < 0.001	518 (96.6)	18 (3.4)	3.9 (1.9–7.9); p < 0.001
Health self-efficacy score									
>=80	1265 (91.9)	111 (8.1)	Ref	1358 (98.7)	18 (1.3)	Ref	1371 (99.6)	5 (0.4)	Ref
<80	515 (77.9)	146 (22.1)	3.2 (2.5–4.2); p < 0.001	627 (94.9)	34 (5.1)	4.1 (2.2–7.3)	635 (96.1)	26 (3.9)	11.2 (4.2–29.3)

OR (95% CI) Odds Ratio (95% Confidence Interval)

Table 3 Logistic regression for the association between low health self-efficacy and lifetime suicide ideation

| | Life-time suicide ideation | | | |
| | Individual adjustment[a] | | Sequential adjustment[b] | |
	OR (95% CI)	χ2 (df) p	OR (95% CI)	χ2 (df) p
Unadjusted	3.2 (2.5–4.2)			
Gender	3.3 (2.5–4.3)	75.8 (1) < 0.001	3.3 (2.5–4.3)	75.8 (1) < 0.001
Age	3.3 (2.5–4.3)	74.4 (1) < 0.001	3.3 (2.5–4.3)	74.4 (1) < 0.001
Education	3.3 (2.5–4.3)	73.9 (1) < 0.001	3.3 (2.5–4.3)	73.9 (1) < 0.001
Marital status	3.1 (2.4–4.1)	70.0 (1) < 0.001	3.2 (2.5–4.3)	71.8 (1) < 0.001
Substance abuse	2.9 (2.3–3.9)	61.6 (1) < 0.001	2.9 (2.3–3.9)	60.4 (1) < 0.001
Psychological distress	2.6 (2.0–3.5)	47.5 (1) < 0.001	2.5 (1.9–3.3)	38.8 (1) < 0.001
Poor self-rated mental health	2.6 (1.9–3.4)	42.6 (1) < 0.001	2.2 (1.6–3.0)	26.9 (1) < 0.001
Poor self-rated physical health	2.5 (1.8–3.3)	39.4 (1) < 0.001	2.0 (1.5–2.8)	20.4 (1) < 0.001

OR (95% CI) Odds Ratio (95% Confidence Interval)
[a]Individual adjustments: adjusted for gender, age, marital status, etc.; [b]sequential adjustments: adjusted for gender, gender + age, gender +age + marital status, etc

Among those with lifetime suicidal ideation, stepwise logistic regression demonstrated an association between low health self-efficacy and future suicide intent (Table 5). Low health self-efficacy was independently associated with future intent even after adjustment of gender, age, education, marital status, substance abuse, psychological distress, poor mental and physical health (OR = 4.8, 95% CI 1.0–22.6). We repeated the analyses with self-efficacy as a continuous variable and the association between self-efficacy score and suicidality remained unaltered.

Discussion

In a large community-based telephone interview in Taiwan, we demonstrated that lower levels of health-related self-efficacy were associated with suicidality (i.e., lifetime suicidal ideation, past suicidal attempts and having future intention of suicide). The study findings were generally typical of the literature globally and for the region. In our sample, 12.6% had suicidal ideation and 2. 7% attempted suicide. Globally, the estimated lifetime prevalence (SE) of suicidal ideation, plan, and attempt in cross-national sample is 9.2% (0.1), 3.1% (0.1), and 2.7% (0.1) [19]. In the year 2010, a weighted prevalence of 18.5% was reported for lifetime suicidal ideation in a nationwide community survey conducted using a computer-aided telephone interview system with residents aged ≥15 years in Taiwan [2].

Our study and others have shown that female gender, low education, people living alone or separated, history of psychiatric disorders and substance abuse were associated with suicidality [20–24]. In particular we found female gender was associated with lifetime suicidal thought but not attempt and this may reflect higher prevalence of depression among women than men [25]. While this may seem paradoxical, women in Asian

Table 4 Logistic regression for the association between low health self-efficacy and suicide attempt

| | Attempted suicide in the past | | | |
| | Individual adjustment[a] | | Sequential adjustment[b] | |
	OR (95% CI)	χ2 (df) p	OR (95% CI)	χ2 (df) p
Unadjusted	4.1 (2.3–7.3)	22.7 (1) < 0.001		
Gender	4.1 (2.3–7.4)	23.1 (1) < 0.001	4.1 (2.3–7.4)	23.1 (1) < 0.001
Age	3.9 (2.2–7.1)	21.5 (1) < 0.001	4.0 (2.2–7.2)	21.9 (1) < 0.001
Education	3.8 (2.2–6.9)	20.9 (1) < 0.001	3.8 (2.1–6.9)	20.5 (1) < 0.001
Marital status	3.7 (2.0–6.7)	19.7 (1) < 0.001	3.7 (2.1–6.6)	18.9 (1) < 0.001
Substance abuse	3.6 (2.0–6.5)	18.4 (1) < 0.001	3.3 (1.8–6.1)	15.7 (1) < 0.001
Psychological distress	3.0 (1.6–5.5)	12.9 (1) 0.001	2.5 (1.4–4.7)	8.5 (1) 0.004
Poor self-rated mental health	2.6 (1.4–4.8)	8.8 (1) 0.003	2.0 (1.0–3.8)	4.4 (1) 0.04
Poor self-rated physical health	2.9 (1.6–5.6)	11.5 (1) 0.001	1.9 (1.0–3.7)	3.4 (1) 0.07

OR (95% CI) Odds Ratio (95% Confidence Interval)
[a]Individual adjustments: adjusted for gender, age, marital status, etc.; [b]sequential adjustments: adjusted for gender, gender + age, gender +age + marital status, etc

Table 5 Logistic regression for the association between low health self-efficacy and future suicide intent

	Future suicide intent			
	Individual adjustment[a]		Sequential adjustment[b]	
	OR (95% CI)	χ2 (df) p	OR (95% CI)	χ2 (df) p
Unadjusted	9.6 (2.2–42.0)	9.1 (1) 0.002		
Gender	9.4 (2.1–41.1)	8.9 (1) 0.003	9.4 (2.1–41.1)	8.9 (1) 0.003
Age	9.6 (2.2–41.7)	9.0 (1) 0.003	9.3 (2.1–40.9)	8.8 (1) 0.003
Education	9.5 (2.2–41.7)	9.0 (1) 0.003	9.3 (2.1–40.6)	8.7 (1) 0.003
Marital status	10.0 (2.3–43.7)	9.4 (1) 0.002	9.5 (2.2–41.8)	8.9 (1) 0.003
Substance abuse	9.6 (2.2–41.9)	9.0 (1) 0.003	9.4 (2.1–41.5)	8.8 (1) 0.003
Psychological distress	6.5 (1.5–29.0)	6.0 (1) 0.01	5.9 (1.3–27.2)	5.4 (1) 0.02
Poor self-rated mental health	7.1 (1.6–31.9)	6.7 (1) 0.01	5.6 (1.2–25.7)	5.0 (1) 0.03
Poor self-rated physical health	7.3 (1.6–33.0)	6.8 (1) 0.009	4.8 (1.0–22.6)	4.9 (1) 0.04

OR (95% CI) Odds Ratio (95% Confidence Interval)

[a]Individual adjustments: adjusted for gender, age, marital status, etc.; [b]sequential adjustments: adjusted for gender, gender + age, gender +age + marital status, etc

countries are more likely to seek treatment help for depression compared to male counter parts [26]. Low-education may result in socio-economic disadvantage, unemployment and low-income and in turn increase suicidal risk [4, 27]. Moreover, living alone is a predictor of suicidality, and it is proposed that the diminished family connectedness interacts with suicidal behaviours [28]. In our study and others, it is summarized that the presence of psychiatric disorders and substance abuse convey the highest risk for suicide [20–24].

We demonstrated an increased risk of lifetime suicidal thought or suicidal attempt with low self-efficacy was independent of perceived mental and physical health. Importantly, among those with lifetime suicidal thought, health-related self-efficacy was an independent predictor of having thoughts for suicide actions in the future. A growing body of evidence supports the relationship between self-efficacy and sense of personal control over behaviour change. Indeed self-efficacy has an important role in patient health outcomes [29, 30]. Self-efficacy has been identified as a significant factor explaining the benefits of treatment and health promoting behavioural change in smoking cessation, alcohol and weight loss and chronic disease self-management [31–33]. Health self-efficacy reflects individual's coping ability and confidence in their ability to take care of their health in different circumstances [16]. As health self-efficacy indicates the perceived ability to challenge and cope with adverse situations and develop a sense of health control, it is possible for health self-efficacy to have a direct or indirect effect (difficulty coping with stress and health problems) on suicidal behaviour [34].

The sensitivity of the association between health self-efficacy and suicidality was confirmed in our subgroup analyses. For example, among those with lifetime suicidal ideation, low health self-efficacy was associated with future suicide intent. Hence, health self-efficacy assessment may be a sensitive cognitive substrate to screen people with predisposed risk factors for suicide. Moreover, health self-efficacy assessment is simple and can be used by health professionals without much stigmatisation associated with binary mental health assessment scales. Increasing self-regulation, planning behaviour, positive feedback and empowerment can increase self-efficacy in carrying out lifestyle changes. There is evidence that mental health self-efficacy influences symptom outcomes when clients use a self-guided mobile phone and web-based psychotherapeutic intervention [35]. However longitudinal studies are needed to confirm the causal associations between the changes in health self-efficacy and suicidal behaviour in the longer term. Future research could also assess the potential of health self-efficacy interventions in reducing suicidal thoughts and further risks of suicide, such as future intent or prior attempts of suicide.

Our study has salient strengths. The CATI survey has been conducted by the TSPC over a decade. The findings were derived from a large sample size randomly selected, thus ensuring representativeness. In this study, we simultaneously measured suicidality outcomes (lifetime/recent suicidal thought, prior attempt and future intent) in a random sample. Given that the topic is sensitive and complex, the responders could reply to these questions more comfortably via telephone interview due to anonymity. We controlled from major confounding factors known to be associated with suicidality, including self-perception of mental health and physical health. This emphasizes that health self-efficacy is an independent construct that is not superimposed or biased by self-perception of health. The main limitation of the study was that the findings were based on cross-sectional analyses, hence the causal inference could not be achieved.

It is possible that participants with lower health-related self-efficacy may have difficulties managing their health and indulge in risky behaviours such as substance abuse. Indeed substance abuse is associated with suicidal behaviours. We had not measured factors such as whether lower health literacy was associated with reduced health-related self-efficacy and suicidal behaviours. On the other hand as we report in our study lower self-efficacy may serve as a marker for suicidal behaviours. Further, telephone interviews have innate limitations. For example, we drew landline numbers based on the registration list in computer directories and did not include mobile phone users, thus the results could only generalize to people who have landlines. However, CATI is a professional technique in collecting research data. Although such interviews may be influenced by participant environmental factors, which the researcher has limited control, structured questions and standard operating procedures developed by the researchers at the TSPC were followed by experienced personnel with specific training, thus ensuring that reliable data were acquired. Moreover, the research team has careful inspection of the yearly results drew from CATI for more than 12 years and published articles elsewhere [2, 18], which provide evidence of the reliability of our study.

Regardless of these limitations, the study has implications for identifying and intervening individuals with suicidal risk. We have shown for the first time an association between health-related self-efficacy and lifetime suicidal thought and behaviour in Taiwan; and that the association was robust and was independent of factors known to be associated with suicidality. The authors concluded that health-related self-efficacy was associated with suicide risks in different time points. Perceived efficacy in health was significantly affected current or prior suicide ideation and future suicide intent. Our study adds to the literature on potentially modifiable factors and that evaluation of the progress of self-efficacy in health may be long-term targets of intervention in suicide prevention strategies.

Abbreviations
CATI: Computer-assisted telephone interview; CIs: Confidence intervals; ORs: Odds ratios; TSPC: Taiwan Suicide Prevention Centre

Acknowledgements
The authors would like to thank their colleagues at Taiwan Suicide Prevention Center for their kind help with administration help.

Funding
The study was supported by the Ministry of Health and Welfare, Executive Yuen, Taiwan (grant number M05B4167).

Authors' contributions
VI and CW contributed to conceiving the original idea to investigate self-efficacy and suicidality, and included questions in the 2015 National Suicide Prevention Survey. VI contributed to the analysis of the research and in the manuscript preparation. CW contributed to the design, conduct of the research and in the manuscript preparation. CM contributed to the critical review and in the manuscript preparation. ML contributed to the funding of the project and the design, conduct and analysis of the research. All authors have read and approved the final version of the manuscript.

Competing interests
The authors declare that they have no competing interests.

Author details
[1]Flinders Rural Health South Australia, Flinders University, Renmark, Australia. [2]School of Nursing, National Taiwan University College of Medicine, Taipei, Taiwan. [3]Taiwan Suicide Prevention Center, Taipei, Taiwan. [4]Rural Clinical School, University of New South Wales, Sydney, Australia. [5]Departments of Psychiatry, National Taiwan University College of Medicine & National Taiwan University Hospital, Taipei, Taiwan. [6]Department of Psychiatry, Shin Kong Wu Ho-Su Memorial Hospital, Taipei, Taiwan.

References
1. Law CK, Yip PS, Chen YY. The economic and potential years of life lost from suicide in Taiwan, 1997-2007. Crisis. 2011;32(3):152–9.
2. Lee JI, Lee MB, Liao SC, Chang CM, Sung SC, Chiang HC, Tai CW. Prevalence of suicidal ideation and associated risk factors in the general population. J Formos Med Assoc. 2010;109(2):138–47.
3. Suominen K, Isometsa E, Suokas J, Haukka J, Achte K, Lonnqvist J. Completed suicide after a suicide attempt: a 37-year follow-up study. Am J Psychiatry. 2004;161(3):562–3.
4. Cheng ATA, Chen THH, Chen C-C, Jenkins R. Psychosocial and psychiatric risk factors for suicide. Case-control psychological autopsy study. Br J Psychiatry. 2000;177(4):360–5.
5. Chen IM, Liao SC, Lee MB, Wu CY, Lin PH, Chen WJ. Risk factors of suicide mortality among multiple attempters: a national registry study in Taiwan. J Formos Med Assoc. 2016;115(5):364–71.
6. Gau SS, Chen YY, Tsai FJ, Lee MB, Chiu YN, Soong WT, Hwu HG. Risk factors for suicide in Taiwanese college students. J Am Coll Heal. 2008;57(2):135–42.
7. Chuang H-L, Huang W-C. A re-examination of the suicide rates in Taiwan. Soc Indic Res. 2007;83(3):465–85.
8. Wasson J, Coleman EA. Health confidence: an essential measure for patient engagement and better practice. Fam Pract Manag. 2014;21(5):8–12.
9. Kaplan RM, Ries AL, Prewitt LM, Eakin E. Self-efficacy expectations predict survival for patients with chronic obstructive pulmonary disease. Health Psychol. 1994;13(4):366–8.
10. Bandura A. Self-efficacy: toward a unifying theory of behavioral change. Psychol Rev. 1977;84(2):191–215.
11. Adriaanse MA, CDW V, DTD DR, Hox JJ, JBF DW. Do implementation intentions help to eat a healthy diet? A systematic review and meta-analysis of the empirical evidence. Appetite. 2011;56(1):183–93.
12. Gwaltney CJ, Metrik J, Kahler CW, Shiffman S. Self-efficacy and smoking cessation: a meta-analysis. Psychol Addict Behav. 2009;23(1):56–66.
13. Warsi A, Wang PS, LaValley MP, Avorn J, Solomon DH. Self-management education programs in chronic disease: a systematic review and methodological critique of the literature. Arch Intern Med. 2004;164(15): 1641–9.
14. Valois RF, Zullig KJ, Hunter AA. Association between adolescent suicide ideation, suicide attempts and emotional self-efficacy. J Child Fam Stud. 2015;24(2):237–48.
15. Feng J, Li S, Chen H. Impacts of stress, self-efficacy, and optimism on suicide ideation among rehabilitation patients with acute pesticide poisoning. PLoS One. 2015;10(2):e0118011.
16. Finney Rutten LJ, Hesse BW, St. Sauver JL, Wilson P, Chawla N, Hartigan DB, Moser RP, Taplin S, Glasgow R, Arora NK. Health self-efficacy among populations with multiple chronic conditions: the value of patient-centered communication. Adv Ther. 2016;33(8):1440–51.
17. Ahmad F, Jhajj AK, Stewart DE, Burghardt M, Bierman AS. Single item measures of self-rated mental health: a scoping review. BMC Health Serv Res. 2014;14(1):398.

18. Wu CY, Lee JI, Lee MB, Liao SC, Chang CM, Chen HC, Lung FW. Predictive validity of a five-item symptom checklist to screen psychiatric morbidity and suicide ideation in general population and psychiatric settings. J Formos Med Assoc. 2016;115(6):395–403.

19. Nock MK, Borges G, Bromet EJ, Alonso J, Angermeyer M, Beautrais A, Bruffaerts R, Chiu WT, de Girolamo G, Gluzman S, et al. Cross-National Prevalence and risk factors for suicidal ideation, plans, and attempts. Br J Psychiatry. 2008;192:98–105.

20. Baxter D, Appleby L. Case register study of suicide risk in mental disorders. Br J Psychiatry. 1999;175(4):322–6.

21. Chang H-J, Yang C-Y, Lin C-R, Ku Y-L, Lee M-B. Determinants of suicidal ideation in Taiwanese urban adolescents. J Formos Med Assoc. 2008;107(2): 156–64.

22. Verona E, Sachs-Ericsson N, Joiner TE Jr. Suicide attempts associated with externalizing psychopathology in an epidemiological sample. Am J Psychiatr. 2004;161(3):444–51.

23. Suominen K, Henriksson M, Suokas J, Isometsa E, Ostamo A, Lonnqvist J. Mental disorders and comorbidity in attempted suicide. Acta Psychiatr Scand. 1996;94(4):234–40.

24. Henriksson MM, Aro HM, Marttunen MJ, Heikkinen ME, Isometsa ET, Kuoppasalmi KI, Lonnqvist JK. Mental disorders and comorbidity in suicide. Am J Psychiatry. 1993;150(6):935–40.

25. Tai SY, Ma TC, Wang LC, Yang YH. A community-based walk-in screening of depression in Taiwan. TheScientificWorldJOURNAL. 2014;2014:184018.

26. Chang H. Psychological distress and help-seeking among Taiwanese college students: role of gender and student status. Br J Guid Couns. 2007;35(3): 347–55.

27. Yen YC, Yang MJ, Yang MS, Lung FW, Shih CH, Hahn CY, Lo HY. Suicidal ideation and associated factors among community-dwelling elders in Taiwan. Psychiatry Clin Neurosci. 2005;59(4):365–71.

28. Purcell B, Heisel MJ, Speice J, Franus N, Conwell Y, Duberstein PR. Family connectedness moderates the association between living alone and suicide ideation in a clinical sample of adults 50 years and older. Am J Geriatr Psychiatry. 2012;20(8):717–23.

29. Bandura A. Health promotion by social cognitive means. Health Educ Behav. 2004;31(2):143–64.

30. Holloway A, Watson HE. Role of self-efficacy and behaviour change. Int J Nurs Pract. 2002;8(2):106–15.

31. Gwaltney CJ, Metrik J, Kahler CW, Shiffman S. Self-efficacy and smoking cessation: a meta-analysis. Psychol Addict Behav. 2009;23(1) https://doi.org/10.1037/a0013529.

32. Byrne S, Barry D, Petry NM. Predictors of weight loss success: exercise vs. dietary self-efficacy and treatment attendance. Appetite. 2012;58(2):695–8.

33. Connor JP, George SM, Gullo MJ, Kelly AB, Young RM. A prospective study of alcohol expectancies and self-efficacy as predictors of young adolescent alcohol misuse. Alcohol Alcoholism (Oxford, Oxfordshire). 2011;46(2):161–9.

34. Kobayashi Y, Fujita K, Kaneko Y, Motohashi Y. Self-efficacy as a suicidal ideation predictor: a population cohort study in rural Japan. Open J Prev Med. 2015;5:61–71.

35. Clarke J, Proudfoot J, Birch M-R, Whitton AE, Parker G, Manicavasagar V, Harrison V, Christensen H, Hadzi-Pavlovic D. Effects of mental health self-efficacy on outcomes of a mobile phone and web intervention for mild-to-moderate depression, anxiety and stress: secondary analysis of a randomised controlled trial. BMC Psychiatry. 2014;14(1):272.

13

Associations of training to assist a suicidal person with subsequent quality of support: results from a national survey of the Australian public

Anthony F. Jorm*[iD], Angela Nicholas, Jane Pirkis, Alyssia Rossetto and Nicola J. Reavley

Abstract

Background: When a person is in severe distress, people in their social network can potentially take action to reduce the person's suicide risk. The present study used data from a community survey to examine whether people who had received training in how to assist a person at risk of suicide had higher quality intentions and actions to provide support.

Methods: A national telephone survey was carried out with 3002 Australian adults on attitudes and intentions toward helping someone in severe distress or at risk of suicide as well as actions taken. Participants were asked about their intentions to assist a hypothetical person in a vignette and about any actions they took to assist a family member or friend in distress over the previous 12 months. Participants were also asked whether they had received professional training, Mental Health First Aid training or other training in how to assist a person at risk of suicide.

Results: Responses covered ten intentions/actions that were recommended in guidelines for the public on how to support a suicidal person and 5 that were recommended against in the guidelines. Scales were created to measure positive and negative intentions to act and positive and negative actions taken. All three types of training were associated with greater positive intentions and actions, and with lesser negative intentions. These associations were largely due to a greater willingness of those trained to talk openly about suicide with a person in distress.

Conclusions: Training in how to support a person at risk of suicide is associated with better quality of support. Such training merits wider dissemination in the community.

Keywords: Suicide, Mental health first aid, Gatekeepers

Background

While mental health and primary care services can play an important role in detecting suicide risk and acting to reduce it, many people at risk of suicide are not in immediate contact with services. Psychological autopsy studies show that less than half of people who die by suicide are in contact with primary care services in the month before their death, and the rate of contact is even lower for specialist mental health care [1, 2]. For this reason, members of a suicidal person's social network may be well placed to detect and act to reduce the person's suicide risk. However, there are a number of barriers to members of a person's social network taking on this role. While about one-third to a half of people who die by suicide explicitly communicate their intent to family members [3], in other cases the indicators of suicidal intent may be unclear and misread by the person's family and friends [4, 5], and thereby not prompt preventive action. People in the social network may also not feel comfortable raising the issue of suicide with the person and alerting others in the social network [4]. They may also respond in a dismissive or disapproving way to

* Correspondence: ajorm@unimelb.edu.au
Centre for Mental Health, Melbourne School of Population and Global Health, The University of Melbourne, 207 Bouverie St, Carlton, VIC 3010, Australia

the person's expressions of suicidal feelings [6], thereby shutting down communication.

There is a need to determine what actions members of a suicidal person's social network can take that are likely to be helpful and also what actions should be avoided. However, it is not feasible to test the preventive effects of specific actions by the public using experimental methods. For this reason, expert consensus has been used to develop suicide first aid guidelines for the public using the Delphi method. Kelly and colleagues [7] recruited 22 professionals, 10 people who had been suicidal in the past and 6 carers of people who had been suicidal in the past and presented them with 114 statements about how to assist someone who is thinking about suicide. These statements were sourced through a systematic search of both professional and lay literature. Thirty of these statements were endorsed at a high level and formed into guidelines. Subsequently, Ross and colleagues [8] re-developed the guidelines using two expert panels, comprising 41 suicide prevention professionals and 35 consumer advocates. The panelists rated 436 statements and endorsed 164 which were used to form updated guidelines. These guidelines provide a standard for improving the support that members of the public provide to suicidal persons in their social network.

When judged against these guidelines, community survey data reveal limitations in the public's ability to act effectively to prevent suicide. In two Australian national surveys, respondents were shown a vignette of a person with depression and suicidal thoughts and asked what they would do if the person was someone they knew and cared about [9, 10]. Coding of open-ended responses showed that while many would listen to the person, provide support and encourage professional help-seeking, very few would assess the person's risk of suicide or act to reduce this.

A range of gatekeeper training programs have been developed to improve the response of the public and professionals to suicidal persons. A review of these programs concluded that gatekeeper training can improve knowledge, beliefs/attitudes, self-efficacy, and reluctance to intervene, but transfer to actual intervention behaviour is largely unstudied [11]. In Australia, a number of training programs have been rolled out to improve the public's ability to assist suicidal persons. Probably the most widespread is Mental Health First Aid (MHFA), which is a 12–14 h course training members of the public in how to provide initial assistance to someone developing a mental health problem or in a mental health crisis, including helping a person with suicidal thoughts or behaviours [12]. MHFA training has been received by over 2% of the Australian population. A meta-analysis of trials evaluating MHFA showed improvements in knowledge, stigmatizing attitudes and helping behaviours

towards people with mental health problems [13]. However, there has not been any specific evaluation of the impact of MHFA training on support given to suicidal persons. Other common programs in Australia are QPR (Question, Persuade, and Refer) and Applied Suicide Intervention Skills Training (ASIST). QPR is a 1.5–2 h course specifically on suicide prevention. Evaluations of QPR have shown improvements in knowledge, self-efficacy and helping behaviour [14]. ASIST is a 2-day program aimed at both professionals and the public. Evaluations of ASIST have found improvements in knowledge, confidence and intervention skills, but mixed results on intervention behaviour [15].

The present study aimed to use Australian national survey data to investigate associations between training in how to assist a suicidal person and actions taken on suicide. The survey investigated Australian community members' attitudes, intentions and behaviours toward helping someone in severe distress or at risk of suicide. As part of this survey, participants were asked about their intentions to assist a hypothetical person in a vignette and about any actions they took to assist a family member or friend in distress over the previous 12 months. Participants were asked about intentions and actions that were either recommended or not recommended in the expert-consensus guidelines developed by Ross and colleagues [8]. Participants were also asked about any training or course they had taken in how to help someone who is suicidal, allowing a comparison between those who had received various types of training and those untrained. It was hypothesized that people who had received training would have higher quality intentions and actions.

Methods

Participants

The survey was commissioned by *beyondblue*, which is an Australian, non-government non-profit organization working to address issues associated with depression and anxiety disorders. The survey was conducted by Roy Morgan Research Ltd. in March 2017. The sample was drawn by a process of random digit dialing of both landlines and mobile telephones covering the whole of Australia. Up to six calls per number were made to establish contact. Interviewers ascertained whether there were residents in the household aged 18 or over and, if there were multiple, selected one for interview using the next-birthday method. Oral consent was obtained from all respondents before commencing the interviews. Computer-assisted telephone interviews were carried out with 3002 people. There are a number of ways to calculate survey response rates. For this survey, the American Association for Public Opinion Research response rate [16] was 3.1% and the simple response rate was 12.2%.

Measures

The survey interview covered sociodemographic characteristics, intentions and confidence to help a person in distress, barriers and enablers, actual helping behaviour, the participant's own suicidal thoughts, help received, attitudes to suicide, exposure to suicide, training in suicide prevention and exposure to suicide prevention messages in the media. The full interview is given in Additional file 1. Only the measures of specific relevance to the aims of the present paper are described in detail below.

Sociodemographics

Participants were asked questions about sociodemographic characteristics, which were coded as follows for the analyses reported here: female gender, age group (18–30, 31–59, 60+), mainly speak a language other than English, education with Bachelor's degree or above and non-urban location.

Helping intentions

Helping intentions were assessed in relation to one of six vignettes of distressed persons that were randomly assigned to participants. The vignettes covered male or female versions of three scenarios: a person with distress and adverse life events, a person with distress and adverse life events but no overt suicidality ("John/Jenny says he/she feels he/she will never be happy again and believes his/her family would be better off without him/her"), and a person with distress and adverse life events with overt suicidality ("John/Jenny says he/she feels s/he will never be happy again and believes his/her family would be better off without him/her. You run into a friend of John's/Jenny's. S/he tells you that John/Jenny told him/her he/she feels desperate and has been thinking of ways to end his/her life"). The six scenarios are given in Additional file 1.

Participants were then asked "How likely is it that you would take the following actions with John/Jenny?" Very unlikely, Unlikely, Neither likely nor unlikely, Likely, Very likely. The actions presented were: "Ask about how he/she is feeling; Listen to John's/Jenny's problems without judgement; Remind him/her what he/she has going for himself/herself*; Ask how you can help; Try to solve John's/Jenny's problems*; Reassure John/Jenny that you know exactly how badly he/she feels*; Help make an appointment with a health professional – for example a GP or counsellor; Call a crisis line – for example, Lifeline; Go to an appointment with a professional with him/her – for example a GP; Ask if he/she has been thinking about killing himself/herself; If John/Jenny told me he/she was thinking about killing himself/herself, I would try to make him/her understand that suicide is wrong*; If John/Jenny told me he/she was thinking about killing himself/herself, I would ask if he/she has a means

to kill herself/himself – for example, pills or a weapon; If John/Jenny told me he/she was thinking about killing himself/herself, I would listen to why he/she wants to die; I would tell him/her how much it will hurt his/her family and friends if he/she were to kill himself/herself*; I would ask if he/she has a plan for suicide – for example a date or how they will die".

Ten of the items above are recommended by expert-consensus guidelines, while 5 are recommended against (the latter are asterisked above) [8]. The 10 recommended items were made into a Positive Intentions scale by averaging the ratings across items to give a score range from 1 (every item rated 'very unlikely') to 5 (every item rated 'very likely'). Similarly, the 5 items recommended against were averaged to give a Negative Intentions scale from 1 to 5.

Helping behaviour

Participants were asked "In the last 12 months, has anyone in your family or close circle of friends experienced a similar level of distress to John/Jenny?" and "Did just one of your family or close friends experience this level of distress in the last 12 months, or more than one?". If the participant knew more than one person, they were told: "Because you know more than one family member or close friend experiencing a similar level of distress, for the next few questions, I want you to think about the one you know BEST". Participants were asked an open-ended question about what they did to help the person and then a series of questions about specific actions taken that paralleled the questions on intentions. The interviewer recorded 'yes' or 'no' for each of the 15 items listed above for measuring intentions.

As for the intentions items above, the 10 recommended items were made into a Positive Actions scale by summing the number of 'yes' responses to give a score range from 0 (no positive actions carried out) to 10 (all positive actions carried out). Similarly, the 5 items recommended against were summed to give a score range from 0 (no negative actions carried out) to 5 (all negative actions carried out).

Exposure to suicide

Participants were asked "Do you know anyone who has died by suicide?", with responses recorded as yes or no.

Training received

Participants were asked "Have you ever completed any training or course in how to help someone who is suicidal?" The interviewer coded responses as professional training, MHFA, ASIST, QPR or other. The commissioning organization *beyondblue* is not associated with any of the training programs evaluated in the present study.

Table 1 Sociodemographic characteristics of the sample ($N = 3002$)

Characteristic	N (%)
Female gender	1785 (59.5%)
Aged 18–30	356 (11.9%)
Aged 31–59	1408 (46.9%)
Aged 60+	1238 (41.2%)
Bachelor's degree or above	1215 (40.5%)
Non-urban location	1254 (41.8%)
Exposed to suicide	1839 (61.3%)

Statistical analysis

Items concerning intentions and actions recommended or not recommended in expert-consensus guidelines were made into scales. Reliability of these scales was quantified with coefficient omega-total using the statistical package R [17].

The associations between type of training received and quality of intentions and actions were examined using simultaneous linear regression in IBM SPSS Statistics 22. Types of training (professional, MHFA, other) were coded as dichotomous variables and used as predictors of scale scores, with adjustment for type of vignette (dummy coded), sociodemographic characteristics and exposure to suicide. The sociodemographic variables and exposure to suicide were used as covariates because they all had associations ($P < 0.05$) with having received at least one type

Table 2 Descriptive statistics and reliabilities (coefficient omega) for the intentions and actions scales

Scale	Mean (SD)	Range	Omega (interval)[a]	Omega (ordinal)[a]
Positive Intentions	4.02 (0.61)	1–5	0.80	0.85
Negative Intentions	3.77 (0.74)	1–5	0.68	0.74
Positive Actions	5.50 (2.29)	0–10	0.75	0.85
Negative Actions	2.71 (1.44)	0–5	0.64	0.76

[a]Omega-total assuming either interval or ordinal level of measurement

of training. Unstandardized regressions coefficients and their 95% CIs are reported for types of training. Effect sizes were measured using Cohen's d by dividing unstandardized regression coefficients by the sample standard deviation, with values of 0.2, 0.5 and 0.8 being regarded as 'small', 'medium' and 'large' respectively.

Where associations were found at $P < 0.05$ for types of training, post-hoc regression analyses were carried out to explore associations with individual intention and action items as the outcome variables. Linear regression was used for associations with the intention items (which were rated on a Likert scale) and binary logistic regression for the action items (which were yes/no). Because these exploratory analyses were post-hoc and involved multiple outcome variables, a conservative Bonferroni approach was used, with alpha divided by the number of items in a scale.

Results

Table 1 shows the sociodemographic characteristics of the sample. Figure 1 shows the breakdown of the sample according to training received. Because the number of participants who had done ASIST and QPR was small), these were combined with the Other group. The categories of training overlapped, because some people had more than one type of training.

Table 2 shows the descriptive statistics on the Positive and Negative Intentions scales and the Positive and Negative Actions scales. This table also gives the omega reliability coefficients for the scales, with values generally being acceptable.

Table 3 shows the inter-correlations among the scales. It can be seen that positive intentions were more highly correlated with positive actions than with negative

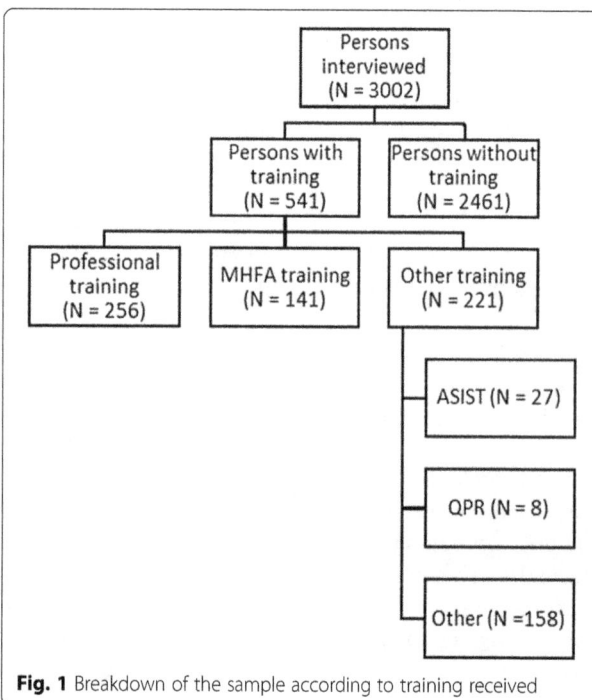

Fig. 1 Breakdown of the sample according to training received

Table 3 Correlations among intentions and actions scales

Scale	Positive intentions	Negative intentions	Positive actions	Negative actions
Positive Intentions	1.00	0.34	0.44	0.26
Negative Intentions		1.00	0.13	0.54
Positive Actions			1.00	0.51
Negative Actions				1.00

For all correlations, $P < 0.001$

Table 4 Unstandardized regression coefficients (and 95% CIs) for associations between type of training and scales measuring intentions and actions[a]

Scale	Professional training	MHFA	Other training
Positive Intentions	0.24 (0.16, 0.31)	0.26 (0.16, 0.36)	0.21 (0.13, 0.29)
Negative Intentions	−0.25 (−0.34, −0.16)	−0.15 (−0.27, −0.02)	−0.16 (−0.26, −0.07)
Positive Actions	0.76 (0.26, 1.26)	0.98 (0.39, 1.57)	0.78 (0.29, 1.28)
Negative Actions	−0.22 (−0.53, 0.10)	0.26 (−0.11, 0.64)	−0.16 (−0.48, 0.16)

[a]Adjusted for sociodemographics, type of vignette presented and exposure to suicide

actions (0.44 vs 0.26). Conversely, negative intentions were more highly correlated with negative actions than with positive actions (0.54 vs 0.13). However, positive intentions were correlated 0.34 with negative intentions, and positive actions were correlated 0.51 with negative actions, even though one set is recommended by experts and the other recommended against, indicating a general tendency to intend to take action or not.

Of the 3002 participants, 1056 knew someone who was distressed in the past 12 months and 935 did something to support the person. Multiple binary regression analyses were carried out to see whether training was a predictor of knowing someone and, among the subgroup that did, whether support was provided. After adjusting for covariates, only MHFA training was associated with knowing someone (OR = 1.51, 95% CI 1.05–2.17, $P = 0.026$). There was no association of training with provision of support.

Multiple linear regression analyses were carried out to explore whether type of training predicted intention and action scale scores. The unstandardized coefficients after adjustment for covariates are shown in Table 4. Table 5 shows the corresponding values of Cohen's d. All types of training were associated with greater positive intentions and actions, with similar effect sizes in the small-to-medium range. Similarly, all types of training were associated with lesser negative intentions, although the effect sizes were greater for professional training (small-to-medium) than for MHFA and other training (small). By contrast, all associations with negative actions were non-significant and less than small.

Table 6 shows post-hoc analyses of associations of training with specific Positive and Negative Intentions items, while Table 7 shows post-hoc analyses of associations with specific Positive Actions items. These

significant associations are with items that involve explicit communication about suicide.

Discussion

The findings show that training in how to help a suicidal person is associated with increased intentions to act in ways recommended by guidelines for the public, and decreased intentions to act in ways recommended against by the guidelines. All three types of training—professional, MHFA and other—had similar small-to-medium associations with positive intentions. However, the association with reduced negative intentions was small-to-medium for professional training, but only small for MHFA and other training. For actions to help a distressed person in the past 12 months, all types of training were associated with taking more actions recommended by the guidelines, with small-to-medium effect sizes. Associations with actions not recommended were not significant. When specific intentions and actions were examined, training was associated specifically with a greater willingness to talk openly about suicide with a distressed person. It should be noted when considering these findings that the associations with professional training were in relation to helping a family member or friend, rather than in the context of helping a client in a professional role.

We are not aware of any previous studies that have examined associations with suicide-relevant training in the context of a community survey. However, a US study used a similar approach in a large cross-sectional survey of behavioural health care staff [18]. This study found that staff who had received training in ASIST, QPR or other suicide-relevant training had greater suicide knowledge and confidence in working with suicidal persons. However, unlike the present study, the US study did not

Table 5 Cohen's d (and 95% CIs) for associations between type of training and scales measuring intentions and actions[a]

Scale	Professional training	MHFA	Other training
Positive Intentions	0.39 (0.26, 0.51)	0.43 (0.26, 0.59)	0.34 (0.21, 0.48)
Negative Intentions	−0.34 (−0.46, −0.22)	−0.20 (−0.36, −0.03)	−0.22 (−0.35, −0.09)
Positive Actions	0.33 (0.11, 0.55)	0.43 (0.17, 0.69)	0.34 (0.13, 0.56)
Negative Actions	−0.15 (−0.37, 0.07)	0.18 (−0.08, 0.44)	−0.11 (−0.33, 0.11)

[a]Adjusted for sociodemographics, type of vignette presented and exposure to suicide

Table 6 Significant associations between type of training and specific intentions[a]

Type of training	Positive intentions that were more likely	Negative intentions that were less likely
Professional	Ask if he/she has been thinking about killing himself/herself. Ask if he/she has the means to kill himself/herself. Ask if he/she has a plan for suicide—for example a date or how they will die.	Reassure you know exactly how badly he/she feels. Would try to make him/her understand that suicide is wrong. Tell him/her how much it will hurt his/her family and friends if he/she were to kill himself/herself.
MHFA	Ask if he/she has been thinking about killing himself/herself. Ask if he/she has the means to kill himself/herself. Ask if he/she has a plan for suicide—for example a date or how they will die.	Would try to make him/her understand that suicide is wrong.
Other	Listen to problems without judgement Ask if he/she has been thinking about killing himself/herself. Ask if he/she has the means to kill himself/herself. Ask if he/she has a plan for suicide—for example a date or how they will die.	Would try to make him/her understand that suicide is wrong.

[a]Significant with Bonferroni-adjusted alpha of 0.05/15 = 0.003

assess whether this greater knowledge and confidence was associated with behaviour.

The present study found associations between intentions to support a hypothetical person in a vignette and supportive actions to a family member or friend in the previous 12 months. The associations showed some specificity, with positive intentions correlating with positive actions and negative intentions with negative actions. While the associations were measured cross-sectionally in the current study, they support the findings from longitudinal studies that mental health first aid intentions predict subsequent mental health first aid actions [19, 20]. These findings indicate that suicide helping intentions can be used as a proxy short-term outcome where it is not feasible to measure behaviour, e.g. at a post-test assessment after a training course.

The major limitation of the study is that the data are cross-sectional, limiting causal inference. Although a variety of potential confounders were adjusted for, it is possible that there are other unmeasured differences between the groups that were not. We also lacked data on how long ago the training was received and, in many cases, information about what the content of the

Table 7 Significant associations between type of training and specific positive actions[a]

Type of training	Positive actions that were more likely
Professional	Ask if he/she has the means to kill himself/herself. Ask if he/she has a plan for suicide—for example a date or how they will die.
MHFA	Ask if he/she has been thinking about killing himself/herself. Ask if he/she has the means to kill himself/herself. Ask if he/she has a plan for suicide—for example a date or how they will die.
Other	Ask if he/she has the means to kill himself/herself. Ask if he/she has a plan for suicide—for example a date or how they will die.

[a]Significant with Bonferroni-adjusted alpha of 0.05/10 = 0.005

training was. If the training was within the past year, then it is possible that it followed rather than preceded any reported behaviour. The only specific type of training we can draw conclusions on is MHFA, which is a broader type of training in how to assist people developing mental health problems or in mental health crisis situations, with assisting a suicidal person being only one component. In fact, the present study is the first to examine suicide-specific outcomes of MHFA training and adds to the evidence from trials that such training increases knowledge, reduces stigmatizing attitudes and improves supportive behaviours towards people with mental health problems [13].

Other limitations are the low response rate and possible biases in the sample. We found that 4.7% of the sample reported having received MHFA training, whereas the population estimate of adults having done MHFA training is 2.6%, indicating an over-representation of people with an interest in mental health.

On the other hand, the methods used in the present study have some strengths. The study examined the effects of training in a real-life community context. In trials to evaluate suicide-relevant training, the measures used generally only cover short-term changes and are often transparent in their purpose and thus potentially subject to biased reporting to please the researcher. In the current study, there was no obvious connection between the purposes of the study and any training received. Participants were told that the study was on "what Australian adults understand about recognising and assisting an individual in severe distress", with the question on training being asked towards the end of the interview.

Conclusions

The findings show that training in how to help someone who is suicidal is associated with better quality intentions and actions towards a distressed person in the social network, in particular a greater willingness to talk openly about suicide. The magnitude of the association was similar for short courses and professional training. If these benefits can be confirmed in controlled trials, it would indicate that such courses merit wider dissemination in the community to increase the support provided to suicidal persons and to reduce the risk of suicide.

Abbreviations

ASIST: Applied Suicide Intervention Skills Training; MHFA: Mental Health First Aid; QPR: Question, Persuade, Refer; SPSS: Statistical Package for the Social Sciences

Acknowledgements

Roy Morgan Research Ltd. carried out the survey.

Funding

The survey was funded by *beyondblue*, which approved the content of the interview and the survey methodology. However, *beyondblue* had no role in the running of the survey, the data analysis, the interpretation of the findings or the writing of this article. AFJ, JP and NJR are supported by National Health and Medical Research Council Fellowships. AN is supported through an Australian Government Research Training Program Scholarship (National Health and Medical Research Council) and an Australian Rotary Health Ian Scott PhD scholarship.

Authors' contributions

AFJ drafted the manuscript and AN, JP, AR and NJR suggested improvements. AFJ, AN, JP, AR and NJR contributed to the development of the interview and management of the project. All authors read and approved the final manuscript.

Competing interests

AFJ is the co-founder of MHFA training and Chair of the Board of MHFA International. AN, JP, AR and NJR have no competing interests.

References

1. Luoma JB, Martin CE, Pearson JL. Contact with mental health and primary care providers before suicide: a review of the evidence. Am J Psychiatry. 2002;159(6):909–16.
2. Stene-Larsen K, Reneflot A. Contact with primary and mental health care prior to suicide: a systematic review of the literature from 2000 to 2017. Scand J Public Health. 2017;1403494817746274. https://doi.org/10.1177/1403494817746274.
3. Isometsa ET. Psychological autopsy studies–a review. Eur Psychiatry. 2001;16(7):379–85.
4. Owens C, Owen G, Belam J, Lloyd K, Rapport F, Donovan J, Lambert H. Recognising and responding to suicidal crisis within family and social networks: qualitative study. BMJ. 2011;343:d5801.
5. Owen G, Belam J, Lambert H, Donovan J, Rapport F, Owens C. Suicide communication events: lay interpretation of the communication of suicidal ideation and intent. Soc Sci Med. 2012;75(2):419–28.
6. Sweeney L, Owens C, Malone K. Communication and interpretation of emotional distress within the friendships of young Irish men prior to suicide: a qualitative study. Health Soc Care Community. 2015;23(2):150–8.
7. Kelly CM, Jorm AF, Kitchener BA, Langlands RL. Development of mental health first aid guidelines for suicidal ideation and behaviour: a Delphi study. BMC Psychiatry. 2008;8:17.
8. Ross AM, Kelly CM, Jorm AF. Re-development of mental health first aid guidelines for suicidal ideation and behaviour: a delphi study. BMC Psychiatry. 2014;14:241.
9. Jorm AF, Blewitt KA, Griffiths KM, Kitchener BA, Parslow RA. Mental health first aid responses of the public: results from an Australian national survey. BMC Psychiatry. 2005;5:9.
10. Rossetto A, Jorm AF, Reavley NJ. Quality of helping behaviours of members of the public towards a person with a mental illness: a descriptive analysis of data from an Australian national survey. Ann General Psychiatry. 2014;(1):2. https://doi.org/10.1186/1744-859X-13-2.
11. Burnette C, Ramchand R, Ayer L. Gatekeeper training for suicide prevention: a theoretical model and review of the empirical literature. Rand Health Q. 2015;5(1):16.
12. Jorm AF, Kitchener BA. Noting a landmark achievement: mental health first aid training reaches 1% of Australian adults. Aust N Z J Psychiatry. 2011;45(10):808–13.
13. Hadlaczky G, Hökby S, Mkrtchian A, Carli V, Wasserman D. Mental health first aid is an effective public health intervention for improving knowledge, attitudes, and behaviour: a meta-analysis. Int Rev Psychiatry. 2014;26(4):467–75.
14. Litteken C, Sale E. Long-term effectiveness of the question, persuade, refer (QPR) suicide prevention gatekeeper training program: lessons from Missouri. Community Ment Health J. 2018;54:282–92.
15. Rodgers PL. Review of the applied suicide intervention skills training program (ASIST): rationale, evaluation results, and directions for future research. Alberta: LivingWorks Education Incorporated Calgary; 2010.
16. Research AAfPO: Standard definitions: final dispositions of case codes and outcome rates for surveys. 9th edn. Oakbrook Terrace: AAPOR; 2016.
17. Dunn TJ, Baguley T, Brunsden V. From alpha to omega: a practical solution to the pervasive problem of internal consistency estimation. Br J Psychol. 2014;105(3):399–412.
18. Silva C, Smith AR, Dodd DR, Covington DW, Joiner TE. Suicide-related knowledge and confidence among behavioral health care staff in seven states. Psychiatr Serv. 2016;67(11):1240–5.
19. Rossetto A, Jorm AF, Reavley NJ. Predictors of adults' helping intentions and behaviours towards a person with a mental illness: a six-month follow-up study. Psychiatry Res. 2016;240:170–6.
20. Yap MBH, Jorm AF. Young people's mental health first aid intentions and beliefs prospectively predict their actions: findings from an Australian national survey of youth. Psychiatry Res. 2012;196(2–3):315–9.

14

Experiences of parenting and clinical intervention for mothers affected by personality disorder: a pilot qualitative study combining parent and clinician perspectives

Ruth Wilson[1], Tim Weaver[2], Daniel Michelson[3] and Crispin Day[4][*] (iD)

Abstract

Background: Evidence-based parenting programmes are recommended for the treatment of child mental health difficulties. Families with complex psychosocial needs show poorer retention and outcomes when participating in standard parenting programmes. The *Helping Families Programme* (HFP) is a 16-week community-based parenting intervention designed to meet the needs of these families, including families with parental personality disorder. This study aimed to explore the help seeking and participatory experiences of parents with a diagnosis of personality disorder. It further aimed to examine the acceptability of referral and intervention processes for the HFP from the perspectives of (i) clinicians referring into the programme; and (ii) referred parents.

Method: Semi-structured interviews were conducted with parents recruited to receive HFP ($n = 5$) as part of a research case series and the referring NHS child and adolescent mental health service (CAMHS) clinicians ($n = 5$). Transcripts were analysed using Interpretive Phenomenological Analysis.

Results: Four themes were identified for parents: (i) the experience of parenthood, (ii) being a parent affected by personality disorder, (iii) experience of the intervention, and (iv) qualities of helping. Three themes emerged for clinicians: (i) challenges of addressing parental need, (ii) experience of engaging parents with personality disorders and (iii) limited involvement during HFP. Comparison of parent and clinician themes led to the identification of two key interlinked themes: (i) concerns prior to receiving the intervention, and (ii) the challenges of working together without a mutual understanding.

Conclusions: This pilot study identifies potentially significant challenges of working with parents affected by personality disorder and engaging them in HFP and other similar interventions. Results have important wider clinical implications by highlighting potential barriers to engagement and participation and providing insights on how these barriers might be overcome. Findings have been used to inform the referral and intervention processes of a pilot RCT and further intervention development.

Keywords: Parenting, Personality disorder, Child behaviour, Child emotional problems

* Correspondence: crispin.1.day@kcl.ac.uk
[4]CAMHS Research Unit, IOPPN, King's College London, Michael Rutter Centre, De Crespigny Park, Camberwell, London SE5 8AZ, UK
Full list of author information is available at the end of the article

Background

One in ten children in developed economies experience emotional, behavioural and other mental health disorders. These disorders have negative impacts on childhood development, academic achievement and social functioning and are associated with subsequent adult mental health difficulties, long-term unemployment and criminal behaviour [1–3]. Parental personality disorder increases the likelihood of child mental health problems and maltreatment. Associated parental problems include increased emotional dysregulation, hostile interpersonal functioning, self-harm and substance misuse [4–6]. Potentially harmful parenting behaviours such as excessive parental control, possessiveness and physical punishment have also been documented [7] that can interfere with child-parent attachment and undermine parents' capacity to provide children with warm, nurturant and consistent parenting.

Families with complex psychosocial needs are likely to experience poorer outcomes from established parenting programmes based on social learning theory [8–11]. Parental mental health has also been shown to moderate the effectiveness of parenting interventions with families showing less improvement in child problem behaviours at the end of treatment [10, 12]. Support for families with complex psychosocial needs is often fragmented, not tailored and personalised, and fails to address the interplay between parenting and specific parental emotional and interpersonal functioning [13–15].

The *Helping Families Programme* (HFP) is a modular parenting programme for parents with complex psychosocial needs, including personality disorder [16, 17]. HFP aims to improve i) child mental health and behavioural problems, ii) parent-child relationships, iii) parental emotion regulation and coping and iv) families' social resources. HFP incorporates validated therapeutic content focussed on parenting, emotional regulation and interpersonal functioning [9, 18–20] with a relational, goal-orientated model of collaborative, therapeutic engagement that reduces parental alienation and stigma [16, 21]. The intervention delivered individually, offers parenting and self-care strategies and aims to develop a shared understanding between parent and clinician about how parents' emotional and interpersonal difficulties impact on their parenting and the child's functioning.

The qualitative research reported here was conducted in order to inform the design and methodology for a subsequent feasibility RCT of the Helping Families Programme [21]. The qualitative study sought to (i) examine the parenting and help-seeking experiences of parents affected by personality disorder, (ii) explore the acceptability of HFP to this population, and (iii) refine the protocol for the subsequent pilot RCT.

Method

Design

A qualitative design informed by Interpretative Phenomenological Analysis (IPA) [22, 23] was used to develop a rich understanding of the subjective lived experiences of participating parents and referring clinicians. IPA's focus on generating meaning and significance from lived experience was important when exploring the acceptability of HFP. Ethical approval was obtained from the NRES Committee London (Camberwell St Giles).

Sites & participants

Participants were recruited from four CAMHS teams in two London NHS trusts. Clinicians were asked to refer parents who were (i) affected by personality disorder, or likely to meet diagnostic criteria, and (ii) had a child (living with them) aged 3–11 years with a behavioural and/or emotional disorder. All referred parents and their referring clinician were eligible for qualitative interview. However, as described elsewhere [24] we screened for adult personality disorder and child mental disorders respectively, and excluded parents with a psychotic disorder, those in another psychoeducational parenting intervention, and those who's child had a neurodevelopmental disorder or was on a child protection plan. Informed consent was obtained for all qualitative interviews.

Participants

Five parents (all mothers, three lone parents) and their referring CAMHS clinicians (n = 5) participated in the qualitative interviews (i.e. 10 interviews). The sample size is consistent with IPA's ideographic focus and the consensus in the literature on samples of this size [25]. *All parents either met research diagnoses or had clinical diagnoses of personality disorder (any) and their children met criteria for a behavioural and/or emotional problem. All children had siblings (range 1–2).*

Interviews

Separate semi-structured topic guides were developed for the parent and clinician interviews. In line with COREQ guidelines [26] we note the interviewer (RW) is a White-British female MA graduate, aged < 30 years, with no clinical responsibility for participants.

The researcher used the topic guides to build rapport and encourage open description of personal experiences [23] of parenting, help-seeking, their participation in HFP (if applicable) and related research processes [22]. Data were collected after participants had completed their participation in the case series. Interviews took place within the family home. Parents were given £10 to reimburse their time.

The referring clinicians topic guide explored their experience of working with the parents, and reflections on the parents involvement in the HFP. Clinicians were interviewed in their work place.

Data analysis

Interviews were audio-recorded and verbatim transcripts obtained for analysis. Parent and clinician data were initially analysed separately and then triangulated to explore the relationship between their subjective experiences.

Data were analysed using the methods of IPA [22, 23] and coded at three levels: (i) the researcher familiarised herself with each transcript attaching descriptive codes containing initial observations and reflections to data, (ii) the researcher developed second-level descriptive labels which were then coded and organised into conceptual categories. Interpretations at this analytic stage were intended to capture the subjective value attributed by participants to emerging categories. For example, the theme 'experience of parenthood' incorporated the sub-codes containing emotional responses (e.g. frustration) and parenting behaviours (e.g. seeking support and negative experiences of parenting programmes). (iii) emergent results were subsequently explored and verified in shared meetings between authors (CD and TW) familiar with the transcripts. The codes, categories and themes emerging from the two respondent groups were examined and potential connections explored.

Results were subject to validation with a parent and a clinician participant. These latter procedures resulted in support for the emergent themes.

Results

Parent themes

The experience of parenthood

Parents reported frequent problematic and distressing interactions with their children and the resulting negative impact on their family life. Parents described difficulties understanding and controlling their child's behaviour.

> *"...I'm hitting my head up against a brick wall because I just don't know what else to do." (Parent 3)*

The daily challenges of a child experiencing difficulties commonly coupled with a feeling of 'helplessness' about how to improve their situation appeared to define participants' experiences of parenthood. Parents often appeared desperate and voiced a willingness to try whatever support was available, despite previous negative experiences of parenting interventions, variously described as 'ineffective', 'inappropriate' or 'patronising'.

Being a parent affected by personality disorder

Being a parent affected by personality disorder appeared to mediate many encounters with professionals. Some parents felt judged and blamed by clinicians. Parents felt professionals assumed that a personality disorder diagnosis automatically meant that they would be a *'bad parent'*.

> *"They were trying to say, 'oh it's down to your parenting, you were this, you were that .... it's you that has given it to him'... I felt like they were blaming me." (Parent 1)*

Consequently, parents felt clinicians did not take their parenting experiences seriously, perceived them to be a function of their interpersonal difficulties and therefore felt 'unheard' and unable to communicate their sense of helplessness.

Parents felt they had acquiesce to professional advice and intervention. Although often feeling pessimistic, they felt that they had to accept help offered on the clinicians terms as they would otherwise be seen as uncooperative.

Experience of the intervention

Despite initial pessimism, after participation in HFP most parents described family life as 'more manageable' and their parenting challenges as 'slightly easier'. Parents' described successfully using various HFP parenting strategies (e.g. boundary setting, use of routines, spending time with the child), reported a greater awareness of the impact of their own parenting behaviour on their child, and expressed more interest and appreciation of their child's own subjective experiences.

> *"If I'm calmer and settled then obviously he's gonna be a bit more calm and settled." (Parent 1)*

As a result, parents felt a greater sense of agency in their parenting behaviour, more confidence and an increased sense of hope.

> *"I can see that it has worked and see the changes." (Parent 2)*

Qualities of helping

Parents identified two key factors that encouraged their engagement in HFP. Parents attached value to perceived therapist personal qualities such as 'encouraging', 'non-judgemental', 'open', 'honest', 'not patronising' and 'patient'. Parents felt listened to, understood and, as a result, encouraged and more in control. Illustrating this one parent described how session content was adjusted to reflect their personal circumstances and problems:

> *"(If) my bipolar (lay description) was really bad or I felt really low and my depression was so bad, it wasn't*

a matter of 'right okay we've still got to do this' ... (It was) let's put this aside; let's concentrate on what you need' " (Parent 3)

These qualities were often described as absent in previous therapeutic interventions from which parents had disengaged.

Clinicians
Challenges addressing parental need
Clinicians described their challenges in meeting the needs of parents affected by personality disorder whose children had behavioural and emotional problems. Clinicians attributed some of these difficulties to systemic issues of funding, workload and 'high thresholds' in specialist services, and the organisational and cultural separation of CAMHS and adult services.

"... they're like two different worlds in what we provide." (Clinician 2).

Clinicians described the clinical challenges involved. Due to their priority focus on the child's difficulties, at times, they felt that parents' own psychological needs could be overlooked. Clinicians also felt less confident in assessing and managing parent's mental health difficulties. Clinicians questioned the use of conventional parenting programmes for parents affected by personality disorder, voicing concerns about the group formats commonly used in parenting programmes and the potential for this to exacerbate parental emotional and interpersonal difficulties. Nevertheless, ongoing concerns about child and family functioning led clinicians to continue to offer support and intervention despite concerns about its limitations.

Engaging parents in HFP
Clinicians expressed concern that personality disorder was a pejorative term that may have a detrimental impact on their therapeutic relationship. Citing previous cases when they had discussed personality and interpersonal functioning with parents and encountered defensiveness or disengagement, clinicians expressed reservations about discussing parental personality disorder in relation to HFP. In suggesting parent referral to another service, a clinician described how she had thought particularly carefully about her use of language to avoid the parent feeling blamed.

"I've worked with her for quite a while and I was aware of the pattern that we'd been having in terms of we suggest a service, we get completely shut down ... there's no way she's actually gonna come round to this" (Clinician 1)

Limited involvement during HFP
Referring clinicians often had little contact with parents once they participated in HFP, due to the limited time they had to follow-up families who were not of immediate concern. Consequently, referring clinicians had limited knowledge of the impact of HFP on parents and their children. They were nevertheless positive about its potential value:

"She's (mother) not got in-touch with me. That's a massive difference." ... " just really for this parent to have someone else to speak to and to understand her ... it's definitely a benefit to her." (Clinician 1)

Triangulation of parent and clinician themes
Parents had negative experiences with previous parenting interventions and clinicians were also aware of this. While parents were willing to participate, they and their referring clinicians felt pessimistic about the potential benefit of HFP prior to engagement.

Parents frequently felt their concerns about their child's difficulties were unheard by previous clinicians. When trying to explain their family difficulties and sense of helplessness, parents felt stigmatised and blamed for their child's problems because of their personality disorder diagnosis. This left parents feeling that their diagnosis 'caused' their children's difficulties and undermined their efforts to obtain suitable help. At the same time, clinicians experienced difficulties in talking openly and effectively with parents affected by personality disorder because they held different views about the nature, cause and understanding of the family difficulties. Resolving these difficulties in ways that heighten parental engagement through a shared understanding was challenging for both parents and clinicians.

Discussion
Our results provide insight into the experiences of parents affected by personality disorder, and the perspectives of the CAMHS clinicians with whom they work. The sample size, though small, is acceptable for a study using IPA. However, caution should be exercised in generalising the findings to other parents affected by personality disorder and other clinicians within and beyond CAMHS.

Analysis identified two negative parent themes related to (a) their sense of helplessness as parents and their resignation and pessimism about the effectiveness of parenting programmes, and (b) the feeling that clinicians in the past had erroneously attributed their family difficulties to their personality disorder. While parents felt desperate for change, based on past negative experiences, they were sceptical about achieving it through parenting interventions. Clinicians expressed similar doubts. Hence there was a shared ambivalence about the value of participation in the HFP intervention. This highlights the crucial role of sensitive and positive parental engagement and the value of developing tailored interventions designed to meet the needs of this population [10].

These findings are consistent with studies reporting stigma felt by parents with significant mental health difficulties [18]. While parenting difficulties may indeed be related to the symptomatic difficulties of the parent [5], in developing useful clinical formulations, other factors known to contribute to parenting difficulties need to be taken into account such as the child's temperament and their own mental health difficulties [10, 27], lone parenthood [13] and social isolation [1, 27]. A comprehensive, ecological formulation that incorporates risk and resilience factors may provide a more accurate and acceptable basis for a shared understanding of child, parenting and family difficulties than a clinical approach that more narrowly focusses on parental mental health. While cautious interpretation is required, parents who did engage with HFP reported subjectively positive outcomes including changes to their parental behaviour, reflective function and emotional regulation.

Clinical implications

Findings highlight potential barriers to engagement and participation for both parents and referring clinicians. To be successful, programmes such as HFP need to overcome this ambivalence and pessimism by engendering hope and motivation in parents and encouraging clinicians in their referral and gatekeeping roles [21]. Programmes also need to address the well documented engagement challenges for this population of parents, including underlying feelings of mistrust and difficulties in relating to others that are likely to interfere with building effective a therapeutic alliance [15].

Parents highlighted the subjective value of clinicians' therapeutic consistency, flexibility, and relationships. These process characteristics may be more difficult to achieve within curricularised, group-based parenting programmes [5]. Offering tailored, individualised approaches, such as HFP, could give clinicians the opportunity to develop genuine open, shared understanding with parents about their difficulties without implying blame and judgement which become a barrier to treatment [21]. Additionally, a tailored, individualised approach would also enable the clinician to be flexible to differences in parenting styles across the spectrum of personality disorder diagnoses which, though beyond the scope of this paper, are well documented within the literature [7].

Research implications

Targeted parenting interventions like HFP need to demonstrate their value to parents and clinicians through clinical outcome research. Though not methodologically robust in themselves, the current findings are consistent with and build upon previously published findings [11] and support the rationale for the pilot RCT currently in progress.

Our findings have informed recruitment strategies for the pilot RCT, which is recruiting parents with significant interpersonal difficulties rather than requiring parents have a formal research diagnosis of personality disorder. Recruitment will be through clinicians working within adult and child mental health services and social care practitioners. Participant and referring clinician information emphasises HFP's use of a flexible, tailored approach based on individual, home-based delivery. Clinicians in referring teams have been encouraged to use the study's findings to focus on, and showing genuine appreciation of, the difficulties parents face in caring for a child experiencing behavioural and emotional difficulties, rather than the ways in which the parents' own interpersonal difficulties may make parenting challenging, or be the cause of and contribute to their child's difficulties. Clinicians have been encouraged to be sensitive to the possible ambivalence that parents may feel and to openly explore the relative merits of involvement in HFP.

The results presented in this paper are based on small cohort of parents and clinicians which may limit generalisability. Parents supported by adult mental health services may have different perspectives on stigma and the role of diagnosis. The subsequent RCT has recruited parents through social care pathways. This will add further exploration and validation to these initial findings. Additional research methods including ethnography [28] and conversation analysis [29] may be useful to understand in greater depth the nature of the interactions between parents and clinicians particularly methods that can increase parent hope and motivation [20]. Also additional research looking at the trans-generational processes in which parental personality disorder impacts on child development through parenting practices [4, 7], including the role of child abuse and associated trauma, is required to further inform the intervention. Finally, the research focused on the experience of primary care-givers and help-seekers. The study did not examine the potential impact of a co-parent despite the sample including two-parent families. This is a limitation of the current study given wider evidence shows positive couple relationships are associated with lower levels of maternal stress and more positive parenting [21].

Conclusions

This study provides new evidence from parents and referring clinicians about the experience of help seeking, parent-focussed support and participation in parenting interventions for parents with personality disorder. The results have implications for therapeutic engagement and intervention with this population of parents and their children who are at increased risk of poorer family outcomes and low engagement in parenting interventions. In response, changes have been made to HFP referral and recruitment procedures prior to conducting a pilot RCT of the intervention.

Abbreviations
CAMHS: Child and adolescent mental health service; HFP: Helping Families Programme; IPA: Interpretative phenomenological analysis; RCT: Randomised control trial

Acknowledgements
We would like to thank our colleagues at the Centre for Parent and Child Support, King's College London and Middlesex University for help in developing this work.

Funding
This study was funded by the National Institute of Health Research, Health Technology Assessment, Project Reference Number: 12/194/01.

Authors' contributions
Author CD was the chief investigator and designed the study. Author RW recruited participants, conducted the interviews and conducted the analysis in consultation with CD and TW. RW conducted the literature review and wrote the manuscript. CD provided extensive input into manuscript revisions. TW consulted on qualitative methodology and provided input into manuscript revisions. DM contributed to study conception and design, and critical revisions of the manuscript. All authors read and approved the final manuscript.

Competing interests
The authors declare that they have no competing interests.

Author details
[1]Community Eating Disorder Service, East London NHS Foundation Trust, London, UK. [2]Department of Mental Health, Social Work and Integrative Medicine, Middlesex University, London, UK. [3]Department of Population Health, Centre for Global Mental Health, London School of Hygiene & Tropical Medicine, London, UK. [4]CAMHS Research Unit, IOPPN, King's College London, Michael Rutter Centre, De Crespigny Park, Camberwell, London SE5 8AZ, UK.

References
1. Davis H, Day C, Cox A, Cutler L. Child and adolescent mental health needs assessment and service implications in an inner city area. Clin Child Psychol Psychiatry. 2000;5:169_88.
2. Fergusson D, Horwood L, Ridder E. Show me the child at seven: the consequences of conduct problems in childhood for psychosocial functioning in adulthood. J Child Psychol Psychiatry. 2005;46:837–49.
3. Loeber R, Farrington D. Young children who commit crime: epidemiology, developmental origins, risk factors, early interventions, and policy implications. Dev Psychopathol. 2000;12:737–62.
4. Dutton DG, Denny-Keys MK, Sells JR. Parental personality disorder and its effects on children: a review of current literature. J Child Custody. 2011;8:268–83.
5. Stepp SD, Whalen DJ, Pilkonis PA, Hipwell AE, Levine MD. Children of mothers with borderline personality disorder: identifying parenting behaviors as potential targets for intervention. Personal Disord. 2011;3(1):76–91.
6. Newman LK, Stevenson CS, Bergman LR, Boyce P. Borderline personality disorder, mother-infant interaction and parenting perceptions: preliminary findings. Aust N Z J Psychiatry. 2007;41:598–605.
7. Johnson JG, Cohen P, Kasen S, Ehrensaft MK, Crawford TN. Associations of parental personality disorders and axis I disorders with childrearing behavior. Psychiatry. 2006;69(4):336–50.
8. Early Intervention Foundation Foundations for Life. What works to support parent child interaction in the early years. London: Early Intervention Foundation; 2016.
9. National Institute for Health and Clinical Excellence (NICE). Antisocial behaviour and conduct disorders in children and young people: recognition and management (Nice guideline CG158). 2013. https://www.nice.org.uk/guidance/cg158.
10. Reyno SM, McGrath PJ. Predictors of parent training efficacy for child externalizing behavior problems: a meta-analytic review. J Child Psychol Psychiatry. 2006;47:99–111.
11. Maliken AC, Fainsilber KL. Exploring the impact of parental psychopathology and emotion regulation on evidence-based parenting interventions: a transdiagnostic approach to improving treatment effectiveness. Clin Child Fam Psychol Rev. 2013;16:173–86.
12. Kazdin AE, Wassell G. Barriers to treatment participation and therapeutic change among children referred for conduct disorder. J Clin Child Psychol. 1999;28:160–72.
13. Armstrong H. Ministerial foreword. In: Reaching out: think family. London: Cabinet Office Social Exclusion Task Force; 2007. http://www.devon.gov.uk/reachingoutthinkfamily.pdf. Accessed 18 Sept 2017.
14. Bee P, Bower P, Byford S, Churchill R, Calam R, Stallard P, et al. The clinical effectiveness, cost-effectiveness and acceptability of community-based interventions aimed at improving or maintaining quality of life in children of parents with serious mental illness: a systematic review. NIHR J Library. 2014; https://doi.org/10.3310/hta18080.
15. McMurran M, Huband N, Overton E. Non-completion of personality disorder treatments: a systematic review of correlates, consequences, and interventions. Clin Psychol Rev. 2010;30:277–87.
16. Day C, Ellis M, Harris L. Helping families programme manual. London: South London & Maudsley NHS Foundation Trust/King's College; 2012.
17. Day C, Kowalenko S, Ellis M, Dawe S, Harnet P, Scott S. The helping families programme: a new parenting intervention for children with severe and persistent conduct problems. Child Adolesc Mental Health. 2011;16:167–71.
18. Ackerson B. Coping with the dual demands of severe mental illness and parenting: the parents' perspective. Fam Soc. 2003;84:109–19.
19. Barlow J, Jarrett P, Mockford C, McIntosh E, Davis H, Stewart-Brown S. Role of home visiting in improving parenting and health in families at risk of abuse and neglect: results of a multicentre randomised controlled trial and economic evaluation. Arch Dis Child. 2007;92:229–33.
20. Newton-Howes G, Weaver T, Tyrer P. Attitudes of staff towards patients with personality disorder in community mental health teams. Aust N Z J Psychiatry. 2008;42:572–7.
21. Davis H, Day C. Working in partnership with parents. 2nd ed. London: Pearson; 2010.
22. Smith J, Osborne M. Interpretive phenomenological analysis. In: Smith J, editor. Qualitative psychology: a practical guide to research methods. London: Sage; 2003. p. 51–80.
23. Smith JA. Semi-structured interviewing and qualitative analysis. Rethinking Methods Psychol. 1995;1:8–26.
24. Day C, Briskman J, Crawford M, Harris L, McCrone P, McMurran M, et al. Feasibility trial of a psychoeducational intervention for parents with personality difficulties: the helping families programme. Contemp Clin Trials Commun. 2017;8:67–74.

25. Brocki JM, Wearden AJ. A critical evaluation of the use of interpretative
     phenomenological analysis (IPA) in health psychology. Psychol Health. 2006;
     21(1):87–108.
26. Tong A, Sainsbury P, Craig J. Consolidated criteria for reporting qualitative
     research (COREQ): a 32-item checklist for interviews and focus groups. Int J
     Qual Health Care. 2007;19(6):349–57.
27. Feinstein EBI. What works to enhance inter-parental relationships and
     improve outcomes for children. Early Intervention Foundation. 2016. http://
     dera.ioe.ac.uk/25869/1/what-works-to-enhance-inter-parental-relationships.
     pdf. Accessed 18 Sept 2017.
28. Hammersley M. Atkinson P. Principles in practice. Routledge: Ethnography; 2007.
29. Hutchby I, Wooffitt R. Conversation analysis. Cambridge: Polity; 2008.

15

Anorexia nervosa-associated pancytopenia mimicking idiopathic aplastic anemia

Masahiro Takeshima[1*] ⓘ, Hiroyasu Ishikawa[1,2], Akihiro Kitadate[3], Ryo Sasaki[4], Takahiro Kobayashi[5], Hiroshi Nanjyo[6], Takashi Kanbayashi[1] and Tetsuo Shimizu[1]

Abstract

Background: Patients with anorexia nervosa (AN) often present with pancytopenia. In most cases described in the literature, AN with pancytopenia demonstrates gelatinous marrow transformation (GMT), which is a typical bone marrow feature of malnutrition. Differentiation of AN-associated pancytopenia from other types of pancytopenia, especially idiopathic aplastic anemia (IAA), has not been studied. We encountered a case of pancytopenia in a patient with AN and relatively poor nutritional status, whose hematological findings mimicked those of IAA, specifically fatty bone marrow and absence of GMT.

Case presentation: The patient was a 32-year-old woman with poorly controlled AN. At 31 years of age, her body mass index (BMI) had fallen from 17.0 kg/m^2 to below 13.8 kg/m^2. The patient presented with ongoing fatigue and thus was examined by a hematologist. Hematological findings were consistent with IAA: peripheral blood tests revealed pancytopenia, whereas the bone marrow displayed fatty replacement without GMT. Despite the absence of bone marrow features typically seen in malnutrition, the patient's hematological abnormalities had manifested after a decrease in body weight. Thus, although the bone marrow findings indicated IAA, we considered that the nutritional etiology of pancytopenia could not be thoroughly ruled out. Using nutritional therapy alone, the hematological abnormalities improved as BMI increased to 16.5 kg/m^2. The final diagnosis was pancytopenia secondary to malnutrition because pancytopenia and fatty bone marrow improved after implementation of nutritional therapy alone.

Conclusions: The present case is the first documented case of AN with pancytopenia for which bone marrow examination confirmed fatty marrow without any evidence of GMT. IAA and pancytopenia secondary to malnutrition can present the same clinical findings. This case is significant because it suggests a need to differentiate between malnutrition and IAA.

Keywords: Anorexia nervosa, Aplastic anemia, Bone marrow, Gelatinous transformation, Pancytopenia

Background

Anorexia nervosa (AN) is associated with various hematological abnormalities, with approximately 3% of cases exhibiting pancytopenia [1]. In almost all cases of AN with pancytopenia reported thus far, bone marrow analyses show atrophy of fat cells and loss of hematopoietic cells, with deposition of an amorphous gelatinous material [2–10]. This phenomenon has been described as gelatinous marrow transformation (GMT) [11, 12]. GMT is often observed in patients with pancytopenia due to malnutrition. However, to the best of our knowledge, the differentiation between malnutrition-associated etiology and other etiologies of pancytopenia in AN was not discussed in previous reports describing patients with AN. We herein report a case of pancytopenia in a patient with poor nutritional status, whose peripheral blood and bone marrow findings indicated idiopathic aplastic anemia (IAA).

---

* Correspondence: m.takeshima@med.akita-u.ac.jp
[1]Department of Neuropsychiatry, Akita University Graduate School of Medicine, 1-1-1,Hondo, Akita City, Akita 010-8543, Japan
Full list of author information is available at the end of the article

Case presentation

A 32-year-old Japanese woman with AN and pancytopenia was admitted to the psychiatric department of our hospital. The patient had no other remarkable medical or familial history. There was no occupational history indicating exposure to organic solvents (e.g., benzene).

The patient started binge eating and purging at 14 years of age. At 16 years of age, she was diagnosed with AN, and had multiple hospitalizations in this regard. The patient's first admission to our department was at 26 years of age, at which time her body mass index (BMI) was 9.5 kg/m^2 (weight, 22 kg; height, 152 cm). The patient had mild, transient bicytopenia with a low white blood cell (WBC) count (3000 cells/μL; reference range, 4000–9000 cells/μL) and a low hemoglobin (Hb) level (10.3 g/dL; reference range, 12.0–15.2 g/dL). These abnormalities improved with nutritional therapy. At the time of discharge, the patient's weight had improved, with a BMI of approximately 17 kg/m^2.

At 32 years of age, the patient's binge eating and purging behavior worsened again, and she began to lose weight. Five months prior to her eventual hospitalization (BMI, 15.0 kg/m^2), no hematological abnormalities were identified. At 46 days prior to the hospitalization, because of ongoing fatigue, she was examined by a hematologist at our hospital. The patient was determined to be underweight, with a body weight of 31.9 kg and a BMI of 13.8 kg/m^2. Peripheral blood analysis confirmed pancytopenia with the following findings: low WBC count, 2500 cells/μL; low neutrophil count, 1010 cells/μL (reference range: 1600–5400 cells/μL); low eosinophil count, 0 cells/μL (reference range: 80–610 cells/μL); low basophil count, 30 cells/μL (reference range: 0–180 cells/μL); normal lymphocyte count, 1280 cells/μL (reference range: 1060–4190 cells/μL); normal monocyte count, 200 cells/μL (reference range: 90–690 cells/μL); low reticulocyte count, 14.4 × 10^3 cells/μL (reference range: 35.0–125.0 × 10^3 cells/μL); low Hb level, 6.1 g/dL; high mean corpuscular volume, 113.9 fL (reference range: 80.0–100.0 fL); and low platelet (Plt) count, 10.6 × 10^4 cells/dL (reference range: 11.7–32.9 × 10^4 cells/dL). Blood biochemistry studies showed low serum levels of folate (3.0 ng/mL; reference range: 4.0–19.9 ng/mL) but normal serum levels of iron and vitamin B12. The etiology of pancytopenia was tentatively suspected to be folate deficiency, and thus the patient was prescribed folate at 10 mg/day. At 28 days prior to hospitalization, the folate level had recovered within normal limits, but the peripheral blood counts had worsened (low WBC count, 2200 cells/μL; low Hb level, 2.5 g/dL; and low Plt count, 8.6 × 10^4 cells/dL).

The patient was temporarily admitted to the hematology department of our hospital for blood transfusions. Laboratory tests yielded negative results for autoimmune disorders (including systemic lupus erythematosus), malignant lymphoma, infectious diseases, hemophagocytic lymphohistiocytosis, and hypersplenism. The patient was offered nutritional therapy to improve her weight but she refused and was therefore discharged following blood transfusions. After discharge, outpatient follow-up was performed by the hematology department. However, the patient's hematologic condition did not improve. Despite receiving blood transfusions twice monthly, the patient was eventually hospitalized once again for severe anemia. The patient believed that her hematological problems were not related with her eating behavior and persistently refused nutritional therapy. Finally, she was admitted to the psychiatric department to receive both hematologic and psychiatric support.

On admission, the patient's body weight was 30 kg and BMI was 13.0 kg/m^2. The vital signs were normal. Physical examination revealed no abnormalities other than bilateral non-pitting edema of the lower legs. The patient received folate (10 mg/day), sertraline (50 mg/day), zolpidem (10 mg/day), and flunitrazepam (2 mg/day). Toxicology analysis was not performed because the patient presented no feature indicating exposure to toxic compounds. Laboratory findings were as follows: low WBC count, 2100 cells/μL; low reticulocyte count, 9.4 × 10^3 cells/μL; low Hb level, 5.7 g/dL; and low Plt count, 4.1 × 10^4 cells/dL. The differential WBC count was normal. Serum levels of iron, folate, vitamin B12, zinc, copper, and ceruloplasmin were within normal ranges. These results did not identify the etiology of the hematological problems. The patient persistently refused nutritional therapy and hoped that some other causes of pancytopenia (other than malnutrition) would be found. On hospitalization day 7, upon obtaining written informed consent from the patient, we performed bone marrow aspiration and biopsy.

Bone marrow aspiration revealed low counts of nucleated cells (5.5 × 10^3 cells/μL; reference range: 100–200 × 10^3 cells/μL) and megakaryocytes (< 15.6 cells/μL; reference range: 50–150 cells/μL). Bone marrow biopsy revealed hypoplasia but no dysplasia and confirmed the presence of fatty replacement with no gelatinous material (Fig. 1). It was notable that the bone marrow displayed fatty marrow findings without any evidence of GMT, which would generally indicate IAA. Moreover, no chromosomal abnormalities or cell surface abnormalities were found upon bone marrow examination. T1-weighted images from thoracolumbar magnetic resonance imaging confirmed homogenous high signal intensity, characteristic of fatty marrow. Detailed examination of peripheral blood and bone marrow findings indicated IAA. However, despite the absence of bone marrow features typically seen in malnutrition, the patient's hematological abnormalities manifested after a decrease in body weight. Thus,

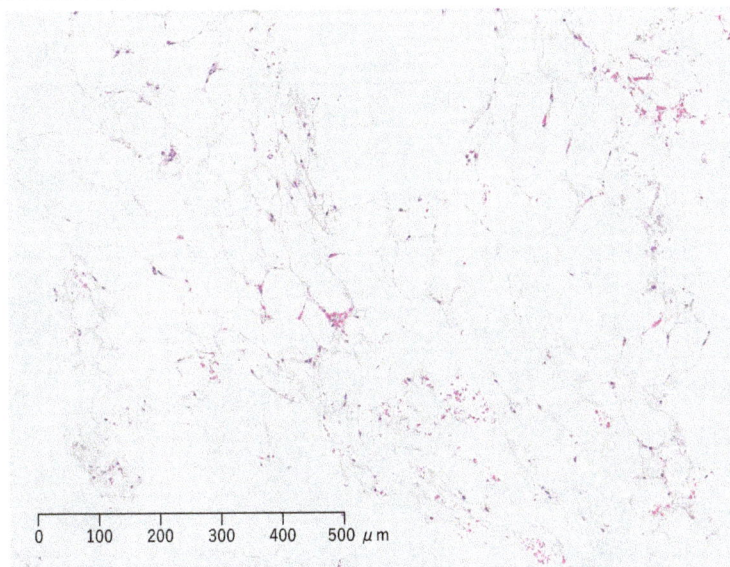

Fig. 1 Bone marrow biopsy of a patient with poorly controlled anorexia nervosa and severe hematological abnormalities. On hospitalization day 7, hematoxylin-eosin staining of the bone marrow sample revealed hematopoietic hypoplasia with increased fatty material but no apparent gelatinous material

although the biopsy findings indicated IAA, we considered that the nutritional etiology of pancytopenia could not be thoroughly ruled out.

After bone marrow aspiration and biopsy, the patient accepted nutritional therapy. At the time of admission, she was given 600 kcal/day intravenously. Energy intake was gradually increased, and the patient received oral nutrition amounting to 3200 kcal/day from hospitalization day 14 until discharge. The patient's caloric intake was strictly managed, which resulted in weight restoration (Table 1). The hematological abnormalities began to improve with the gradual increase in caloric intake. By hospitalization day 11, the patient's condition had improved to the point where she no longer required transfusions. On hospitalization day 28, the patient's weight was

38.1 kg, and her BMI was 16.5 kg/m^2. Pancytopenia had also improved (Table 1), and thus the patient was discharged the following day. Bone marrow aspiration and biopsy performed 2 weeks after discharge yielded normal findings. Because both blood and bone marrow findings improved after implementation of nutritional therapy alone, the final diagnosis was pancytopenia secondary to malnutrition.

Discussion and conclusions

To the best of our knowledge, no other literature reports have described patients with AN who present with peripheral blood and bone marrow findings consistent with IAA. In the present case, pancytopenia is believed to have been caused by malnutrition. Thus, the present

Table 1 Laboratory data prior to and throughout the course of hospitalization in the present case

Day	−46	−28[a]	−25[b]	0[c]	+ 7	+ 14	+ 21	+28[d]	Unit	Normal range
WBC count	**2500**	**2200**	**2400**	**2100**	**1200**	**2400**	**3000**	4200	cells/μL	4000–9000
Hb	**6.1**	**2.5**	**7.1[e]**	**5.7[e]**	**4.2**	**9.6[e]**	**8.3**	**8.3**	g/dL	12.0–15.2
MCV	113.9	122.0	95.8	92.4	95.7	95.2	96.7	98.5	fL	80.0–100.0
Reticulocyte count	**14.4**	N.A.	**13.2**	**9.4**	**24.3**	52.4	69.4	115.1	×10^3 cells/μL	35.0–125.0
Plt count	**10.6**	**8.6**	**8.5**	**4.1**	**7.5**	**11.1**	14.5	22.6	×10^4 cells/dL	11.7–32.9
BMI	13.8	12.9	N.A.	13.0	13.7	15.0	15.8	16.5	kg/m^2	18.5–24.9

The hematological abnormalities improved by nutritional therapy alone
Bold font indicates abnormally low values
WBC white blood cell, *Hb* hemoglobin, *MCV* mean corpuscular volume, *Plt* platelet, *BMI* body mass index, *N.A* not available
[a]Admission to the hematology department
[b]Discharge from the hematology department
[c]Admission to the psychiatric department
[d]Discharge from the psychiatric department
[e]Value measured within a week of last transfusion

Table 2 Summary of bone marrow findings in previously reported patients with anorexia nervosa and pancytopenia

Age	Sex	BMI (kg/m^2)	Hematopoietic cells in the bone marrow	Gelatinous material in the bone marrow	Fat cells in the bone marrow	Year of publication	Reference
32	F	13	hypocellular	(−)	increase	2018	present case
16	F	ND	hypocellular	(+)	decrease	2016	[7]
33	F	12.3	hypocellular	(+)	decrease	2013	[4]
18	F	12.1	hypocellular	(+)	lack	2013	[3]
28	M	18.2	hypocellular	(+)	increase	2004	[9]
28	F	12.3	hypocellular	(+)	lack	2003	[6]
20	F	10.7	hypocellular	(+)	decrease	1998	[10]
17	F	11.4	hypocellular	(−)	lack	1993	[15]
36	F	10.2	hypocellular	(+)	lack	1987	[8]
17	ND	ND	hypocellular	(+)	lack	1981	[5]
62	ND	ND	hypocellular	(+)	lack	1981	[5]
14	ND	ND	hypocellular	(+)	decrease	1981	[5]
18	F	ND	hypocellular	(+)	decrease	1979	[1]

In most cases described in the literature, anorexia nervosa with pancytopenia demonstrated gelatinous marrow transformation
BMI body mass index, *F* female, *M* male, *ND* not described

case is the first documented case of AN with pancytopenia for which bone marrow examination confirmed fatty marrow without GMT. Therefore, it was necessary to differentiate the actual cause of pancytopenia from IAA, as analysis of peripheral blood and bone marrow led to the suspicion of IAA [13]. However, because blood and bone marrow findings improved after implementation of nutritional therapy alone, the final diagnosis was revised to pancytopenia secondary to malnutrition. These findings are significant because they suggest a potential need to differentiate between malnutrition and IAA.

Bone marrow pathology findings were also distinctive in the present case. Although cytopenia was severe, bone marrow examination did not indicate GMT, which is thought to be the most critical bone marrow finding among patients with eating disorders. A significant correlation has been reported among BMI, WBC count, and red blood cell count in patients with eating disorders, as well as between weight loss and the extent of bone marrow abnormalities [14]. Therefore, it was difficult to establish our patient's diagnosis, as there was discrepancy between the results of bone marrow and blood tests.

Nearly all reported cases of eating disorders accompanied by pancytopenia included findings of gelatinous bone material [2–10] (Table 2). Upon examining patients with eating disorders, Abella et al. [14] classified bone marrow findings into four degrees of severity: normal, hypoplastic or aplastic without gelatinous degeneration, hypoplastic or aplastic with partial or focal gelatinous degeneration, and hypoplastic or aplastic with complete

gelatinous degeneration of the bone marrow. Although the patients described by Abella et al. did not have pancytopenia, it is notable that those with hypoplastic or aplastic marrow without gelatinous degeneration exhibited increased bone marrow fat fraction owing to increased adipocyte diameter [14]. In the present case, bone marrow findings were consistent with a hypoplastic or aplastic disorder (without gelatinous degeneration), as defined by Abella et al. [14]. Therefore, in such cases, abnormal bone marrow findings related to malnutrition cannot be differentiated based on the presence of fatty marrow, which is a typical bone marrow feature of IAA. Caution is therefore necessary, to avoid the potential pitfalls of a diagnosis based on hematologic parameters alone.

An accurate differential diagnosis of pancytopenia is crucial for selection of the most appropriate treatment. Should a case like the one described here be misdiagnosed as IAA, standard treatments such as immunotherapy and bone marrow transplant may be implemented, which would place an unnecessary burden on the patient. In cases where it is difficult to distinguish between IAA and pancytopenia due to malnutrition, we recommend a course of treatment focused on nutritional therapy, as well as careful follow-up.

Abbreviations
AN: Anorexia nervosa; BMI: Body mass index; GMT: Gelatinous marrow transformation; Hb: Hemoglobin; IAA: Idiopathic aplastic anemia; Plt: Platelet; WBC: White blood cell

Acknowledgements
We would like to thank Editage (www.editage.jp) for English language editing.

Authors' contributions
MT, RS, and AK treated the patient. MT and HI wrote the paper. TK1, HN, TK2, and TS critically reviewed the diagnostic results and contributed to manuscript preparation. All authors read and approved the final version of the manuscript.

Consent for publication
Written informed consent for publication of this case report was obtained from the patient. A copy of the signed written consent to publish is available for review by the editor of this journal.

Competing interests
The authors declare that they have no competing interests.

Author details
[1]Department of Neuropsychiatry, Akita University Graduate School of Medicine, 1-1-1,Hondo, Akita City, Akita 010-8543, Japan. [2]Department of Neuropsychiatry, Nakadori Rehabilitation Hospital, 6-1-58, Nakadori, Akita City, Akita 010-0001, Japan. [3]Division of Hematology/Oncology, Department of Medicine, Kameda General Hospital, 929 Higashi-chou, Kamogawa City, Chiba 296-8602, Japan. [4]Department of Neuropsychiatry, Akita City Hospital, 4-30, Matsuoka-machi, Kawamoto, Akita City, Akita 010-0933, Japan. [5]Department of Hematology, Nephrology and Rheumatology, Akita University Graduate School of Medicine, 1-1-1, Hondo, Akita City, Akita 010-8543, Japan. [6]Division of Clinical Pathology, Akita University Graduate School of Medicine, 1-1-1, Hondo, Akita City, Akita 010-8543, Japan.

References
1. Devuyst O, Lambert M, Rodhain J, Lefebvre C, Coche E. Haematological changes and infectious complications in anorexia nervosa: a case-control study. Q J Med. 1993;86:791–9.
2. Amrein PC, Friedman R, Kosinski K, Ellman L. Hematologic changes in anorexia nervosa. JAMA. 1979;241:2190–1.
3. Mohamed M, Khalafallah A. Gelatinous transformation of bone marrow in a patient with severe anorexia nervosa. Int J Haematol. 2013;97:157–8.
4. Morii K, Yamamoto T, Kishida H, Okushin H. Gelatinous transformation of bone marrow in patients with anorexia nervosa. Intern Med. 2013;52:2005–6.
5. Myers TJ, Perkerson MD, Witter BA, Granville NB. Hematologic findings in anorexia nervosa. Conn Med. 1981;45:14–7.
6. Nishio S, Yamada H, Yamada K, Okabe H, Okuya T, Yonekawa O, et al. Severe neutropenia with gelatinous bone marrow transformation in anorexia nervosa: a case report. Int J Eat Disord. 2003;33:360–3.
7. Schafernak KT. Gelatinous transformation of the bone marrow from anorexia nervosa. Blood. 2016;127:1374.
8. Steinberg SE, Nasraway S, Peterson L. Reversal of severe serous atrophy of the bone marrow in anorexia nervosa. JPEN J Parenter Enteral Nutr. 1987;11:422–3.
9. Vande Zande VL, Mazza JJ, Yale SH. Hematologic and metabolic abnormalities in a patient with anorexia nervosa. WMJ. 2004;103:38–40.
10. Younis E, Jarrah N, Abdeen G, Raqqad A, Tarawneh M, Ajlouni K. Anorexia nervosa with pancytopenia. Ann Saudi Med. 1998;18:478–9.
11. Hütter G, Ganepola S, Hofmann WK. The hematology of anorexia nervosa. Int J Eat Disord. 2009;42:293–300.
12. Shergill KK, Shergill GS, Pillai HJ. Gelatinous transformation of bone marrow: rare or underdiagnosed? Autops Case Rep. 2017;7:8–17.
13. Killick SB, Bown N, Cavenagh J, Dokal I, Foukanel T, Hill A, et al. Guidelines for the diagnosis and management of adult aplastic anaemia. Br J Haematol. 2016;172:187–207.
14. Abella E, Feliu E, Granada I, Millá F, Oriol A, Ribera JM, et al. Bone marrow changes in anorexia nervosa are correlated with the amount of weight loss and not with other clinical findings. Am J Clin Pathol. 2002;118:582–8.
15. Fukudo S, Tanaka A, Muranaka M, Sasaki M, Iwahashi S, Nomura T, et al. Case report: reversal of severe leukopenia by granulocyte colony-stimulating factor in anorexia nervosa. Am J Med Sci. 1993;305:314–7.

The impact of child maltreatment on non-suicidal self-injury: data from a representative sample of the general population

Rebecca C. Brown[1]* , Stefanie Heines[1], Andreas Witt[1], Elmar Braehler[2,3], Joerg M. Fegert[1], Daniela Harsch[1] and Paul L. Plener[1,4]

Abstract

Background: Child maltreatment is an identified risk factor for Non-Suicidal Self-Injury (NSSI). The aim of the current study was to investigate effects of different types of maltreatment, and mediating effects of depression and anxiety on NSSI in the general population.

Methods: A representative sample of the German population, comprising $N = 2498$ participants (mean age = 48.4 years (SD = 18.2), 53.3% female) participated in this study. Child maltreatment was assessed using the Childhood Trauma Questionnaire (CTQ),NSSI was assessed with a question on lifetime engagement in NSSI, depressive symptoms were assessed by the Patient Health Questionnaire (PHQ-2) and anxiety symptoms by the General Anxiety Disorder questionnaire (GAD-2).

Results: Lifetime prevalence of NSSI in this sample was 3.3, and 30.8% reported at least one type of child maltreatment. Participants in the NSSI group reported significantly more experiences of child maltreatment. Emotional abuse was endorsed by 72% of all participants with NSSI. A path analytic model demonstrated an unmediated direct effect of emotional neglect, a partially mediated effect of emotional abuse, and a fully mediated effect of sexual abuse and physical neglect by depression and anxiety on NSSI.

Conclusions: Especially emotional neglect and abuse seem to play a role in the etiology of NSSI above and beyond depression and anxiety, while sexual and physical abuse seem to have a rather indirect effect.

Keywords: Child maltreatment, Non-suicidal self-injury, NSSI, Child abuse and neglect

Background

Child maltreatment (emotional, physical, and sexual abuse, as well as physical and emotional neglect) has shown to be associated with a large variety of different mental- and physical health problems throughout the lifespan [1, 2]. The experience of at least one type of child maltreatment was reported by around 30% of the general population of Germany in two independent studies [3, 4]. Different mental health problems like depressive disorders, suicide attempts, and drug abuse have been identified as long-term consequences of child maltreatment [1]. Furthermore, child maltreatment has been identified as risk-factor for Nonsuicidal Self-Injury (NSSI) and self-harm in several studies (for review see [5]). NSSI is defined as the deliberate damaging of the surface of the skin (e.g. cutting, scratching, or burning) without suicidal intent [6]. Studies investigating NSSI in the general population have found NSSI to be very common among adolescents, with international lifetime prevalence rates of around 18% [7]. However, studies from adult populations indicate that NSSI is less prevalent in mid- to late adulthood. A study from the general population in the US using random digit dialing reported a

* Correspondence: rebecca.brown@uniklinik-ulm.de
[1]Department of Child and Adolescent Psychiatry/Psychotherapy, University of Ulm, Steinhoevelstr, 5, 89075 Ulm, Germany
Full list of author information is available at the end of the article

lifetime prevalence of 5.9 and 0.9% within the last year [8]. These results correspond well to a recent study of a representative sample of the German general population, finding a lifetime prevalence of 3 and 0.3% within the last year [9].

Several studies have investigated the relationship between child maltreatment and NSSI, however mainly in adolescent samples. So far, most consistent evidence has been found for emotional abuse and neglect to be related to the engagement in NSSI. In a systematic review of the literature, Lang and Sharma-Patel [5] found consistent evidence for emotional neglect to predict NSSI. A very recent study [10] reported a direct association of emotional abuse and NSSI, while the effect of sexual and physical abuse was mediated completely by emotion expressivity (i.e. difficulties in expressing emotions appropriately) and emotion coping (ability to cope with negative emotions).

These results are in line with mixed results on sexual and physical abuse in previous studies. In a meta-analysis including 45 studies on the association of child sexual abuse and self-injury, Klonsky and Moyer [11] found a modest relationship between child sexual abuse and NSSI. It has been shown in several other studies, that the association between NSSI and sexual abuse was (almost) completely mediated by factors like low self-esteem [12], dissociation [13], alexithymia [14], self-criticism [15], and posttraumatic stress symptoms [16]. A more recent systematic review [17] reported similar outcomes. Regarding physical abuse, results from studies are also rather mixed, with some results pointing towards a significant relationship [18, 19], while others did not find significant associations [10, 20]. One study [15] also found a significant effect of physical neglect on NSSI in a sample of adolescents.

These rather mixed results might be due to several mediating and moderating factors in the relationship between child abuse and neglect and engagement in NSSI. According to the Developmental Psychopathology Framework [21], especially negative experiences with primary caregivers can lead to deficits in emotion regulation and neurophysiological dysregulation, which can then in turn lead to engaging in maladaptive coping-strategies, like NSSI. However, this relationship seems to be of a rather complex nature, as different types of maltreatment may lead to impairment of different aspects of emotion regulation and might therefore have differential impact on NSSI [22].

While NSSI can occur without further psychopathology [23], it mostly co-occurs with other symptoms and disorders, such as depression and anxiety [24, 25]. Furthermore, a large body of research found depression and anxiety to be risk-factors for NSSI (for review see [26]), but these are also known to occur as a consequence of child maltreatment [1]. These factors might therefore also play a mediating role between the experience of child maltreatment and engaging in NSSI. A study by Glassman and colleagues, for example, found depression to be mediating the effect of child maltreatment on NSSI [15].

In summary, most studies testing the association of child maltreatment and NSSI were conducted in rather young clinical or convenience samples, while data from representative samples in adult populations are still scarce. Analyses of samples in the general population are important, as NSSI but also child maltreatment might be overrepresented in clinical and convenience samples. By recruiting a random, representative sample of the general population, evidence of results from previous studies including selective samples can be strengthened and new conclusions on the effects of child maltreatment on NSSI across the lifespan in a non-clinical population can be drawn. The aim of the current study was to investigate the association of different types of child maltreatment and NSSI in a sample of the general population of Germany. In detail, the differential impact of perceived severity and type of maltreatment, as well as a possible mediation of depressive and anxiety symptoms were of interest. It was hypothesized that (1) having experienced any type of child maltreatment would lead to a higher vulnerability for engaging in NSSI, (2) a cumulating effect of different types of child maltreatment on lifetime NSSI would be found, (3) especially emotional abuse and neglect would directly affect NSSI, and (4) that physical abuse and –neglect, as well as sexual abuse, would be mediated by depression and anxiety symptoms.

Methods

Using a random route procedure, a representative sample of the German population was acquired by a demographic consulting company (USUMA, Berlin, Germany) between September and November 2016. Households of every third residence in a randomly chosen geographical area were invited to participate in the study. Households were approached by door to door in person recruitment. In multi-person households, participants were randomly selected using a Kish-Selection-Grid. After initial recruitment contact, research staff scheduled a time convenient for the participant to complete questionnaires. Inclusion criteria were a minimum age of 14 and sufficient knowledge of the German language. Of 4902 designated addresses, 2510 households participated in the study. Main reasons for non-participation were that participants were not present or refusal to participate. Responses were anonymous. In a first step, socio-demographic information was gathered in an interview-format by research staff. All other information was obtained via paper and pencil questionnaires, with research staff being available for questions.

The study was conducted in accordance with the Declaration of Helsinki, and fulfilled the ethical guidelines of the International Code of Marketing and Social Research Practice of the International Chamber of Commerce and of the European Society of Opinion and Marketing Research. All participants (and in case of minorstheir caregivers, 3.4% of the sample) gave informed written consent. The study was approved by the Ethics Committee of the Medical Department of the University of Leipzig.

Measures

The prevalence of five types of child maltreatment was assessed using the 28 item brief version of the Childhood Trauma Questionnaire (CTQ) [27, 28]. The CTQ is a screening measure for the assessment of child maltreatment. It contains five subscales each assessed by five items, including sexual, (e.g. "someone tried to make me do sexual things or watch sexual things") emotional, (e.g. "people in my family said hurtful or insulting things to me") and physical abuse (e.g. "I was punished with a belt, a board, a cord, or some other hard object"),as well as emotional, (e.g. "I felt loved" (reversed)) and physical neglect (e.g. "I didn't have enough to eat"). Additionally, three items assess whether participants tend to trivialize problematic experiences within their family (e.g. "There was nothing I would have wished to be different in my family"). Good psychometric properties of the German version of the CTQ were demonstrated by Klinitzke and colleagues [27], with internal consistencies ranging between Cronbach's Alpha = .62 (physical neglect) and Cronbach's Alpha = .96 (sexual abuse) for all subscales. The intra-class coefficient for an interval of six weeks was 0.77 for the overall scale and between 0.58 and 0.81 for subscales. In the current sample, internal consistencies were Cronbach's Alpha = .55 for physical neglect, Cronbach's Alpha = .82 for emotional neglect and emotional abuse, respectively, Cronbach's Alpha = .83 for physical abuse, and Cronbach's Alpha = .91 for sexual abuse. Based on norm data by Bernstein and colleagues [29], severity scores for each subscale can be calculated, ranging from "none -minimal", "minimal-moderate", "moderate-severe", to "severe-extreme". These categories were used in the current study, when calculating χ^2 tests between participants with or without NSSI. Continuous scores of each scale of the CTQ were entered in the path analytic model.

Lifetime prevalence of NSSI was assessed by a question ("Have you ever intentionally harmed yourself, without the intention to die?"), which was taken from the Self-Injurious Thoughts and Behavior Interview (SITBI, [30]) in its validated German version (Fischer et al., 2014).

The use of a paper and pencil version of the SITBI in its German version has been shown to provide reliable results in a former study [9].

Depressive symptoms were assessed with the German version of the screening tool Patient Health Questionnaire (PHQ-2), focusing on the depressive symptoms 'low mood' and 'loss of interest'. Scores can reach values from 0 to 6, with a cut-off of values higher than 3 leading to values of sensitivity of 87% and specificity of 78% for major depression [31]. The internal consistency in the current sample was Cronbach's Alpha = .81. Anxiety symptoms were screened for using the GAD-2 (General Anxiety Disorder questionnaire). Like the PHQ-2, the questionnaire consists of two items, with possible values from 0 to 6 and a cut-off of 3. This cut-off is sensitive for screening for generalized anxiety disorders (86%), panic disorders (76%), social anxiety disorder (70%) and moderately for PTSD (59%). It is specific for all four types of anxiety disorders mentioned above (81–83%), with an internal consistency of Cronbach's alpha = .82 (Cronbach's alpha = .79 in the current sample) [32].

Participants

Of the $N = 2510$ participants, $n = 12$ participants were excluded due to missing data on NSSI. Participants were on average 48.4 years old (SD = 18.2) and 53.3% were female. The sample was representative for the German population with regard to age and gender. Of the entire sample, 21.7% reported to have completed high-school with 'Abitur', which qualifies for entering university, 5.3% reported to be currently unemployed, 54.5% lived with a partner, and 3.2% reported a place of birth outside of Germany. Average depression and anxiety scores of the entire sample were under the clinical cut-off of 3. A detailed description of participants with regard to child maltreatment and psychiatric symptoms by age group can be seen in Table 1.

Statistical analyses

Statistical analyses were conducted using SPSS version 21 and MPlus Version 7.31. Differences between the co-occurrence of child maltreatment and NSSI, and differences in the severity of child maltreatment were calculated using χ^2 tests. Different types of child maltreatment were were weakly to moderately inter-correlated ($r = 0.27$ for emotional neglect and sexual abuse to $r = 0.65$ for emotional and physical neglect). For this reason, a path analytic model for the relationship of different types of child maltreatment as independent variables (continuous scores, and allowing for inter-correlation of those variables) with NSSI as the dependent variable and depression and anxiety scores (continuous scores) as mediating variables was calculated using MPlus. Model fit was calculated via the

Table 1 Experience of child maltreatment and psychiatric symptoms of participants divided by age groups

	14–19 years	20–29 years	30–39 years	40–49 years	50–59 years	60–69 years	70+ years
Child maltreatment							
Emotional abuse	5.7% (N = 8)	5.7% (N = 19)	6.9% (N = 27)	9.1% (N = 36)	7.8% (N = 38)	3.6% (N = 14)	5.7% (N = 20)
Physical abuse	7.1% (N = 10)	4.2% (N = 14)	6.1% (N = 24)	5.5% (N = 22)	8.2% (N = 40)	6.2% (N = 24)	8.9% (N = 31)
Sexual abuse	5.0% (N = 7)	4.2% (N = 14)	6.9% (N = 27)	11.1% (N = 44)	9.2% (N = 45)	7.0% (N = 27)	6.3% (N = 22)
Emotional neglect	6.4% (N = 9)	12.7% (N = 42)	12.4% (N = 49)	13.1% (N = 52)	17.9% (M = 87)	10.9% (n = 42)	14.3% (N = 50)
Physical neglect	5.7% (N = 8)	16.9% (N = 56)	17.5% (N = 69)	18.7% (N = 74)	22.6% (N = 110)	20.9% (N = 81)	45.8% (N = 160)
Psychiatric symptoms							
Anxiety	6.4% (N = 9)	6.3% (N = 21)	7.6% (N = 30)	8.8% (N = 35)	10.7% (N = 52)	4.8% (N = 19)	6.1% (N = 21)
Depression	7.9% (N = 11)	6.4% (N = 21)	6.4% (N = 25)	8.3% (N = 33)	9.3% (N = 45)	5.1% (N = 20)	7.8% (N = 27)
NSSI	7.8% (N = 11)	7.5% (N = 25)	5.1% (N = 20)	3.5% (N = 14)	1.6% (N = 8)	0.8% (N = 3)	0.6% (N = 2)

Child maltreatment: at least moderate to severe level. Anxiety and depression levels: GAD-2 and PHQ-2 scores above clinical cut-off, NSSI: lifetime engagement NSSI

weighted root mean square residual (WRMR), which is best used for modelling categorical variables [33]. A WRMR< .90 implies good model fit for continuous and categorical variables [34]. As the NSSI and non-NSSI group differed significantly concerning age and gender, age and gender were included as covariates in the model. Standardized coefficients of the model are reported.

Results

A total of 83 participants (3.3%) reported lifetime engagement in NSSI. Concerning child abuse, 30.8% reported having experienced at least one type of child maltreatment, with 16.8% reporting one type of maltreatment and 14.0% of the overall sample reported several types of maltreatment. The most common type of at least moderate to severe maltreatment was physical neglect (22.4%), followed by emotional neglect (13.2%), sexual abuse (7.6%), physical abuse (6.7%), and emotional abuse (6.5%). For further details on maltreatment data see Witt et al. [4].

Differences between participant in the NSSI and the non-NSSI group

It was hypothesized that (1) having experienced any type of child maltreatment would lead to a higher vulnerability for engaging in NSSI, (2) a cumulating effect of different types of child maltreatment on lifetime NSSI would be found. Around two thirds (65.1%) of participants in the NSSI group reported having experienced at least one type of child maltreatment. This was significantly different from 29.7% of participants in the non-NSSI group ($\chi^2 = 46.93$, $p < .001$). Furthermore, 48.2% of participants in the NSSI group reported having experienced multiple types of child maltreatment, while this was true for 12.8% of the non-NSSI group ($\chi^2 = 83.38$, $p < .001$).

With regards to different types of child maltreatment, participants with NSSI generally reported higher levels of child maltreatment in all areas (see Fig. 1). At least moderate to severe emotional abuse was reported by 42.2% of participants in the NSSI group vs. 5.3% in the non-NSSI group ($\chi^2 = 223.5$, $p < .001$). Physical abuse of at least moderate to severe level was reported by 32.2% of the NSSI group vs. 5.9% in the non-NSSI group ($\chi^2 = 93.9$, $p < .001$). Regarding sexual abuse, 28.9% in the NSSI group reported at least moderate to severe levels, while this was true for 6.7% in the non-NSSI group ($\chi^2 = 130.5$, p < .001). Concerning neglect, 33.7% in the NSSI group vs. 12.6% in the non-NSSI group reported moderate to severe emotional neglect ($\chi^2 = 11.9$, $p < .05$), while 36.2% in the NSSI group reported moderate to severe physical neglect vs. 22.0% in the non-NSSI group ($\chi^2 = 111.3$, p < .001). Further details on severity of neglect in association with NSSI can be seen in Fig. 1.

Participants with NSSI indicated significantly higher, yet on average not clinically relevant, scores of depression and anxiety symptoms. Furthermore, participants reporting NSSI were significantly younger and more likely to be female (for details see Table 2).

Path analytic model of child maltreatment related to NSSI, mediated by depression and anxiety scores

It was further hypothesized that (3) especially emotional abuse and neglect would directly affect NSSI, and (4) that physical abuse and –neglect, as well as sexual abuse, would be mediated by depression and anxiety symptoms.

The path analytic modelshowed good model fit (weighted root mean square residual (WRMS = .001, df = 59). Emotional abuse (estimated direct effect = 0.14, $p < .001$) and emotional neglect (estimated direct effect = 0.11, $p = .001$) were the only types of child maltreatment that showed significant direct effects on NSSI, while physical abuse (estimated direct effect

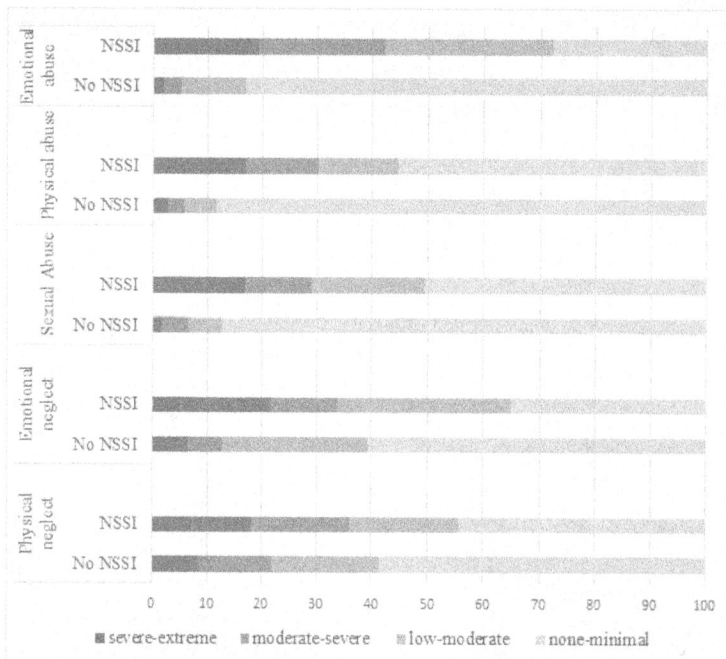

Fig. 1 Different types of maltreatment by severity in association with lifetime engagement in NSSI. *Note*: displayed are percentages of participants meeting CTQ-scores in corresponding categories (severe-extreme to none-minimal)

= .05, *p* = .15), sexual abuse (estimated direct effect = .05, *p* = .08), and physical neglect (estimated direct effect = − 0.02, *p* = .75) did not. The effect of emotional neglect was not significantly mediated by depression or anxiety scores. The effect of emotional abuse was partially mediated by depression scores (specific indirect effect:=0.03, *p* = .02) and anxiety scores (specific indirect effect = 0.04, *p* = .01). Effects of sexual abuse and physical neglect were fully mediated by depression and anxiety scores, as direct effects of both variables on NSSI were non-significant, but indirect effects were(total indirect effect = 0.03, *p* = .009 for sexual abuse and total indirect effect: =0.02, *p* = .007 for physical neglect). Physical neglect was not significantly related to NSSI, depression or anxiety scores (for details see Fig. 2).

Discussion

As former studies have reported conflicting results regarding the relationship between different types of abuse and neglect and NSSI, the aim of the current study was to investigate these associations as well as mediating effects of depression and anxiety on NSSI in the general population. In this representative sample of the German population, around 3% of all participants reported lifetime engagement in NSSI, and around 30% reported having experienced at least one form of child maltreatment. Among those participants with a lifetime history of NSSI, around 65% reported at least one type of maltreatment. Around 50% reported multiple types of maltreatment, while this was only true for around 12% of the general population. Overall, participants with a history of NSSI showed higher levels of severity of child

Table 2 Relevant characteristics of participants

	Total (N = 2498)	NSSI (n = 83)	No NSSI (n = 2415)	Chi²/T	Phi/ Cohen's d
Age					
Mean (SD)	48.4 (18.2)	34.9 (14.4)	48.9 (18.2)	−6.93**	0.77
Range	14–94	15–79	14–94		
Gender				10.83*	0.07
Female (%)	1333 (53.4)	59 (71.1)	1274 (52.8)		
Male (%)	1165 (46.6)	24 (28.9)	1141 (47.2)		
Depression Score	0.69 (1.16)	2.26 (1.68)	0.64 (1.10)	12.71**	1.44
Anxiety Score	0.69 (1,14)	2.33 (1.78)	0.64 (1.07)	13.60**	1.54

**p < .001, *p < .05

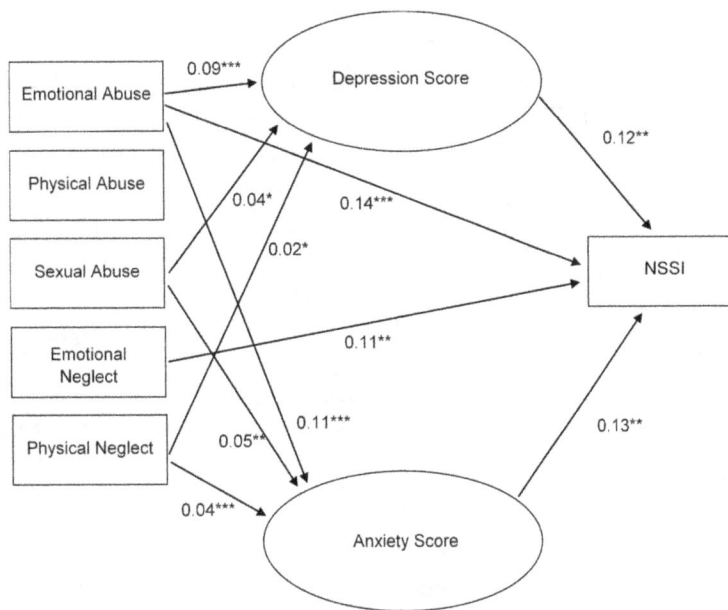

Fig. 2 Path analytic model of child maltreatment related to NSSI with depression and anxiety scores as mediating factors. *Note*: For reasons of comprehensibleness, only significant associations are displayed in the graph. *$p < .05$, **$p < .01$, ***$p < .001$

maltreatment for all maltreatment subtypes (emotional, physical, and sexual abuse, emotional and physical neglect). However, a path analytic model showed only emotional neglect and abuse to be directly associated with NSSI, while the effect of sexual abuse and physical neglect were fully mediated by depression and anxiety symptoms.

Findings of this study are in line with previous findings reporting long-term negative mental health outcomes of child maltreatment [1]. Except physical abuse, all types of child maltreatment were significantly associated with higher depression and anxiety scores, as well as (sometimes indirectly) lifetime engagement in NSSI. This is the first study to report such long-term negative outcomes in a representative sample of the general population.

The association of child maltreatment and NSSI is especially obvious when considering that around two thirds of participants with NSSI reported child maltreatment, and 50% reported more than one type of maltreatment (of at least moderate to severe level). This could also point towards a dose-impact effect, meaning that the experience of several types of maltreatment might increase the likelihood of adverse long-term effects. A previous study also assessing child maltreatment using the CTQ [15], examined the relationship of child maltreatment with NSSI in the past year in a sample of 86 adolescents. Interestingly, even though the age difference between this sample and our sample was quite large, and NSSI within the past year vs. lifetime NSSI were assessed, results of both studies are rather similar. Results of the current study therefore add to the literature

by showing that child maltreatment does not only have a rather short-term effect on NSSI during adolescence, but may have an effect on NSSI later on in life.

The types of maltreatment being directly associated with NSSI were a history of emotional abuse and neglect (72 and 65% of participants with NSSI reported at least mild-moderate emotional abuse and neglect, respectively, and 42 and 32% at least moderate-severe levels). This direct impact was still significant in the presence of depression or anxiety symptoms, while the effect of emotional abuse was partially mediated by depression and anxiety scores. Results concerning emotional abuse are in line with previous studies [10, 15, 35] and support theoretical approaches like the Developmental Psychopathology Network [21] or the Biopsychosocial Model by Marsha Linehan [36], both linking adverse childhood experiences with primary caregivers with the development of dysfunctional emotion regulation and thus developing dysfunctional coping skills like NSSI.

With regard to sexual abuse and physical neglect, the current study found support for those factors to play a role in the etiology of NSSI. However, these effects were fully mediated by the presence of depressive and anxiety symptoms. These results add on to findings (for review see [11, 17]) presenting sexual abuse as rather having an indirect than a direct effect on the development of NSSI. In previous studies, this effect was also mediated by factors like dissociation, self-esteem, or alexithymia, which were not assessed in the current study [12–15]. The fact that NSSI is most often engaged in as a dysfunctional emotion regulation strategy might explain why emotional abuse and –neglect were directly associated with NSSI, as they may more directly effect a persons' ability to regulate emotions. On the other hand, physical types of abuse (like sexual or physical abuse) might only indirectly effect emotion regulation, for example in a person consequently developing symptoms of an affective disorder. This may have been one reason for effects of physical and emotional abuse being fully mediated by anxiety and depressive symptoms in the current study. However, assessment of other mediating factors, known to be linked to child maltreatment will be necessary before drawing further conclusions.

Limitations

NSSI was only assessed by one question, which may have had an impact on the reliability of the assessment of NSSI. However, prevalence rates of NSSI in this study are in line with results of a previous, separate representative sample of the German population, reporting prevalence of lifetime NSSI of also around 3% [9]. While in the previous sample, NSSI was assessed much more rigorously by using the whole Self-Injurious-Thoughts-and-Behaviors Interview and assessing methods and functions of NSSI, the single assessment question in this study seemed to have been quite reliable as it yielded comparable rates. Furthermore, as this was a cross-sectional design assessing data in retrospect and in self-report, the possibility of memory bias regarding NSSI and child maltreatment has to be kept in mind when interpreting results. Regarding differential effect of types of maltreatment, one should be aware of the rather high rate of co-occurrence of different types of maltreatment. However, by entering all types of maltreatment into a path analytic model, this inter-correlation was accounted for. Furthermore, no corrections were made to protect against violation of assumptions in statistical tests due to the discrepant cell sizes between the two levels of the dichotomous outcome variable for NSSI.

Conclusions

Child maltreatment, and especially emotional abuse and neglect, seem to play a significant role in the etiology of NSSI, above and beyond depressive and anxiety symptoms. Results of this study also have implications for preventative and therapeutic interventions. As particularly emotional abuse and neglect are oftentimes not detected (as they do not lead to physical indications like bruises and does not lead to a diagnosis of Posttraumatic Stress Disorder, as criterion A is not met), professionals working with children should be

aware of its long-term consequences. This implies both, offering parenting training and supervision as preventative measures, and assessing and addressing emotional abuse and neglect in the treatment of NSSI. As impairment in emotion regulation seems to be a significant mediator of the effect between child maltreatment and NSSI, but is a complex concept to explore [22], it should be a focus in future studies. Future studies will also need to focus on outcomes of different types of child abuse and neglect on NSSI in a longitudinal design.

Abbreviations
CTQ: Child Trauma Questionnaire; NSSI: Non-suicidal self-injury

Authors' contributions
RCB drafted the manuscript and was involved in statistical analyses and interpretation of data. AW performed statistical analyses in MPlus. SH was involved in interpretation of data. PLP and JMF made substantial contributions to conception and design of the study. EB and DH were involved in acquisition of data. AWSH, EB, JMF, DH, and PLP were involved in revising the manuscript critically for important intellectual content. All authors gave final approval of the version to be published and all authors agreed to be accountable for all aspects of the work in ensuring that questions related to the accuracy of integrity of any part of the work are appropriately investigated and resolved.

Competing interests
All authors declare to have no competing interests. JMF has received research funding from the EU, DFG (German Research Foundation), BMG (Federal Ministry of Health), BMBF (Federal Ministry of Education and Research), BMFSFJ (Federal Ministry of Family, Senior Citizens, Women and Youth), German armed forces, several state ministries of social affairs, State Foundation Baden-Württemberg, Volkswagen Foundation, European Academy, Pontifical Gregorian University, RAZ, CJD, Caritas, Diocese of Rottenburg-Stuttgart. Moreover, he received travel grants, honoraria and sponsoring for conferences and medical educational purposes from DFG, AACAP, NIMH/NIH, EU, Pro Helvetia, Janssen-Cilag (J&J), Shire, several universities, professional associations, political foundations, and German federal and state ministries during the last five years. Every grant and every honorarium has to be declared to the law office of the University Hospital Ulm. Professor Fegert holds no stocks of pharmaceutical companies. PLP has received research funding from the German Federal Institute for Drugs and Medical Devices (BfARM), the German Federal Ministry of Education and Research (BMBF), VW-Foundation, Baden-Württemberg Stiftung, Lundbeck and Servier. He received a speaker's honorarium from Shire. He is a member of the Editorial Board for BMC Psychiatry. Professor Plener holds no stocks of pharmaceutical companies.

Author details
[1]Department of Child and Adolescent Psychiatry/Psychotherapy, University of Ulm, Steinhoevelstr, 5, 89075 Ulm, Germany. [2]Department of Psychosomatic Medicine and Psychotherapy, University Medical Center of the Johannes Gutenberg University of Mainz, Langenbeckstraße 1, 55131 Mainz, Germany. [3]Department of Medical Psychology and Medical Sociology, University of Leipzig, Leipzig, Germany. [4]Department of Child and Adolescent Psychiatry, Medical University of Vienna, Waehringerguertel 18-20, 1090 Vienna, Austria.

References

1. Norman RE, Byambaa M, De R, Butchart A, Scott J, Vos T. The long-term health consequences of child physical abuse, emotional abuse, and neglect: a systematic review and meta-analysis. PLoS Med. 2012;9(11):e1001349.
2. Weber S, Jud A, Landolt MA. Quality of life in maltreated children and adult survivors of child maltreatment: a systematic review. Qual Life Res. 2016; 25(2):237–55.
3. Iffland B, Brahler E, Neuner F, Hauser W, Glaesmer H. Frequency of child maltreatment in a representative sample of the German population. BMC Public Health. 2013;13(980):1471–2458.
4. Witt A, Brown RC, Plener PL, Braehler E, Fegert JM. Child maltreatment in Germany: prevalence rates in the general population. Child Adolescent Psychiatry Mental Health. 2017;(11). https://doi.org/10.1186/s13034-017-0185-0
5. Lang CM, Sharma-Patel K. The relation between childhood maltreatment and self-injury: a review of the literature on conceptualization and intervention. Trauma Violence Abuse. 2011;12(1):23–37.
6. Lloyd-Richardson EE, Perrine N, Dierker L, Kelley ML. Characteristics and functions of non-suicidal self-injury in a community sample of adolescents. Psychol Med. 2007;37(8):1183–92.
7. Muehlenkamp JJ, Claes L, Havertape L, Plener PL. International prevalence of adolescent non-suicidal self-injury and deliberate self-harm. Child Adolesc Psychiatry Ment Health. 2012;6:10.
8. Klonsky ED. Non-suicidal self-injury in United States adults: prevalence, sociodemographics, topography and functions. Psychol Med. 2011;41(9):1981
9. Plener PL, Allroggen M, Kapusta ND, Brahler E, Fegert JM, Groschwitz RC. The prevalence of nonsuicidal self-injury (NSSI) in a representative sample of the German population. BMC Psychiatry. 2016;16(1):353.
10. Thomassin K, Shaffer A, Madden A, Londino DL. Specificity of childhood maltreatment and emotion deficit in nonsuicidal self-injury in an inpatient sample of youth. Psychiatry Res. 2016;244:103–8.
11. Klonsky ED, Moyer A. Childhood sexual abuse and non-suicidal self-injury: meta-analysis. Br J Psychiatry. 2008;192(3):166–70.
12. Low G, Jones D, MacLeod A, Power M, Duggan C. Childhood trauma, dissociation and self-harming behavior: a pilot study. Br J Med Psychol. 2000;73:269–78.
13. Yates TM, Carlson EA, Egeland B. A prospective study of child maltreatment and self-injurious behavior in a community sample. Dev Psychopathol. 2008;20(2):651–71.
14. Paivio SC, McCulloch CR. Alexithymia as a mediator between childhood trauma and self-injurious behaviors. Child Abuse Negl. 2004;28(3):339–
15. Glassman LH, Weierich MR, Hooley JM, Deliberto TL, Nock MK. Child maltreatment, non-suicidal self-injury, and the mediating role of self-criticism. Behav Res Ther. 2007;45(10):2483–90.
16. Weierich MR, Nock MK. Posttraumatic stress symptoms mediate the relation between childhood sexual abuse and nonsuicidal self-injury. J Consult Clin Psychol. 2008;76(1):39–44.
17. Maniglio R. The role of child sexual abuse in the etiology of suicide and non-suicidal self-injury. Acta Psychiatr Scand. 2011;124(1):30–41.
18. Goncalves S, Machado B, Silva C, Crosby RD, Lavender JM, Cao L, Machado PP. The moderating role of purging behaviour in the relationship between sexual/physical abuse and nonsuicidal self-injury in eating disorder patients. Eur Eat Disord Rev. 2016;24(2):164–8.
19. Wan Y, Chen J, Sun Y, Tao F. Impact of childhood abuse on the risk of non-suicidal self-injury in mainland Chinese adolescents. PLoS One. 2015;10(6): e0131239.
20. Auerbach RP, Kim JC, Chango JM, Spiro WJ, Cha C, Gold J, Esterman M, Nock MK. Adolescent nonsuicidal self-injury: examining the role of child abuse, comorbidity, and disinhibition. Psychiatry Res. 2014;220(1–2):579
21. Yates TM. The developmental psychopathology of self-injurious behavior: compensatory regulation in posttraumatic adaptation. Clin Psychol Rev. 2004;24:35–74.
22. Muehlenkamp JJ, Kerr PL, Bradley AR, Adams Larsen M. Abuse subtypes and nonsuicidal self-injury: preliminary evidence of complex emotion regulation patterns. J Nerv Ment Dis. 2010;198(4):258–63.
23. Stanford S, Jones MP. Psychological subtyping finds pathological, impulsive, and 'normal' groups among adolescents who self-harm. J Child Psychol Psychiatry. 2009;50(7):807–15.
24. Asarnow JR, Porta G, Spirito A, Emslie G, Clarke G, Wagner KD, Vitiello B, Keller M, Birmaher B, McCracken J, et al. Suicide attempts and nonsuicidal self-injury in the treatment of resistant depression in adolescents: findings from the TORDIA study. J Am Acad Child Adolesc Psychiatry. 2011;50(8):772–81.
25. In-Albon T, Ruf C, Schmid M. Proposed diagnostic criteria for the DSM-5 of nonsuicidal self-injury in female adolescents: diagnostic and clinical correlates. Psychiatry J. 2013;2013:159208.
26. Fox KR, Franklin JC, Ribeiro JD, Kleiman EM, Bentley KH, Nock MK. Meta-analysis of risk factors for nonsuicidal self-injury. Clin Psychol Rev. 2015;42:156–67.
27. Klinitzke G, Romppel M, Hauser W, Brahler E, Glaesmer H. The German version of the childhood trauma questionnaire (CTQ): psychometric characteristics in a representative sample of the general population. Psychother Psychosom Med Psychol. 2012;62(2):47–51.
28. Wingenfeld K, Spitzer C, Mensebach C, Grabe HJ, Hill A, Gast U, Schlosser N, Hopp H, Beblo T, Driessen M. The German version of the childhood trauma questionnaire (CTQ):preliminary psychometric properties. Psychother Psychosom Med Psychol. 2010;60(8):1.
29. Bernstein MJ, Claypool HM. Social exclusion and pain sensitivity: why exclusion sometimes hurts and sometimes numbs. Personal Soc Psychol Bull. 2012;38(2):185–96.
30. Nock MK, Holmberg EB, Photos VI, Michel BD. Self-injurious thoughts and behaviors interview: development, reliability, and validity in an adolescent sample. Psychol Assess. 2007;19(3):309–17.
31. Loewe B, Kroenke K, Grafe K. Detecting and monitoring depression with a two-item questionnaire (PHQ-2). J Psychosom Res. 2005;58(2):163–71.
32. Kroenke K, Spitzer RL, Williams JB, Monahan PO, Lowe B. Anxiety disorders in primary care: prevalence, impairment, comorbidity, and detection. Ann Intern Med. 2007;146(5):317–25.
33. Brown T. Confirmatory factor analyses for applied research. New York: Guildford; 2006.
34. Yu CY. Evaluating cutoff criteria of model fit indices for latent variable models with binary and continuous outcomes (Vol. 30). Los Angeles: University of California, Los Angeles; 2002.
35. Kaess M, Parzer P, Mattern M, Plener PL, Bifulco A, Resch F, Brunner R. Adverse childhood experiences and their impact on frequency, severity, and the individual function of nonsuicidal self-injury in youth. Psychiatry Res. 2013;206(2–3):265–72.
36. Linehan MM. Dialectical behavior therapy for treatment of borderline personality disorder: implications for the treatment of substance abuse. NIDA Res Monogr. 1993;137:201–16.

telephone, if it was not possible for the participant to come in.

80.8% ($n = 59$) of these individuals provided data for the 3 month follow-up assessment, 75.3% ($n = 55$) for the 6 month and 53.4% ($n = 39$) for the 12 month follow-up assessment. 46.6% ($n = 34$) of individuals provided data for all three follow-up assessments, 26% ($n = 19$) for two follow-up assessments, 16.4% ($n = 12$) for one follow-up assessment and 11% ($n = 8$) for none of the follow-up assessments.

Interventions
Clinical care for participants included psychotropic medication and/or psychological therapies/counselling: of those participants who were assessed at baseline, 50.7% ($n = 37$) were taking antidepressant medication and an additional 5.5% ($n = 4$) were prescribed antipsychotic and/or mood stabilising medication. Additionally, 52.1% ($n = 38$) of participants were receiving counselling or some sort of therapy (e.g. cognitive-behavioural or -analytic therapy) and 32.9% ($n = 24$) had been assessed or referred for therapy.

Measures
Participants completed an interview and self-report assessment on the following measures at all four time points:

Comprehensive Assessment of At-Risk Mental States (CAARMS)
The CAARMS [4] is a semi-structured interview designed to determine the at-risk mental state for psychosis. The four subscales unusual thought content (e.g. delusional mood, overvalued ideas), non-bizarre ideas (e.g. suspiciousness, grandiosity), perceptual abnormalities (e.g. distortions, illusions, hallucinations), and disorganised speech (e.g. difficulties with speech and communication) quantify severity (0 = absent/never-6 = psychotic and severe) and frequency (0 = absent/never-6 = continuous) of psychotic experiences. A combination of intensity and frequency ratings allows for the determination of whether individuals meet criteria for being at UHR for psychosis and for determining onset of first episode psychosis (FEP). A score of at least three for both intensity and frequency on at least one subscale (with exception of at least four for intensity for disorganised speech) indicates UHR status, if coupled with a decline in functioning or chronic low functioning. The CAARMS indicates UHR status if symptoms were present over the last 12 months. An overall inter-rater reliability of 0.85 has been reported and CAARMS criteria displayed good concurrent (e.g. with the Brief Psychotic Rating Scale) and predictive validity (e.g. higher risk of transition to psychosis in individuals with an at-risk mental state) [4].

Criteria for FEP are met if participants score a 6 on intensity and at least a 4 for frequency on non-bizarre ideas, unusual thought content or disorganised speech or a 5–6 on intensity and a 4–6 on frequency for perceptual abnormalities.

Social and Occupational Functioning Assessment Scale (SOFAS)
The SOFAS has been derived from the Global Assessment Scale [24] which is a modestly reliable and valid measure of psychiatric disturbance [25], and provides a rating of overall psychological functioning on a scale from 0 to 100 [26]. The SOFAS is usually used to rate an individual's current functioning, however highest and lowest functioning ratings for the past 12 months were employed to determine a drop in functioning. The researcher rated the score on the SOFAS based on information provided in the interview for the Global Functioning: Social and Role Scales. The SOFAS has been included in the Diagnostic and Statistical Manual for Psychiatric Disorders IV-TR [27] to overcome short-comings of existing measures of individuals' functioning [28].

Classification based on psychotic experiences
At each time point participants were classified into individuals at UHR for psychosis as opposed to those who did not fulfil UHR criteria ("non-UHR"). A further distinction was made concerning the relevance of the functioning criterion for the definition of UHR status: individuals with psychotic experiences with both an intensity and frequency of at least three on the CAARMS, but without a 30% drop in functioning or chronic low functioning (SOFAS score ~ 50 during the past 12 months) were referred to as "psychotic experiences without functional decline" (as opposed to UHR who experienced either this described drop in functioning or chronic low functioning). All combinations of an intensity and frequency of less than three on all sub-scales were considered as "no significant psychotic experiences", regardless of functioning. Hence, an additional three-group comparison was conducted with individuals at UHR, individuals with psychotic experiences without functional decline and individuals with no significant psychotic experiences.

Quick Inventory of Depressive Symptoms (QIDS)
The QIDS [29] is a 16-item, semi-structured interview to gauge severity of depressive symptoms over the past 7 days. Items are scored 0–3 and total scores range from 0 to 27. A meta-analysis reported concurrent validity, e.g. with the Hamilton Rating Scale for Depression ranging from 0.72 to 0.79 and a Cronbach's α ranging from 0.65 to 0.87 [30]. Cronbach's α in this sample ranging from 0.61 to 0.78 across time points.

Overall Anxiety Severity and Impairment Scale (OASIS)

The OASIS [31] is a brief five-item self-report questionnaire of severity and impairment across multiple anxiety disorders and sub-threshold anxiety. It captures frequency and intensity of anxiety, avoidance behaviour and interference of anxiety with everyday life and relationships. Total scores range from 0 to 20. The OASIS showed convergence with major anxiety measures (e.g. for social, posttraumatic stress, and generalised anxiety), a Cronbach's α of 0.84 for the five items [31], and one-month re-test reliability of 0.82 [32].

Kessler psychological distress scale (K-10)

The K-10 [33] is a 10-item self-report questionnaire assessing psychological distress via questions about depressive and anxiety symptoms in the past 30 days. Items are rated on a five-point scale with total scores ranging from 10 to 50. The K-10 is a moderately reliable instrument (kappa ranging from 0.42 to 0.74) [34] and demonstrates good concurrent validity with other instruments such as the General Health Questionnaire and current diagnosis of anxiety and affective disorders [35]. Cronbach's α in this sample ranged from 0.88 to 0.89 across time points.

Psychosocial functioning

The Global Functioning: Social [36] and Role [37] Scales are semi-structured interviews and were used to index current social and role functioning, providing overall scores from 1 to 10, with 10 indicating superior functioning and 1 extreme dysfunction. Inter-rater reliability ranged from 0.85 to 0.95, and the social functioning scale was significantly correlated with social contacts ($r = 0.70$) and role functioning with work and school functioning ($r = 0.57$) [38].

Quality of life

Perceived quality of life was assessed using the World Health Organisation Quality of Life (WHOQoL) [39] self-reported item "Thinking about your life in the last four weeks, how would you rate your quality of life", on a five-point scale from 1 ("very poor") to 5 ("very good") retrieved from the 26-item measure WHO-BREF. All four domains of quality of life of the WHO-BREF correlated significantly with this item, whereby psychological and environmental domains were more strongly associated as compared to social and physical domains. This indicates that the item that we used not only demonstrated face validity but also represents the WHO-BREF, which is characterised by good to excellent psychometric properties, well [40].

Statistical analysis

An independent samples t-test was used to compare UHR and non-UHR individuals for age. For analysis of categorical data, such as gender, ethnicity, occupation and highest education, χ^2 tests were used to evaluate group differences. To increase robustness of findings, binary linear regression analyses were conducted to identify whether or not attending any of the three follow-up assessments was related to high or low scores in any of the clinical or functioning measures or quality of life at the respective prior assessment.

As there was incomplete data at all four time points (34 individuals who completed all assessments), mixed linear modelling was implemented using four time points (baseline, three, six and 12 months) for both the UHR vs non-UHR comparison and classification of no significant psychotic experiences, UHR, and psychotic experiences without functional decline for the dependent variables QIDS, OASIS, K-10, social and role functioning, and WHOQoL score. Group and time (and their interaction) were specified as fixed effects in the model as we assumed that individual-specific effects were correlated with both factors. Bonferroni post-hoc tests were used to compare QIDS, K-10, OASIS, and WHOQoL scores between UHR, individuals with psychotic experiences without functional decline and no significant psychotic experiences within the mixed linear modelling analyses.

Results

Demographics and UHR vs non-UHR group comparisons at baseline

At baseline, 56.2% ($n = 41$) of participants presented with no significant psychotic experiences, 19.2% ($n = 14$) were experiencing psychotic experiences without functional decline, whereas another 19.2% ($n = 14$) of individuals were at UHR. Four participants fulfilled CAARMS criteria for a FEP (5.5%) and were therefore excluded from the remainder of the study, leaving a final sample of 69 participants. Out of the final sample of 69 individuals, the 14 individuals with psychotic experiences without functional decline (20.3%) and 41 individuals with no significant psychotic experiences (59.4%) formed the non-UHR group, as opposed to the UHR group ($n = 14$; 20.3%).

Transition to FEP according to CAARMS rating was monitored and recorded for two participants at the three-month follow-up assessment and an additional participant at the six-month follow-up assessment for those individuals who took part in the respective assessments. No further transitions were recorded for the 12-month follow-up assessment (overall transition rate of 3/69 of whole sample: 4%; overall transition rate of 3/15 individuals identified as UHR at baseline: 27%).

The total sample ($n = 69$, 48 females, 69.6%) had a $M_{age} \pm SD$ of 20.8 ± 2.6 years and was predominantly White-British. At baseline, there were no significant group differences on demographic variables between UHR and non-UHR individuals (see Table 1).

Table 1 Baseline demographic information for the total sample, and comparing UHR and non-UHR at baseline

	Total sample (n = 69)	UHR (n = 14)	Non-UHR (n = 55)	Test statistics
Age (M ± SD) in years	20.8 ± 2.6	20.8 ± 3.1	20.7 ± 2.5	t (67) = 0.12, p = 0.91
Gender (m/f)	21/48	5/9	16/39	X^2 (1) = 0.23, p = 0.63
Ethnicity				
White[a]	58	12	46	
Asian[b]	3	1	2	
Black[c]	2	0	2	X^2 (3) = 0.88, p = 0.83
Mixed-race[d]	6	1	5	
Occupation				
University student[e]	18	1	17	
College/A-Levels	20	3	17	
Unemployed	11	2	9	X^2 (4) = 7.70, p = 0.10
Employed[f]	17	7	10	
Homemaker	3	1	2	
Highest qualification				
University[g]	6	1	5	
A-Levels[h]	31	4	27	X^2 (3) = 2.91, p = 0.41
GSCE[i]	26	8	18	
No qualification	6	1	5	

UHR ultra-high risk, *M* mean, *SD* standard deviation, *m* male, *f* female
[a]White-British & White-Other
[b]Asian-Pakistani, Asian-Bangladeshi & Other Asian
[c]Black-African
[d]Mixed-Race White-Black-Caribbean
[e]Undergraduate and postgraduate university students
[f]Working full or part-time
[g]Bachelor or Master degree
[h]A-Levels, National Vocational Qualification (NVQ) Level 4, or equivalent
[i]General Certificate of Secondary Education (GCSE, year-10 equivalent) or NVQ level 1 or 2

None of the clinical or functioning measures or quality of life were associated with non-attendance at three, six and 12 months follow, except for lower OASIS scores at 3 month follow-up that predicted non-attendance at 6 month follow-up (6 month follow-up attendance, n = 45, OASIS M ± SD: 7.9 ± 3.9; 6-months follow-up non-attendance, n = 6, OASIS M ± SD: 3.3 ± 3.1; p = 0.036).

Longitudinal UHR vs non-UHR group comparisons
Statistical comparisons revealed that there were no differences between those individuals that were included in the baseline analyses and those who did not take part at three, six or 12 month follow-up concerning any clinical baseline measures or classification as UHR and non-UHR (all p > 0.05). UHR vs non-UHR classification at three, six, and 12-month follow-up was conducted in accordance with procedure of baseline classification, yet with ratings from each respective assessment. Due to the small number of transitions (n = 3) and the fact that transition to FEP was determined on the basis of the CAARMS as a classification tool and not on clinical criteria or eligibility for treatment with early intervention services, data was handled as "non-UHR" in all three follow-up cases due to no drop in or chronic low functioning (and as "psychotic experiences without functional decline" for the three-group comparison in 3.3). However, additional mixed linear modelling was conducted that excluded the three transitioned cases, to investigate robustness of findings.

Ten individuals were classified as UHR at 3 month (16.9%), nine at 6 month (16.3%) and ten at 12-month follow-up (25.6%). Three individuals (4.3%) were classified as UHR at all their assessments, 44 (63.8%) were classified as non-UHR at all their assessments, and 22 (31.9%) changed UHR status at least once during the follow-up period. Linear mixed effects modelling was conducted with time (baseline, three, six and 12 months) and group (UHR vs non-UHR) factors, where group affiliation allowed for change across the four time points (e.g. from non-UHR at baseline to UHR at 3 months or vice versa). Analyses revealed significant group differences between UHR and non-UHR across the four time points for the following: QIDS (F (1, 132.26) = 15.27, p < 0.001), K-10 (F (1, 114.91) = 12.64, p = 0.001), role functioning (F (1, 159.87) = 21.52, p < 0.001) and WHO-QoL (F (1, 160.54) = 7.68, p = 0.006). UHR individuals demonstrated overall higher QIDS scores, and K-10 scores and lower role functioning and WHOQoL scores. Significant time effects were found for the QIDS (F (3, 65.30) = 6.43, p = 0.001), OASIS (F (3, 59.54) = 5.58, p = 0.002), K-10 (F (3, 54.44) = 5.48, p = 0.002) and WHOQoL (F (3, 79.72) = 2.87, p = 0.042) indicating a tendency for improvement in symptomatology and quality of life over time in the group as a whole. No interaction effects were found. When analyses were repeated without the three cases who transitioned to psychosis over the follow-up period, results from linear mixed effects modelling remained qualitatively very similar, except that all significant time effects disappeared. Measures of central tendency for QIDS, OASIS, K-10, social and role functioning and WHOQoL scores across the four time points between UHR and non-UHR individuals are illustrated in Fig. 1.

Classification into UHR, psychotic experiences without functional decline and no significant psychotic experiences from baseline to follow-up
Statistical comparisons revealed that there were no differences between those individuals that were included in the baseline analyses and those who did not take part at

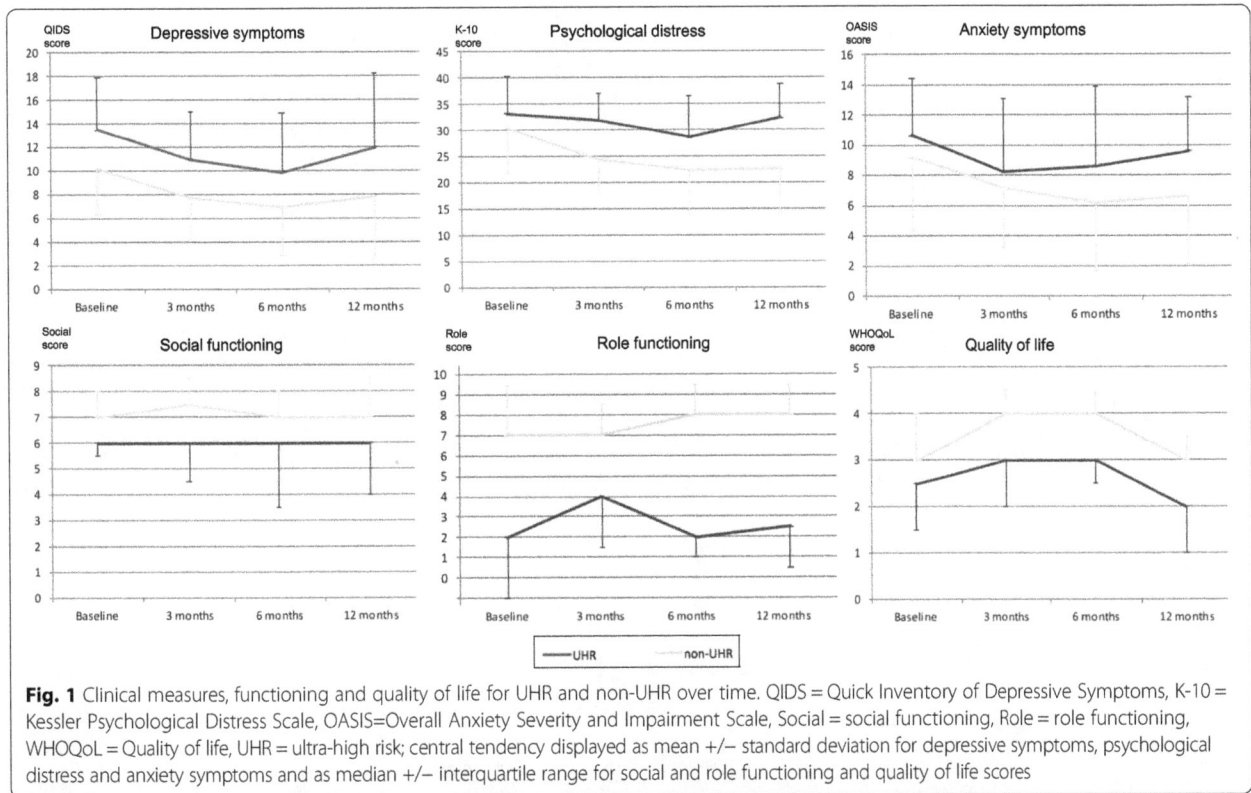

Fig. 1 Clinical measures, functioning and quality of life for UHR and non-UHR over time. QIDS = Quick Inventory of Depressive Symptoms, K-10 = Kessler Psychological Distress Scale, OASIS=Overall Anxiety Severity and Impairment Scale, Social = social functioning, Role = role functioning, WHOQoL = Quality of life, UHR = ultra-high risk; central tendency displayed as mean +/– standard deviation for depressive symptoms, psychological distress and anxiety symptoms and as median +/– interquartile range for social and role functioning and quality of life scores

three, six or 12 month follow-up concerning any clinical baseline measures or classification as UHR, psychotic experiences without functional decline and no significant psychotic symptoms (all $p > 0.05$).

Fourteen (23.7%) individuals were classified as psychotic experiences without functional decline at baseline, 13 (22.0%) at 3 month, 6 (10.9%) at 6 month and nine (23.1%) at 12-month follow-up. Overall, there was a variety of trajectories concerning the three-group classification from baseline and across the three follow-up time points, with the majority of individuals presenting as UHR or psychotic experiences without functional decline for at least one time point ($n = 42$, 60.9%). Linear mixed effects modelling revealed significant group differences between individuals with no significant psychotic experiences, UHR and psychotic experiences without functional decline across the four time points for the following: QIDS (F (2, 125.48) = 11.90, $p < 0.001$), OASIS (F (2, 123.99) = 4.69, $p = 0.011$), K-10 (F (2, 97.22) = 11.14, $p < 0.001$), and WHOQoL (F (2, 157.77) = 6.51, $p = 0.002$). Time effects were found for QIDS (F (3, 63.63) = 5.82, $p = 0.001$), OASIS (F (3, 58.38) = 3.73, $p = 0.016$), K-10 (F (3, 53.15) = 3.99, $p = 0.012$) and WHOQoL (F (3, 79.50) = 3.22, $p = 0.027$). No interaction effects were found. When analyses were repeated without the three cases that transitioned over the follow-up period, results from linear mixed effects modelling remained similar. Figure 2

illustrates this three-group comparison for QIDS and OASIS, K-10, and WHOQoL at all four time points.

Bonferroni post hoc tests indicated a difference between those with no psychotic experiences as compared to those with psychotic experiences without functional decline and as compared to UHR individuals (except for OASIS score between those with no psychotic experiences and UHR individuals and for WHOQoL score between those with and without psychotic experiences), but no differences between individuals at UHR as compared to those with psychotic experiences without functional decline (see Table 2).

Discussion

In the present study we examined the role of psychotic experiences in predicting current and future psychopathology, psychosocial functioning and quality of life in a sample of young, help-seeking individuals with mental health problems. Although participants were recruited from general (not UHR-specific) services, one fifth were classified as UHR for psychosis and an additional one fifth had significant psychotic experiences without functional decline at entry to the study, comparable to the rate in similar studies (e.g. [41]). Mostly consistent with our hypotheses, UHR individuals reported higher levels of depressive symptoms and psychological distress, and lower levels of role functioning and quality of life

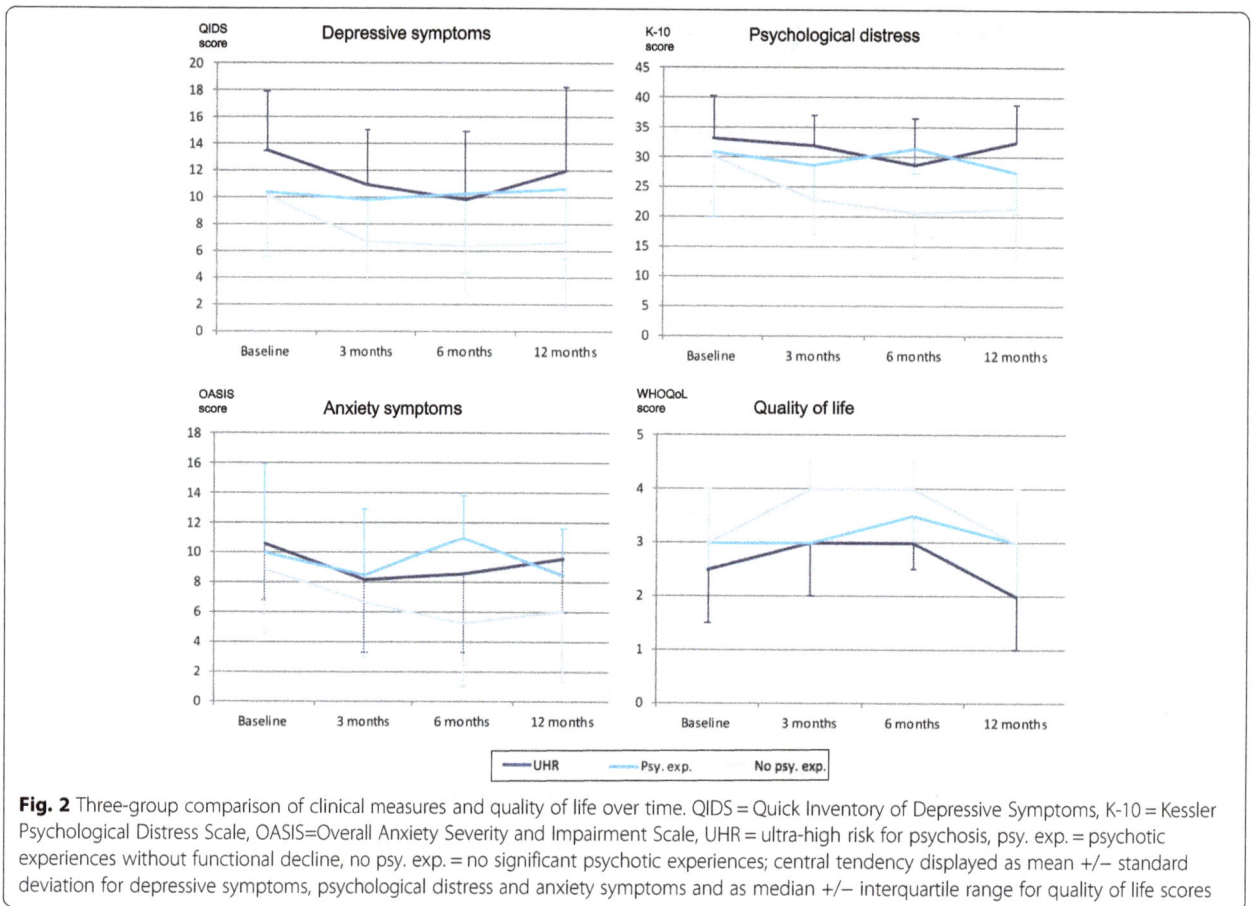

Fig. 2 Three-group comparison of clinical measures and quality of life over time. QIDS = Quick Inventory of Depressive Symptoms, K-10 = Kessler Psychological Distress Scale, OASIS=Overall Anxiety Severity and Impairment Scale, UHR = ultra-high risk for psychosis, psy. exp. = psychotic experiences without functional decline, no psy. exp. = no significant psychotic experiences; central tendency displayed as mean +/− standard deviation for depressive symptoms, psychological distress and anxiety symptoms and as median +/− interquartile range for quality of life scores

compared to non-UHR individuals. As opposed to our hypotheses, no differences were reported for anxiety symptoms or social functioning. When we explored the predictive value of the functioning criterion for definition of UHR status, as predicted, there were no significant differences in all measures between individuals at UHR and those with psychotic experiences without functional decline.

There were no group differences between UHR and non-UHR individuals on anxiety symptoms, and social functioning, although the UHR group showed significantly higher depressive symptoms and substantially lower levels of role functioning than non-UHR individuals. This may likely be explained by the nature of the UHR status and the drop in functioning or chronic low functioning being driven by low levels of role functioning. It is possible that low role functioning is particularly characteristic for this sample comprising of UHR individuals not specifically help-seeking for psychotic experiences but for general mental health problems. Most UHR studies report psychosocial functioning combined (e.g. [10, 21, 22]), however, studies that examined social and role functioning separately using the same measure, found similar levels of social functioning and higher

levels of role functioning as compared to the current study (e.g. [38]). Role functioning may therefore be a particularly important target for early intervention, for example, in terms of vocational and educational interventions in addition to symptom-oriented psychotherapy. Vocational rehabilitation was found to be effective in chronic schizophrenia [42], and has recently been introduced to individuals with a FEP in a randomised controlled trial [43], yet there may be a need for such interventions even earlier in the course of illness.

The finding of higher depressive symptoms and psychological distress, and lower role functioning and quality of life in UHR individuals as compared to non-UHR individuals is in accordance with Wigman et al. [44] who found that clients with non-psychotic psychiatric disorders but additional psychotic experiences showed lower global functioning than those without psychotic experiences. Psychotic experiences have also been shown to predict depressive symptoms in the future [45], yet it has to be acknowledged that there is also contrary evidence indicating a cross-sectional association only [13]. These findings are also consistent with the idea that psychotic experiences are associated with more severe mental health problems [12, 46].

Table 2 Bonferroni post-hoc tests for three-group comparison

Measure Contrast	Bonferroni test p-value
QIDS	
No psy. exp. vs psy. exp.	0.011[*]
No psy. exp. vs UHR	< 0.001[***]
Psy. exp. vs UHR	0.639
K-10	
No psy. exp. vs psy. exp.	0.029[*]
No psy. exp. vs UHR	< 0.001[***]
Psy. exp. vs UHR	0.664
OASIS	
No psy. exp. vs psy. exp.	0.015[*]
No psy. exp. vs UHR	0.153
Psy. exp. vs UHR	1.00
WHOQoL	
No psy. exp. vs psy. Exp.	0.251
No psy. exp. vs UHR	0.002[**]
Psy. exp. vs UHR	0.427

QIDS Quick Inventory of Depressive Symptoms, OASIS Overall Anxiety Severity and Impairment Scale, K-10 Kessler Psychological Distress Scale, no psy. exp no significant psychotic experiences, psy. exp psychotic experiences without functional decline, UHR ultra-high risk for psychosis
[*]$p < 0.05$, [**]$p < 0.01$, [***]$p < 0.001$

UHR status was assessed at each follow up assessment and not only at baseline. This is especially important considering the dynamics of clinical presentation. Indeed, almost one third of individuals changed from UHR to non-UHR (or vice versa) at least once over the follow-up period of only 12 months. This indicates that UHR is not a static concept and clinicians should be aware of the potential for rapid changes in symptomatology.

A considerable amount of the UHR literature has focused on transition to psychosis as the primary outcome. However, it is not only the prediction of transition to psychosis that is key to ensuring young people with mental health problems receive the care they need – focusing on other psychopathology is equally important considering outcomes of those individuals who do not transition to psychosis. Lin et al. [10] followed non-transitioned UHR individuals and found that more than two thirds experienced non-psychotic disorders over the follow-up period of up to 14 years, with 90% presenting with non-psychotic disorders at baseline. This study supports a shift of emphasis from categorical outcomes (e.g. transition to psychosis or assignment of clinical diagnosis) to a more holistic approach of mental health outcomes. In the current sample only 4% transitioned to psychosis, but many experienced ongoing significant psychopathology.

This current study illustrated the distribution of clinical symptoms and quality of life of individuals at UHR and those with psychotic experiences without functional decline and participants with no significant psychotic experiences. Post-hoc tests revealed no significant differences between individuals at UHR and those with psychotic experiences without functional decline. Thus we found no evidence for an exacerbation in clinical symptomatology if functional decline or chronic low functioning was present. Whereas the inclusion of functional decline for UHR status definition serves its purpose to increase specificity of prediction of psychosis [21], it may not be a robust marker for prediction of clinical deterioration or a decrease in quality of life. However, the current results should be interpreted with caution considering the small group sizes.

Lastly, individuals who took part in this study were recruited from both a primary and secondary mental health service in the UK. It is plausible that individuals presenting to secondary mental health services are more impaired concerning their mental health and psychosocial functioning as those presenting to primary care services, considering that the UK operates on general practioner referral who are likely to have more conservative thresholds of what constitutes a psychiatric case as opposed to countries that operate on self-referral for mental health issues [47]. However, actual access to secondary care may be more driven by cost of and capacity for service provision than need for clinical care or illness severity: examination of transition protocols from child to adolescent mental health services revealed that only one quarter of cases that were deemed suitable for transition, actually 'graduated' to an adult mental health service, leaving a service gap especially for 16 and 17 year olds where mental health services are disproportionately expensive [48].

There were several limitations to the current study. The study was characterised by reasonably high attrition rates and the cohort was followed-up over only 12 months, although these first 12 months appear to be the most relevant time period, including the highest number of actual transitions to a FEP [49]. Although the sample was quite small (in particular the numbers of individuals at UHR and those with psychotic experiences without functional decline), the participants provided detailed and comprehensive psychopathological information. The sample comprised a very heterogeneous clinical presentation (including heterogeneous treatment and care setting for help-seeking which we were not able to control for in our analyses) with participants differing widely from none to severe symptom presentation across diagnostic categories. However, the presented findings are not fixed to diagnostic categories during the early stages of mental health, constituting a different approach to mental health that aims to circumvent issues around comorbidity [50] and the question of the existence of natural boundaries between mental disorders [51].

Conclusions

The current study explored the role of psychotic experiences and being at UHR for psychosis in youth who were seeking help for common, non-psychotic mental health problems. Individuals at UHR for psychosis demonstrated significantly higher levels of depressive symptoms and psychological distress, and lower role functioning and quality of life, as compared to non-UHR individuals. Therefore, in addition to symptom-orientated psychotherapy, it may be important to also focus on individuals' compromised role functioning, and consider using vocational and educational rehabilitation in these early stages of mental health problems. Lastly, functional decline and chronic low functioning did not exacerbate clinical symptomatology and may therefore not be a robust marker for prediction of clinical deterioration or a decrease in quality of life.

Abbreviations

ANOVA: Analysis of variance; CAARMS: Comprehensive assessment of at-risk mental states; FEP: First episode of psychosis; K-10: Kessler psychological distress scale; OASIS: Overall anxiety severity and impairment scale; QIDS: Quick inventory of depressive symptoms; SOFAS: Social and occupational functioning assessment scale; UHR: Ultra-high risk; WHOQoL: World Health Organisation Quality of Life

Acknowledgments

The authors would like to thank all participants and staff involved in the conduct of this study.

Funding

AL is supported by an NHMRC Early Career Fellowship (#1148793).

Authors' contributions

KH drafted the manuscript, coordinated input from other authors and submitted the manuscript. KH, AL, LC, AR and AL contributed to data collection. All other authors contributed substantially to the draft and all authors approved final submission.

Competing interests

The authors declare that they have no competing interests.

Author details

[1]School of Psychology, University of Birmingham, Edgbaston, Birmingham, UK. [2]Institute for Mental Health, University of Birmingham, Edgbaston, Birmingham, UK. [3]Telethon Kids Institute, Perth, Australia. [4]Orygen, the National Centre of Excellence in Youth Mental Health, Melbourne, Australia. [5]Centre for Youth Mental Health, University of Melbourne, Melbourne, Australia. [6]Institute of Clinical Sciences, University of Birmingham, Edgbaston, Birmingham, UK. [7]Warwick Medical School, University of Warwick, Coventry, UK. [8]Department of Psychology, University of Sheffield, Sheffield, UK.

References

1. Patel V, Flisher AJ, Hetrick S, McGorry P. Mental health of young people: a global public-health challenge. Lancet. 2007;369:1302–13.
2. Gore FM, Bloem PJN, Patton GC, Ferguson J, Joseph V, Coffey C, Sawyer SM, Mathers CD. Global burden of disease in young people aged 10–24 years: a systematic analysis. Lancet. 2011;377:2093–102.
3. McGorry P, Hickie I, Yung A, Pantelis C, Jackson H. Clinical staging of psychiatric disorders: a heuristic framework for choosing earlier, safer and more effective interventions. Aust N Z J Psychiatry. 2006;40:616–22.
4. Yung AR, Yuen HP, McGorry PD, Phillips LJ, Kelly D, Dell'Olio M, Francey SM, Cosgrave EM, Killackey E, Stanford C, et al. Mapping the onset of psychosis: the comprehensive assessment of at-risk mental states. Aust N Z J Psychiatry. 2005;39:964–71.
5. Yung AR, Buckby JA, Cosgrave EM, Killackey EJ, Baker K, Cotton SM, McGorry PD. Association between psychotic experiences and depression in a clinical sample over 6 months. Schizophr Res. 2007;91:246–53.
6. Rosen JL, Miller TJ, D'Andrea JT, McGlashan TH, Woods SW. Comorbid diagnoses in patients meeting criteria for the schizophrenia prodrome. Schizophr Res. 2006;85:124–31.
7. Lin A, Wood SJ, Nelson B, Brewer WJ, Spiliotacopoulos D, Bruxner A, Broussard C, Pantelis C, Yung AR. Neurocognitive predictors of functional outcome two to 13 years after identification as ultra-high risk for psychosis. Schizophr Res. 2011;132:1–7.
8. Yung AR, Phillips LJ, Yuen HP, Francey SM, McFarlane CA, Hallgren M, McGorry PD. Psychosis prediction: 12-month follow up of a high-risk ("prodromal") group. Schizophr Res. 2003;60:21–32.
9. Addington J, Cornblatt B, Cadenhead K, Cannon T, McGlashan T, Perkins D, Seidman L, Tsuang M, Walker E, Wood S, et al. At clinical high risk for psychosis: outcome for nonconverters. Am J Psychiatry. 2011;168:800–5.
10. Lin A, Wood SJ, Nelson B, Beavan A, McGorry PD, Yung AR. Outcomes of nontransitioned cases in a sample at ultra-high risk for psychosis. Am J Psychiatry. 2015;172:249–58.
11. Varghese D, Scott J, Welham J, Bor W, Najman J, O'Callaghan M, Williams G, McGrath J. Psychotic-like experiences in major depression and anxiety disorders: a population-based survey in young adults. Schizophr Bull. 2011; 37:389–93.
12. Wigman JTW, van Nierop M, Vollebergh WAM, Lieb R, Beesdo-Baum K, Wittchen HU, van Os J. Evidence that psychotic symptoms are prevalent in disorders of anxiety and depression, impacting on illness onset, risk, and severity–implications for diagnosis and ultra-high risk research. Schizophr Bull. 2012;38:247–57.
13. Wigman JTW, Lin A, Vollebergh WAM, van Os J, Raaijmakers QAW, Nelson B, Baksheev G, Yung AR. Subclinical psychosis and depression: co-occurring phenomena that do not predict each other over time. Schizophr Res. 2011; 130:277–81.
14. Rössler W, Hengartner MP, Ajdacic-Gross V, Haker H, Gamma A, Angst J. Sub-clinical psychosis symptoms in young adults are risk factors for subsequent common mental disorders. Schizophr Res. 2011;131:18–23.
15. Kelleher I, Keeley H, Corcoran P, Lynch F, Fitzpatrick C, Devlin N, Molloy C, Roddy S, Clarke MC, Harley M, et al. Clinicopathological significance of psychotic experiences in non-psychotic young people: evidence from four population-based studies. Br J Psychiatry. 2012;201:26–32.
16. Kelleher I, Lynch F, Harley M, Molloy C, Roddy S, Fitzpatrick C, Cannon M. Psychotic symptoms in adolescence index risk for suicidal behaviour: findings from two population-based case-control clinical interview studies. Arch Gen Psychiatry. 2012;69:1277–83.
17. McGorry PD, van Os J. Redeeming diagnosis in psychiatry: timing versus specificity. Lancet. 2013;381:343–5.
18. Brodbeck J, Goodyer IM, Abbott RA, Dunn VJ, St Clair MC, Owens M, Jones PB, Croudace TJ. General distress, hopelessness—suicidal ideation and worrying in adolescence: concurrent and predictive validity of a symptom-level bifactor model for clinical diagnoses. J Affect Disord. 2014;152–154: 299–305.
19. Caspi A, Houts RM, Belsky DW, Goldman-Mellor SJ, Harrington H, Israel S, Meier MH, Ramrakha S, Shalev I, Poulton R, et al. The p factor: one general psychopathology factor in the structure of psychiatric disorders? Clin Psychol Sci. 2014;2:119–37.
20. Weiser M, van Os J, Davidson M. Time for a shift in focus in schizophrenia: from narrow phenotypes to broad endophenotypes. Br J Psychiatry. 2005; 187:203–5.
21. Yung AR, Nelson B, Stanford C, Simmons MB, Cosgrave EM, Killackey E, Phillips LJ, Bechdolf A, Buckby J, McGorry PD. Validation of "prodromal" criteria to detect individuals at ultra high risk of psychosis: 2 year follow-up. Schizophr Res. 2008;105:10–7.
22. Salokangas RKR, Ruhrmann S, von Reventlow HG, Heinimaa M, Svirskis T, From T, Luutonen S, Juckel G, Linszen D, Dingemans P, et al. Axis I diagnoses and transition to psychosis in clinical high-risk patients EPOS

project: prospective follow-up of 245 clinical high-risk outpatients in four countries. Schizophr Res. 2012;138:192–7.

23. Velthorst E, Nelson B, Wiltink S, de Haan L, Wood SJ, Lin A, Yung AR. Transition to first episode psychosis in ultra high risk populations: does baseline functioning hold the key? Schizophr Res. 2013;143:132–7.

24. Endicott J, Spitzer R, Fleiss J, Cohen J. The global assessment scale: a procedure for measuring overall severity of psychiatric disturbance. Arch Gen Psychiatry. 1976;33:766–71.

25. Jones SH, Thornicroft G, Coffey M, Dunn G. A brief mental-health outcome scale - reliability and valididy of the global assessment of functioning (GAF). Br J Psychiatry. 1995;166:654–9.

26. Goldman HH, Skodol AE, Lave TR. Revising axis V for DSM-IV: a review of measures of social functioning. Am J Psychiatry. 1992;149:1148–56.

27. American Psychiatric Association. Diagnostic and statistical manual of mental disorders: DSM-IV-TR. Washington, DC: Author; 2000.

28. Burns T, Patrick D. Social functioning as an outcome measure in schizophrenia studies. Acta Psychiatr Scand. 2007;116:403–18.

29. Rush AJ, Trivedi MH, Ibrahim HM, Carmody TJ, Arnow B, Klein DN, Markowitz JC, Ninan PT, Kornstein S, Manber R, et al. The 16-item quick inventory of depressive symptomatology (QIDS), clinician rating (QIDS-C), and self-report (QIDS-SR): a psychometric evaluation in patients with chronic major depression. Biol Psychiatry. 2003;54:573–83.

30. Reilly TJ, MacGillivray SA, Reid IC, Cameron IM. Psychometric properties of the 16-item quick inventory of depressive symptomatology: a systematic review and meta-analysis. J Psychiatr Res. 2015;60:132–40.

31. Campbell-Sills L, Norman SB, Craske MG, Sullivan G, Lang AJ, Chavira DA, Bystritsky A, Sherbourne C, Roy-Byrne P, Stein MB. Validation of a brief measure of anxiety-related severity and impairment: the Overall Anxiety Severity and Impairment Scale (OASIS). J Affect Disord. 2009;112:92–101.

32. Norman SB, Hami Cissell S, Means-Christensen AJ, Stein MB. Development and validation of an Overall Anxiety Severity and Impairment Scale (OASIS). Depress Anxiety. 2006;23(4):245–9.

33. Kessler RC, Andrews G, Colpe LJ, Hiripi E, Mroczek DK, Normand SLT, Walters EE, Zaslavsky AM. Short screening scales to monitor population prevalences and trends in non-specific psychological distress. Psychol Med. 2002;32:959–76.

34. Dal Grande E, Taylor A, Wilson D. South Australian Health and Wellbeing Survey, December 2000, Population Research and Outcomes Study Unit. In: Department of Health, South Australia; 2002.

35. Andrews G, Slade T. Interpreting scores on the Kessler psychological distress scale (K10). Aust N Z J Public Health. 2001;25:494–7.

36. Auther A, Smith C, Cornblatt B. Global functioning: social scale (GF: social). Zucker-Hillside Hospital: Glen Oaks; 2006.

37. Niendam TA, Bearden CE, Johnson JK, Cannon TD. Global Functioning: Role Scale (GF: Role). Los Angeles: University of California; 2006.

38. Cornblatt B, Auther A, Niendam T, Smith C, Zinberg J, Bearden C, Cannon T. Preliminary findings for two new measures of social and role functioning in the prodromal phase of schizophrenia. Schizophr Bull. 2007;33:688–702.

39. WHO. Study protocol for the World Health Organization project to develop a Quality of Life assessment instrument (WHOQOL). Qual Life Res. 1993;2:153–9.

40. Skevington SM, Lotfy M, O'Connell KA. The World Health Organization's WHOQOL-BREF quality of life assessment: psychometric properties and results of the international field trial. A report from the WHOQOL group. Qual Life Res. 2004;13:299–310.

41. Purcell R, Jorm AF, Hickie IB, Yung AR, Pantelis C, Amminger GP, Glozier N, Killackey E, Phillips LJ, Wood SJ, et al. Demographic and clinical characteristics of young people seeking help at youth mental health services: baseline findings of the transitions study. Early Interv Psychiatry. 2014.

42. Bio DS, Gattaz WF. Vocational rehabilitation improves cognition and negative symptoms in schizophrenia. Schizophr Res. 2011;126:265–9.

43. Killackey E, Allott K, Cotton SM, Jackson H, Scutella R, Tseng YP, Borland J, Proffitt TM, Hunt S, Kay-Lambkin F, et al. A randomized controlled trial of vocational intervention for young people with first-episode psychosis: method. Early Interv Psychiatry. 2013;7:329–37.

44. Wigman JTW, Devlin N, Kelleher I, Murtagh A, Harley M, Kehoe A, Fitzpatrick C, Cannon M. Psychotic symptoms, functioning and coping in adolescents with mental illness. BMC Psychiatry. 2014;14:97.

45. Sullivan SA, Wiles N, Kounali D, Lewis G, Heron J, Cannon M, Mahedy L, Jones PB, Stochl J, Zammit S. Longitudinal associations between adolescent psychotic experiences and depressive symptoms. PLoS One. 2014;9:e105758.

46. Stochl J, Khandaker GM, Lewis G, Perez J, Goodyer IM, Zammit S, Sullivan S, Croudace TJ, Jones PB. Mood, anxiety and psychotic phenomena measure a common psychopathological factor. Psychol Med. 2015;45:1483–93.

47. Goldberg D, Huxley P. Mental illness in the community: the pathway to psychiatric care. London & New York: Routledge Taylor & Francis Group; 2012.

48. Singh SP, Paul M, Ford T, Kramer T, Weaver T. Transitions of care from child and adolescent mental health services to adult mental health services (TRACK study): a study of protocols in greater London. BMC Health Serv Res. 2008;8:135.

49. Nelson B, Yuen HP, Wood SJ, Lin A, Spiliotacopoulos D, Bruxner A, Broussard C, Simmons M, Foley DL, Brewer WJ, et al. Long-term follow-up of a group at ultra high risk ("prodromal") for psychosis the PACE 400 study. JAMA Psychiatry. 2013;70:793–802.

50. Clark LD, Watson D, Reynolds S. Diagnosis and classification of psychopathology: challenges to the current system and future directions. Annu Rev Psychol. 1995;46:121–53.

51. Kendell R, Jablensky A. Distinguishing between the validity and utility of psychiatric diagnoses. Am J Psychiatry. 2003;160:4–12.

18

Injuries prior and subsequent to index poisoning with medication among adolescents: a national study based on Norwegian patient registry

Ping Qin[1*] ⓘ, Shihua Sun[2], Anne Seljenes Bøe[1], Barbara Stanley[1,3] and Lars Mehlum[1]

Abstract

Background: Adolescents treated for self-poisoning with medication have a high prevalence of mental health problems and constitute a high-risk population for self-harm repetition. However, little is known about whether this population is also prone to injuries of other forms.

Methods: Data were extracted from the Norwegian Patient Registry to include all incidents of treated injuries in adolescents aged 10–19 years who were treated for self-poisoning with medication during 2008–2011. This longitudinal approach allowed for the inclusion of injuries of various forms both before and after the index poisoning with medication. Gender differences and associations of injuries with recorded deliberate self-harm or psychiatric comorbidity at index poisoning were analysed. Forms of injury and psychiatric illnesses were coded according to the ICD-10 system.

Results: 1497 adolescents treated for self-poisoning with medication were identified from the source database, including 1144 (76.4%) girls and 353 (23.6%) boys. For these 1497 adolescents a total of 2545 injury incidents were recorded in addition to the index poisoning incidents, consisting of 778 injury incidents taking place before the index poisoning and 1767 incidents taking place subsequently. Altogether 830 subjects (55.4%) had an injury treated either before or after the index poisoning. Injuries to the hand and wrist as well as injuries to the head, neck and throat were predominant in males. Females were more likely to repeat poisoning with medication, particularly those with psychiatric disorders.

Conclusion: Adolescents treated for poisoning with medication represent a high-risk population prone to both prior and subsequent injuries of other forms, and should be assessed for suicidal intent and psychiatric illness.

Keywords: Self-injurious behaviour, Medication poisoning, Adolescence, Emergency health services, Population study

Background

Non-fatal injuries are the leading cause of disability among children and adolescents worldwide [1]. Although accidental injuries account for a large proportion of such incidents in the population under 18 years in most countries, self-inflicted injuries are also prevalent [1]. It is well-documented that adolescents with a history of self-poisoning with medication are at a high risk for repetition of self-poisoning and even death by suicide [2–8]. However, little is known to what extent these adolescents are prone to injuries of other types before and after the medication poisoning episode.

According to community studies [9–11], self-cutting is more prevalent than self-poisoning among adolescents. A switch of injury method is observed in individuals who repeatedly injure themselves [6, 12]. Multiple methods used in repeated injuries have been found to predict suicide attempts [13]. At the same time, there are gender

* Correspondence: ping.qin@medisin.uio.no
[1]National Centre for Suicide Research and Prevention, Institute of Clinical medicine, University of Oslo, Sognsvannsveien 21, N-0372 Oslo, Norway
Full list of author information is available at the end of the article

differences in the incidence as well type of injuries among adolescents [14–17]. While male adolescents have higher overall rates of injuries of all types than their female peers [1, 18, 19], female adolescents show a higher incidence in self-inflicted injuries [11, 20–23]. Moreover, male adolescents are prone to violent injuries because of prevalent risk behaviors such as competitive sports and alcohol consumption [16, 24]. They also tend to use more violent methods, than their female peers, when harming themselves deliberately [11, 12, 23, 25, 26], although there were reports less conclusive [27–29].

In spite of interesting findings, previous studies on adolescent injury have often been based on data from local hospital records or cross-sectional surveys, lacked the details on types of injury, or focused on either accidental or intentional injuries alone [1]. Moreover, no large-scale study, to our awareness, has examined explicitly whether adolescents with self-poisoning are also prone to other forms of injuries, either prior or subsequent to the poisoning. In order to address this gap in the literature, we examined medical records of all external injuries treated in emergency and hospital services among adolescents aged 10–19 years who were treated for medication poisoning in Norway. Our specific objectives are: (1) to examine injuries being treated prior and subsequent to the index medication poisoning by form of injuries and comorbid diagnoses of deliberate self-harm and psychiatric illness, (2) to profile gender differences in specific forms of injuries, and (3) to explore possible associations of prior and subsequent injury incidents with comorbidities of deliberate self-harm and psychiatric disorder diagnosed at the index poisoning. Our hypothesis is that adolescents with a history of medication poisoning are prone to injuries of other forms.

Methods

Study population

The study was based on all adolescents aged 10–19 years in Norway. Subjects of focus were adolescents who were identified from the Norwegian Patient Registry (NPR) as having received acute treatment for self-poisoning with medication from 2008 through 2011. The Norwegian version of the Tenth Revision of the International Statistical Classification of Diseases (ICD-10) has been used for medical diagnoses in the NPR. Identification of adolescents into study cohort was carried out in accordance with a previous study focusing on poisoning with medications [8]. Briefly, adolescents who were admitted with a primary diagnosis of poisoning by therapeutic medicaments and biological substances, coded as T4n or T50 in the Norwegian classification system, were included into the cohort and the date of their first poisoning was regarded as the index date in the present study. For this cohort of adolescents, we retrieved incident records for external injuries of all forms (S00-T65) both prior and subsequent to the first recorded treatment because of poisoning with medication, i.e., the index poisoning in the present study. Records of injuries that occurred on the same day or the day after the previous incident were excluded in order to avoid possible duplicate reports of the same incident.

Study variables

Variables of interest included all external injuries (S00-T65) that led to medical treatment in emergency and hospital services before and after the index medication poisoning. Injury diagnoses were further categorized by specific body regions according to the ICD-10 system as shown in the Tables 1, 2, 3. Injuries with a code of S60 (Superficial injury of wrist and hand) and S61 (Open wound of wrist and hand) were identified because of high relevance to self-cutting behavior. Poisonings by non-medicational substances (T51-T65) and subsequent poisoning with medication (T4n-T50) were considered separately.

Moreover, a supplemental diagnosis confirming intentionality in an injury, coded as X6n in the NPR, was regarded as a recorded deliberate self-harm. We should note, however, data describing the circumstances and the cause of injury were often insufficient in patient records, this diagnosis, i.e. deliberate self-harm (X6n), has been heavily underreported in the patient registry in Norway [30]. Psychiatric comorbidity was defined by having a diagnosis of psychiatric illnesses, coded in F0-F9, either in the primary or secondary diagnoses.

Statistical analysis

Number of injuries prior and subsequent to the index medication poisoning was counted and distribution by specific types of injury and by gender was explored through descriptive analysis. The associations of injuries with comorbid diagnoses of deliberate self-harm and psychiatric disorder at index poisoning were analyzed. x^2 test was used to detect statistical differences between groups. Odds Ratios (OR) with 95% Confidence Intervals (CI) were estimated through general Logistic regression models. The analysis was conducted separately for each specific group of injuries and moreover by sex. The significance level was set to 0.05 and only tests being statistically significant were reported. All analyses were carried out on SPSS 22.0 or SAS 9.4 software for Windows.

Results

A total of 1497 adolescents aged 10–19 years received medical treatment because of self-poisoning with medication from 2008 through 2011. These adolescents comprised

Table 1 Characteristics of injuries before and after the index poisoning with medication, a gender comparison

Characteristics	Total $N = 1497$ n (%)	Female $N = 1144$ n (%)	Male $N = 353$ n (%)	Female/Male OR[a] (95% CI)
Any type of injury or poisoning (Yes)				
Before the index poisoning	431 (28.8)	312 (27.3)	119 (33.7)	0.7 (0.6–1.0)
After the index poisoning	586 (39.1)	457 (39.9)	129 (36.5)	NS*
Injuries to the head, neck, and throat (S00-S29) (Yes)				
Before the index poisoning	107 (7.2)	72 (6.3)	35 (10.0)	0.6 (0.4–0.9)
After the index poisoning	119 (8.0)	82 (7.2)	37 (10.5)	0.7 (0.4–1.0)
Injuries to the abdomen, lower back, lumbar spine and pelvis (S30-S39) (Yes)				
Before the index poisoning	214 (14.3)	146 (12.8)	68 (19.3)	0.6 (0.5–0.8)
After the index poisoning	224 (15.0)	172 (15.0)	52 (14.7)	NS
Injuries to the shoulder, arm and elbow (S40-S59) (Yes)				
Before the index poisoning	105 (7.0)	83 (7.3)	22 (6.2)	NS
After the index poisoning	117 (7.8)	105 (9.2)	12 (3.4)	2.9 (1. 6–5.3)
Injuries to the wrist and hand (S60-S69) (Yes)				
Before the index poisoning	133 (10.2)	83 (7.3)	50 (14.2)	0.5 (0.3–0.7)
After the index poisoning	139 (9.3)	97 (8.5)	42 (11.9)	NS
Superficial and open wound injuries to the wrist and hand (S60-S61) (Yes)				
Before the index poisoning	63 (4.2)	38 (3.3)	25 (7.1)	0.5 (0.3–0.8)
After the index poisoning	83 (5.5)	61 (5.3)	22 (6.2)	NS
Injuries to the hip, leg, and foot (S70-S99) (Yes)				
Before the index poisoning	144 (9.6)	106 (9.3)	38 (10.8)	NS
After the index poisoning	146 (9.8)	111 (7.4)	35 (9.9)	NS
Burns, corrosions, and frostbite (T20-T35) (Yes)				
Before the index poisoning	9 (0.6)	7 (0.6)	2 (0.6)	NS
After the index poisoning	10 (0.7)	9 (0.8)	1 (0.3)	NS
Poisonings by non-medicational substances (T51-T65) (Yes)				
Before the index poisoning	73 (4.9)	60 (5.2)	13 (3.7)	NS
After the index poisoning	32 (2.1)	25 (2.2)	7 (2.0)	NS
Poisoning by medications and biological substances (T40-T50) (Yes)				
After the index poisoning	317 (21.2)	274 (24.0)	43 (12.2)	2.3 (1.6–3.2)
Comorbid diagnosis of deliberate self-harm (X6n) (Yes)				
Before the index poisoning	22 (1.5)	18 (1.6)	4 (1.1)	NS
After the index poisoning	184 (12.3)	166 (14.5)	18 (5.1)	3.2 (1.9–5.2)
Comorbid diagnosis of psychiatric disorder (F) (Yes)				
Before the index poisoning	23 (1.5)	14 (1.2)	9 (2.6)	NS
After the index poisoning	189 (12.6)	162 (14.2)	27 (7.7)	2.0 (1.3–3.1)

[a]The analysis was conducted separately for each specific group of injuries; *NS* Not Significant

1144 (76.4%) girls and 353 (23.6%) boys with a female to male ratio of 3.24. Most of them (89.8%) were between 15 and 19 years old at the time of the index poisoning.

Exposure to injuries during the study period

Of the 1497 adolescents, 431 (28.8%) individuals were treated at least once for external injuries before the index medication poisoning, and 586 (39.1%) cases had at least one treatment because of injuries after the index poisoning during the observation period. In total, 830 (55.4%) adolescents (55.1% of females and 56.7% of males) received hospital treatment at least on one occasion because of injuries or poisoning either before or after the index poisoning. Altogether 2545 injury incidents, in addition to the index poisoning with medication, were recorded, including 778 injury incidents of

Table 2 Influence of comorbid diagnoses of deliberate self-harm and psychiatric disorder at the index poisoning

Subject Group	Deliberate Self-harm at Index Poisoning			Psychiatric Disorders at Index Poisoning		
	Yes n (%)	No n (%)	OR[a] (95% CI)	Yes n (%)	No n (%)	OR[†] (95% CI)
All Subjects: (N = 1497)	668	829		508	989	
Gender						
Female	548 (82.0)	596 (71.9)	1.8 (1.4–2.3)	387 (76.2)	757 (76.5)	NS
Male	120 (18.0)	233 (29.1)		121 (23.8)	232 (23.5)	
Any type of injury or poisoning (S00-T65) (Yes)						
Before the index poisoning	203 (30.4)	228 (27.5)	NS	170 (33.5)	261 (26.4)	1.4 (1.1–1.8)
After the index poisoning	271 (40.6)	315 (38.0)	NS	219 (43.1)	367 (37.1)	1.3 (1.0–1.6)
Injuries to the wrist and hand (S60-S69) (Yes)						
Before the index poisoning	61 (9.1)	72 (8.7)	NS	60 (11.8)	73 (7.4)	1.7 (1.2–2.4)
After the index poisoning	60 (9.0)	79 (9.5)	NS	50 (9.8)	89 (9.0)	NS
Poisoning by medications or other substances (T4n-T65) (Yes)						
Before the index poisoning	27 (4.0)	46 (5.6)	NS	31 (6.1)	42 (4.3)	NS
After the index poisoning	166 (24.9)	163 (19.7)	1.4 (1.1–1.7)	142 (28.0)	187 (18.9)	1.7 (1.3–2.1)
Other injuries (Yes)						
Before the index poisoning	154 (23.1)	163 (19.7)	NS	115 (22.6)	202 (20.4)	NS
After the index poisoning	134 (20.1)	191 (23.0)	NS	100 (19.7)	225 (22.8)	NS
Deliberate self-harm (X6n) (Yes)						
Before the index poisoning	13 (2.0)	9 (1.1)	NS	13 (2.6)	9 (0.9)	2.9 (1.2–6.7)
After the index poisoning	120 (18.0)	64 (7.7)	2.6 (1.9–3.6)	87 (17.1)	97 (9.9)	1.9 (1.4–2.6)
Comorbid psychiatric disorder (F) (Yes)						
Before the index poisoning	11 (1.7)	12 (1.5)	NS	12 (24)	11 (1.1)	NS
After the index poisoning	101 (15.1)	88 (10.6)	1.5 (1.1–2.0)	110 (21.7)	79 (8.0)	3.2 (2.3–4.4)

[a]The analysis was conducted separately for each specific group of injuries; NS = Not significant

other types before the index poisoning and 1767 injuries of all types after the index poisoning.

Figure 1 shows the distribution of the number of injuries prior and subsequent to the index poisoning in the study population. Before the index poisoning, one third (33.7%) of male and over a quarter (27.3%) of female adolescents in the cohort had at least one injury treatment, while the corresponding percentages subsequent to the index poisoning were 36.5 and 40.0%, respectively. Many individuals had only one additional injury other than the index poisoning (19.9% of males and 16.6% of females before the index poisoning, and 20.4% males and 19.0% of females after); However, 14.2% of the male and 12.6% of the female subjects had 2 to 4 injury incidents, and 8.4% of females and 2.0% of males had at least 5 incidents subsequent to the index poisoning with medication.

Form of injuries before and after the index poisoning

The most frequently recorded injury form prior to the index poisoning was injury to the abdomen, lower back, lumbar spine and pelvis (S30-S39), present in 214 (14.3%) individuals and 12.8% of females and 19.3% of males in the cohort

(Table 1). The most common form of injury subsequent to the index poisoning was poisoning with medication and biological substances (T4n-T50), present in 317 (21.1%) individuals and 24.0% of females and 12.2% of males, respectively. The second most frequent injury subsequent to index poisoning was injury to the abdomen, lower back, lumbar spine and pelvis (S30-S39), present in 15.0% of all adolescents in the cohort, 15.0% of the females and 14.7% of the males.

Gender differences in injuries before and after the index poisoning

Table 1 also shows the recorded injuries in male and female adolescents separately. Before the index poisoning, female adolescents had significantly fewer injuries than male adolescents (OR = 0.7, 95% CI: 0.6–1.0). Significant sex differences were seen in certain types of injuries such as injury to the head, neck and throat (S00-S29), injury to the abdomen, lower back, lumbar spine and pelvis (S30-S39), and injury to the wrist and hand (S60-S69), all with a male predominance. Sixty-three (4.2%) individuals had superficial or open wound injuries to the wrist and hand (S60-S61) before the index poisoning; and males

Table 3 Influences of comorbid diagnoses of deliberate self-harm and psychiatric disorder at the index poisoning in males and females

Subject Group	Deliberate Self-harm at Index Poisoning			Psychiatric Disorder at Index Poisoning		
	Yes n (%)	No n (%)	OR[†] (95% CI)	Yes n (%)	No n (%)	OR[a] (95% CI)
Males (N = 353)	120 (34.0)	233 (66.0)		121 (34.3)	232 (65.7)	
Any type of injury or poisoning (S00-T65) (Yes)						
Before the index poisoning	48 (40.0)	71 (30.5)	NS	44 (36.4)	75 (32.3)	NS
After the index poisoning	44 (36.7)	85 (36.5)	NS	49 (40.5)	80 (34.5)	NS
Injuries to the wrist and hand (S60-S69) (Yes)						
Before the index poisoning	17 (14.2)	33 (14.2)	NS	23 (19.0)	27 (11.6)	NS
After the index poisoning	14 (11.7)	28 (12.0)	NS	20 (16.5)	22 (9.48)	NS
Poisoning by medications or other substances (T40-T65) (Yes)						
Before the index poisoning	3 (2.5)	10 (4.3)	NS	4 (3.3)	9 (3.9)	NS
After the index poisoning	20 (16.7)	28 (12.0)	NS	22 (18.2)	26 (11.2)	NS
Other injuries (Yes)						
Before the index poisoning	34 (28.3)	47 (20.2)	NS	27 (22.3)	54 (23.3)	NS
After the index poisoning	20 (16.7)	50 (21.5)	NS	18 (14.9)	52 (22.4)	NS
Deliberate self-harm (X6n) (Yes)						
Before the index poisoning	1 (0.8)	3 (1.3)	NS	2 (1.7)	2 (0.9)	NS
After the index poisoning	12 (10.0)	6 (2.6)	4.2 (1.5–11.5)	11 (9.1)	7 (3.0)	3.2 (1.2–8.5)
Comorbid psychiatric disorder (Fn) (Yes)						
Before the index poisoning	2 (1.7)	7 (3.0)	NS	3 (2.5)	6 (2.6)	NS
After the index poisoning	12 (10.0)	15 (6.4)	NS	19 (15.7)	8 (3.5)	5.2 (2.2–12.3)
Females (N = 1144)	548 (47.9)	596 (52.1)		387 (33.8)	757 (66.2)	
Any type of injury or poisoning (S00-T65) (Yes)						
Before the index poisoning	155 (28.3)	157 (26.3)	NS	126 (32.6)	186 (24.6)	1.5 (1.1–1.9)
After the index poisoning	227 (41.4)	230 (38.6)	NS	170 (43.9)	287 (37.9)	1.3 (1.0–1.7)
Injuries to the wrist and hand (S60-S69) (Yes)						
Before the index poisoning	44 (8.0)	39 (6.5)	NS	37 (9.6)	46 (6.1)	1.6 (1.0–2.6)
After the index poisoning	46 (8.4)	51 (8.6)	NS	30 (7.8)	67 (8.9)	NS
Poisoning by medications or other substances (T40-T65) (Yes)						
Before the index poisoning	24 (4.4)	36 (6.0)	NS	27 (7.0)	33 (4.4)	NS
After the index poisoning	146 (26.6)	135 (22.7)	NS	120 (31.0)	161 (21.3)	1.7 (1.3–2.2)
Other injuries (Yes)						
Before the index poisoning	120 (21.9)	116 (19.5)	NS	88 (22.7)	148 (19.6)	NS
After the index poisoning	114 (20.8)	141 (23.7)	NS	82 (21.2)	173 (22.9)	NS
Deliberate self-harm (X6n) (Yes)						
Before the index poisoning	12 (2.2)	6 (1.0)	NS	11 (2.8)	7 (0.9)	3.1 (1.2–8.2)
After the index poisoning	108 (19.7)	58 (9.7)	2.3 (1.6–3.2)	76 (19.6)	90 (11.9)	1.8 (1.3–2.5)
Comorbid psychiatric disorder (Fn) (Yes)						
Before the index poisoning	9 (1.6)	5 (0.8)	NS	9 (2.3)	5 (0.7)	3.6 (1.2–10.8)
After the index poisoning	89 (16.2)	73 (12.2)	NS	91 (23.5)	71 (9.4)	3.0 (2.1–4.2)

[a]The analysis was conducted separately for each specific group of injuries; NS = Not significant

were significantly more likely than females to have this type of injury (female:male OR = 0.5, 95% CI: 0.3–0.8). At the same time, females were over twice likely to repeat poisoning with medication (T4n-T50) (24.0% vs. 12.2%; OR = 2.3, 95% CI: 1.6–3.2) after the index poisoning. They were also almost three times more likely to have

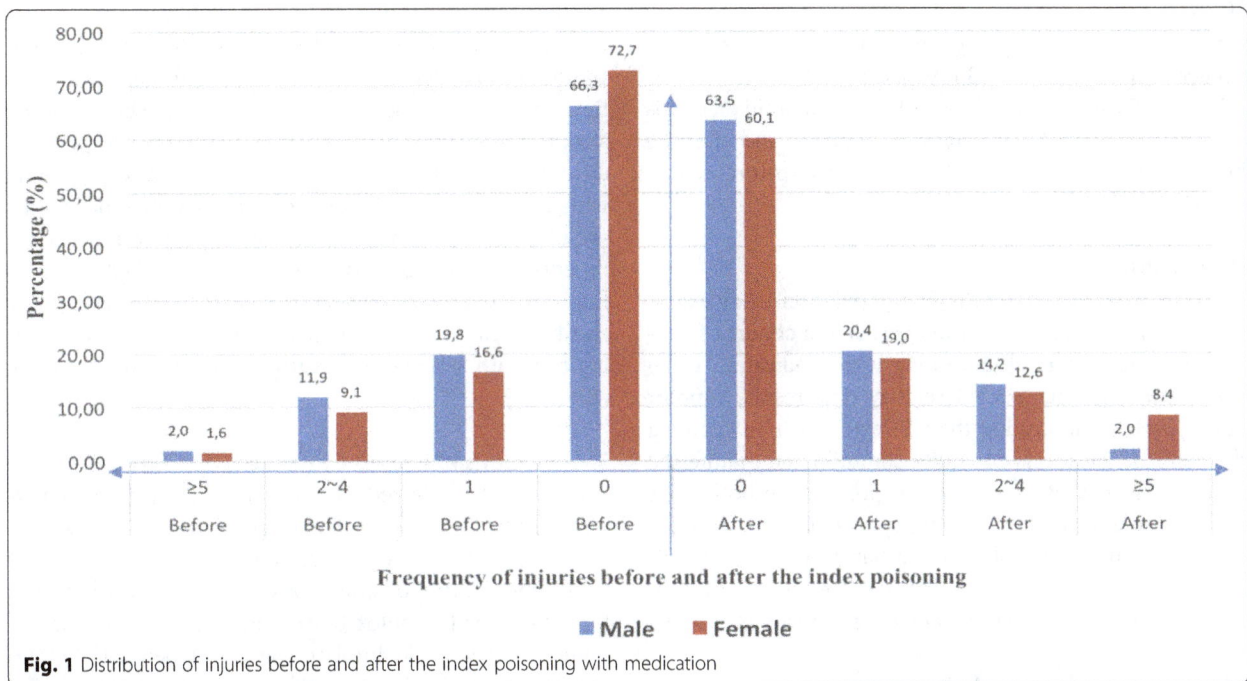

Fig. 1 Distribution of injuries before and after the index poisoning with medication

subsequent injures to the shoulder, arm and elbow (S40-S59) (OR = 2.9, 95% CI: 1.6–5.3).

Moreover, female adolescents were more likely than the males to receive a supplemental diagnosis of deliberate self-harm (OR = 3.2, 95% CI: 1.9–5.2) and also a comorbid diagnosis of psychiatric disorder (OR = 2.0, 95% CI: 1.3–3.1) in connection with their subsequent injuries within the observation period.

Influence of a recorded deliberate self-harm and psychiatric disorders at index poisoning

At the index poisoning with medication, 668 (44.6%) adolescents received a supplementary diagnosis of deliberate self-harm with a significantly higher presentation in females than males (OR = 1.8, 95% CI: 1.4–2.3). 508 (33.9%) individuals received a comorbid diagnosis of psychiatric disorder with no significant gender difference.

Table 2 presents the injury history of all individuals and Table 3 separates males and females according to whether they were diagnosed with deliberate self-harm or psychiatric disorder at the index poisoning. When both sexes were included (Table 2), a recorded diagnosis of deliberate self-harm at the index poisoning increased the likelihood of receiving a supplementary diagnosis of deliberate self-harm (OR = 2.6, 95% CI: 1.9–3.6), as well as a comorbid psychiatric diagnosis at subsequent injuries (OR = 1.5, 95% CI: 1.1–2.0). Furthermore, such a diagnosis was also significantly associated with an increased risk of having subsequent poisoning incidents (OR = 1.4, 95% CI: 1.1–1.7).

Individuals diagnosed with a psychiatric comorbidity at index poisoning had significantly more injuries both prior and subsequent to index poisoning (OR = 1.4, 95% CI: 1.1–1.8 (before); OR = 1.3, 95% CI: 1.0–1.6 (after)). These adolescents were also more likely to have injuries to wrist and hand before the index poisoning (OR = 1.7, 95% CI: 1.2–2.4 for S60-S69; OR = 2.1, 95% CI: 1.3–3.5 for S60-S61), poisoning with medication after the index poisoning (OR = 1.7, 95% CI: 1.3–2.1), and to receive a diagnosis of deliberate self-harm both before (OR = 2.9, 95% CI: 1.2–6.7) and after (OR = 1.9, 95% CI: 1.4–2.6) index poisoning. Individuals receiving a comorbid psychiatric diagnosis at index poisoning were three times more likely to receive a psychiatric diagnosis at subsequent injuries (OR = 3.2, 95% CI: 2.3–4.4).

When males and females were analyzed separately (Table 3), a supplementary diagnosis of deliberate self-harm at the index poisoning was positively associated with a diagnosis of deliberate self-harm given in subsequent injuries in both sexes (OR = 4.2, 95% CI: 1.5–11.5 for males and OR = 2.3, 95% CI: 1.6–3.2 for females). A comorbid diagnosis of psychiatric disorder at index poisoning was positively associated with the presence of comorbid diagnoses of deliberate self-harm (OR = 3.2, 95% CI: 1.2–8.5) and psychiatric disorder (OR = 5.2, 95% CI: 2.2–12.3) at subsequent injuries among male adolescents.

Female adolescents who received a comorbid diagnosis of psychiatric disorders at index poisoning were more likely to receive treatment for both prior (OR = 1.5, 95% CI: 1.1–1.9) and subsequent (OR = 1.3, 95% CI: 1.0–1.7) injuries of any form. Specifically, they more often had prior injuries to the wrist and hand (S60-S69) (OR = 1.6, 95% CI: 1.0–2.6) and subsequent poisoning with medication and other substances

(T40-T65) (OR = 1.7, 95% CI: 1.3–2.2). More notably, these females were most likely to get a supplemental diagnosis of deliberate self-harm (OR = 3.1, 95% CI: 1.2–8.2 (before); OR = 1.8, 95% CI: 1.3–2.5(after)) as well as a comorbid diagnosis of psychiatric disorder at injuries both before and after the index poisoning (OR = 3.6, 95% CI: 1.2–10.8 (before); OR = 3.0, 95% CI: 2.1–4.2 (after)).

Discussion

To our knowledge, this is the first population study examining external injuries of various forms in a cohort of adolescents treated for self-poisoning with medication using data from a national patient registry. The results support our hypothesis indicating that: 1) external injury among the cohort adolescents was quite common and manifested itself in a variety of injuries, 2) the presence of both prior and subsequent injuries was highly associated with a comorbid diagnosis of deliberate self-harm or psychiatric illness at index poisoning, and that 3) there were significant gender differences in injury incidents and form of injuries.

Commonness of injuries of other forms

External injuries were prevalent in our cohort of adolescents, with over half of them having at least one injury before or after the index poisoning. About 30% of these adolescents had a record of treatment because of injuries in forms other than medication poisoning before the index poisoning – an insightful detail which has not been reported in related studies. In the meantime, nearly 40% of the cohort adolescents were treated for injuries of various forms after the index incident of medication poisoning.

The commonness of injuries of other forms, seen in our cohort both before and after the index poisoning, supports the notion in previous studies [12] that methods of injury change during repeat episodes of self-harm. Our data showed that injury to hand and wrist was rather common, presenting in over 10% of the adolescents prior to the index poisoning and 9.3% of them subsequently to the index poisoning. This is probably an underestimation of the true number of such injuries since we have only analyzed hospital treated injuries. Poisoning, on the other hand, was the most frequent injury subsequent to the index poisoning.

Our finding that less than half of the adolescents in the cohort received a comorbid diagnosis of deliberate self-harm at their index poisoning was clearly an underreporting of this diagnosis in the patient registry, as compared with the rates reported by studies [30–33] in which the intentionality of poisoning was additionally reviewed. Similarly, the 33.9% psychiatric comorbidity found in the present study is much lower than the report that approximately 8 in 10 adolescents who self-harm have psychiatric disorders [34]. Despite of

possible underreporting, the relatively higher rates of deliberate self-harm and psychiatric disorders at index poisoning in females than males are consistent with the findings from previous research [2, 31]. The observed strong associations of deliberate self-harm and psychiatric comorbidity being diagnosed at index poisoning with both prior and subsequent injuries of other forms are also in high concordance with studies on self-harm repetition among adolescents [3, 11, 12, 35–38]. These findings underscore the importance of assessment of mental status and intentionality for adolescents presenting to health services for treatment because of poisoning and injury.

Specific forms of injuries by gender

The present study did not detect a highly distinct pattern of injuries between males and females in the cohort, but several findings separated the genders.

Common forms of injury observed in males, both before and after the index poisoning, was injury to the abdomen, lower back, lumbar spine and pelvis (S30-S39) and injury to the head, neck and throat (S00-S29). Females on the other hand showed predominance of injury to the shoulder, arm and elbow (S40-S59). We cannot ascertain, however, whether this illustrates a difference in preferred method of self-injury or simply reflects gender differences in forms of non-intentional injuries likely happening in daily life.

Interestingly, males in the cohort stood out as having significantly more injuries to the hand and wrist prior to the index poisoning. Community studies on self-cutting suggest that this behaviour was more frequent in females than males [29, 39], whereas a male predominance was reported in hospital treated injuries to the hand and wrist [40, 41]. It is therefore possible that females may be overrepresented in hand and wrist injuries not treated in hospital services (community studies), while males are overrepresented in such injuries presenting to hospital [40]. A possible explanation to this could be that injuries of self-cutting on hands and wrists in female adolescents are less often severe and thus go untreated but in male adolescents are more often severe and thus are treated.

Female adolescents diagnosed with a psychiatric disorder at index poisoning seemed to be particularly vulnerable to having sustained injuries both before and after the index poisoning and to receiving a supplemental diagnosis of deliberate self-harm (X6n) on these occasions. They were more often treated for injuries to the wrist and hand before the index poisoning and for repeat poisoning after the index poisoning. These findings support the argument of a possible switch of methods used for self-harm in this group of adolescents [12, 40, 42].

Males in our cohort were significantly more likely than females to have a prior injury to the wrist and hand

(S60-S61) for which no comorbid diagnosis of deliberate self-harm (X6n) was given. This is an interesting finding given the high likelihood of such injury being a deliberate action. Females, on the other hand, were more likely to repeat poisoning with medication and also to receive comorbid diagnoses of deliberate self-harm and psychiatric disorder at their subsequent injuries. A possible reason for this could be that adolescents, especially boys, often attend sport activities, so their injuries on hand and wrist are commonly perceived as accidental instead of deliberate. Another possible explanation for the discrepancy might be that, from a clinical point of view, poisoning with medication occurs more often with intention as compared to injury to the hand or wrist (having in mind that these injuries can be superficial). This is in line with previous research [40, 43] stating that suicidal intent is higher in individuals who self-poison compared to individuals who self-injure. Regardless of the reason, the low rate of deliberate self-harm being given to injuries to the hand and wrist might constitute a problem, because self-injury, particularly self-cutting, is associated with not only risk of repetition, but also risk of suicide completion in adolescents, particularly in males [6, 40, 42]. In the meantime, the higher rate of psychiatric diagnoses for female compared to male adolescents following index poisoning may imply an under-reporting by males of psychological distress and, consequently, an under-treatment of male mental ill-health.

Limitations and strengths

The data obtained for the present study ensured the accuracy of episodic hospital contacts because of injury, but did not contain personal profiles such as socioeconomic status, detailed information on psychiatric diagnosis and other health related records that may have provided interesting insights. Also, for injuries treated in emergency clinics, the assessment of psychiatric illness and deliberate self-harm was not systematically carried out. This may impose an underestimation of the true prevalence of such comorbidities among injury incidents and limit the possibility to fully distinguish between self-inflicted injuries and injuries inflicted by others. Furthermore, since many mild injuries do not lead to medical care, this study could not generalize to those who do not present to emergency or hospital services after injury and does in no way reflect the incidence and frequency of injuries or deliberate self-harm among adolescents. In addition, data on type of medication used in self-poisoning was not available. It would have been of great value to identify whether the medications were prescribed or purchased over the count so that to inform strategies of control to prevent future self-poisoning.

Despite of these limitations, the present study has several strengths. It is, to our knowledge, the first one that has examined a large cohort of adolescents with medication poisoning for their external injuries of various forms. Unlike studies relying on self-reports and clinical records, this study is based on precise data of patient records with a standardized diagnostic classification of injuries and comorbidities. The longitudinal nature of the data has enabled the possibility of looking into the details both retrospectively and prospectively.

Conclusion

This study shows that adolescents with medication poisoning represent a high-risk group prone to both prior and subsequent injuries of various forms in need of hospital treatment. Possible switches in injury methods as well as gender differences in injury incidents and forms were observed. A male predominance of injuries to hand and wrist was found together with an increased likelihood of subsequent poisoning in females. Comorbid diagnoses of deliberate self-harm and psychiatric illness at index poisoning correlated strongly with prior as well as subsequent injuries in the cohort adolescents, especially among the females. With growing evidence for a positive effect of psychosocial assessment for patients treated for self-harm on repetition reduction [7], the present study further pinpoints that evaluation of mental health status and intentionality should be implemented to the utmost extent among adolescents presenting to health services because of self-poisoning or injuries.

Abbreviations
CI: Confidence Intervals; ICD-10: the Tenth Revision of the International Statistical Classification of Diseases; NPR: Norwegian Patient Registry; NS: Not significant; OR: Odds Ratio

Authors' contributions
PQ, BS and LM conceived the idea of study. SS and PQ analyzed the data. SS and ASB prepared the drafts of report. SS, ASB, LM, BS and PQ contributed to the interpretation of data and the critical revision. PQ finalized the manuscript. All authors read and approved the final manuscript.

Consent for publication
Not applicable.

Competing interests
The authors declare that they have no competing interests.

Author details
[1]National Centre for Suicide Research and Prevention, Institute of Clinical medicine, University of Oslo, Sognsvannsveien 21, N-0372 Oslo, Norway. [2]Department of Epidemiology, Shandong University School of Public Health and Shandong University Center for Suicide Prevention Research, Jinan, China. [3]Department of Psychiatry, Columbia University College of Physicians and Surgeons, New York, NY, USA.

References

1. Sminkey L. World report on child injury prevention. Injury prevention. 2008; 14(1):69.
2. Zakharov S, Navratil T, Pelclova D. Suicide attempts by deliberate self-poisoning in children and adolescents. Psychiatry Res. 2013;210(1):302–7.
3. Rodham K, Hawton K, Evans E. Reasons for deliberate self-harm: comparison of self-poisoners and self-cutters in a community sample of adolescents. J Am Acad Child Adolesc Psychiatry. 2004;43(1):80–7.
4. Reith DM, et al. Adolescent self-poisoning: a cohort study of subsequent suicide and premature deaths. Crisis. 2003;24(2):79–84.
5. Law BM, Shek DT. Self-harm and suicide attempts among young Chinese adolescents in Hong Kong: prevalence, correlates, and changes. J Pediatr Adolesc Gynecol. 2013;26(3 Suppl):S26–32.
6. Hawton K, et al. Repetition of self-harm and suicide following self-harm in children and adolescents: findings from the multicentre study of self-harm in England. J Child Psychol Psychiatry. 2012;53(12):1212–9.
7. Bergen H, et al. Psychosocial assessment and repetition of self-harm: the significance of single and multiple repeat episode analyses. J Affect Disord. 2010;127(1–3):257–65.
8. Fadum EA, et al. Self-poisoning with medications in adolescents: a national register study of hospital admissions and readmissions. Gen Hosp Psychiatry. 2014;36(6):709–15.
9. Hawton K, et al. Deliberate self harm in adolescents: self report survey in schools in England. BMJ. 2002;325(7374):1207–11.
10. Ystgaard M, et al. Deliberate self harm in adolescents. Tidsskr Nor Laegeforen. 2003;123(16):2241–5.
11. Madge N, et al. Deliberate self-harm within an international community sample of young people: comparative findings from the Child & Adolescent Self-harm in Europe (CASE) study. J Child Psychol Psychiatry. 2008;49(6):667–77.
12. Miller M, et al. Method choice in nonfatal self-harm as a predictor of subsequent episodes of self-harm and suicide: implications for clinical practice. Am J Public Health. 2013;103(6):E61–8.
13. Nock MK, et al. Non-suicidal self-injury among adolescents: diagnostic correlates and relation to suicide attempts. Psychiatry Res. 2006;144(1):65–72.
14. Dukes RL, Stein JA, Zane JI. Gender differences in the relative impact of physical and relational bullying on adolescent injury and weapon carrying. J Sch Psychol. 2010;48(6):511–32.
15. Beautrais AL. Gender issues in youth suicidal behaviour. Emerg Med (Fremantle). 2002;14(1):35–42.
16. Jelalian E, et al. Risk taking, reported injury, and perception of future injury among adolescents. J Pediatr Psychol. 1997;22(4):513–31.
17. Engstrom K, Laflamme L. Socio-economic differences in intentional injuries: a national study of Swedish male and female adolescents. Acta Psychiatr Scand Suppl. 2002;412:26–9.
18. Malta DC, et al. Factors associated with injuries in adolescents, from the National Adolescent School-based Health Survey (PeNSE 2012). Rev Bras Epidemiol. 2014;17(Suppl 1):183–202.
19. Mytton J, et al. Unintentional injuries in school-aged children and adolescents: lessons from a systematic review of cohort studies. Inj Prev. 2009;15(2):111–24.
20. Brunner R, et al. Life-time prevalence and psychosocial correlates of adolescent direct self-injurious behavior: a comparative study of findings in 11 European countries. J Child Psychol Psychiatry. 2014;55(4):337–48.
21. Fortune SA, Hawton K. Suicide and deliberate self-harm in children and adolescents. Paediatrics and Child Health. 2007;17(11):443–7.
22. Kidger J, et al. Adolescent self-harm and suicidal thoughts in the ALSPAC cohort: a self-report survey in England. BMC Psychiatry. 2012;12:69.
23. Muehlenkamp JJ, et al. International prevalence of adolescent non-suicidal self-injury and deliberate self-harm. Child Adolesc Psychiatry Ment Health. 2012;6:10.
24. Chau N, et al. Determinants of school injury proneness in adolescents: a prospective study. Public Health. 2008;122(8):801–8.
25. McPhedran S, Baker J. Suicide prevention and method restriction: evaluating the impact of limiting access to lethal means among young Australians. Arch Suicide Res. 2012;16(2):135–46.
26. Portzky G, De Wilde EJ, van Heeringen K. Deliberate self-harm in young people: differences in prevalence and risk factors between the Netherlands and Belgium. Eur Child Adolesc Psychiatry. 2008;17(3):179–86.
27. Morey C, et al. The prevalence of self-reported deliberate self harm in Irish adolescents. BMC Public Health. 2008;8:79.

28. Hawton K, Harriss L, Rodham K. How adolescents who cut themselves differ from those who take overdoses. European Child & Adolescent Psychiatry. 2010;19(6):513–23.
29. Laukkanen E, et al. The prevalence of self-cutting and other self-harm among 13- to 18-year-old Finnish adolescents. Soc Psychiatry Psychiatr Epidemiol. 2009;44(1):23–8.
30. Mellesdal L, et al. Self-harm induced somatic admission after discharge from psychiatric hospital–a prospective cohort study. European Psychiatry. 2014; 29(4):246–52.
31. White AM, et al. Hospitalizations for suicide-related drug poisonings and co-occurring alcohol overdoses in adolescents (ages 12-17) and young adults (ages 18-24) in the United States, 1999-2008: results from the Nationwide inpatient sample. Suicide Life Threat Behav. 2013;43(2):198–212.
32. Hovda KE, et al. Acute poisonings treated in hospitals in Oslo: a one-year prospective study (I): pattern of poisoning. Clin Toxicol. 2008;46(1):35–41.
33. Lipnik-Štangelj M. Hospitalizations due to poisonings in Slovenia–epidemiological aspects. Wien Klin Wochenschr. 2010;122:54–8.
34. Hawton K, et al. Psychiatric disorders in patients presenting to hospital following self-harm: a systematic review. J Affect Disord. 2013;151(3):821–30.
35. Shek DT, Yu L. Self-harm and suicidal behaviors in Hong Kong adolescents: prevalence and psychosocial correlates. Sci World J. 2012;2012:932540.
36. Sansone RA, et al. Multiple psychiatric diagnoses and self-harm behavior. Int J Psychiatry Clin Pract. 2005;9(1):41–4.
37. Bjarehed J, Lundh LG. Deliberate self-harm in 14-year-old adolescents: how frequent is it, and how is it associated with psychopathology, relationship variables, and styles of emotional regulation? Cogn Behav Ther. 2008;37(1):26–37.
38. Mars B, et al. Clinical and social outcomes of adolescent self harm: population based birth cohort study. BMJ. 2014;349:g5954.
39. Ross S, Heath N. A study of the frequency of self-mutilation in a community sample of adolescents. Journal of Youth and Adolescence. 2002;31(1):67–77.
40. Hawton K, et al. Self-cutting: patient characteristics compared with self-poisoners. Suicide Life Threat Behav. 2004;34(3):199–208.
41. Lilley R, et al. Hospital care and repetition following self-harm: multicentre comparison of self-poisoning and self-injury. Br J Psychiatry. 2008;192(6): 440–5.
42. Owens D, et al. Switching methods of self-harm at repeat episodes: findings from a multicentre cohort study. J Affect Disord. 2015;180:44–51.
43. Haw C, et al. Suicidal intent and method of self-harm: a large-scale study of self-harm patients presenting to a general hospital. Suicide Life Threat Behav. 2015;45(6):732–46.

19

Re-development of mental health first aid guidelines for supporting Aboriginal and Torres Strait islanders who are experiencing suicidal thoughts and behaviour

Gregory Armstrong[1*] [iD], Natalie Ironfield[2], Claire M. Kelly[3], Katrina Dart[3], Kerry Arabena[4], Kathy Bond[3], Nicola Reavley[2] and Anthony F. Jorm[2]

Abstract

Background: Suicide is a leading cause of death among Indigenous Australians. Friends, family and frontline workers (for example, teachers, youth workers) are often best positioned to provide initial assistance if someone is suicidal. Culturally appropriate expert consensus guidelines on how to provide mental health first aid to Australian Aboriginal and Torres Strait Islander persons who are experiencing suicidal thoughts or behaviour were developed in 2009. This study describes the re-development of these guidelines to ensure they contain the most current recommended helping actions.

Methods: The Delphi consensus method was used to elicit consensus on potential helping statements to be included in the guidelines. These statements describe helping actions that Indigenous community members and non-Indigenous frontline workers can take, and information they should have, to help someone who is experiencing suicidal thoughts or displaying suicidal behaviour. A panel was formed, comprising 27 Aboriginal and Torres Strait Islander people who have expertise in Indigenous suicide prevention. The panellists were presented with the helping statements via online questionnaires and were encouraged to suggest re-wording of statements and any additional helping statements that were not included in the original questionnaire. Statements were only accepted for inclusion in the guidelines if they were endorsed by ≥90% of panellists as essential or important.

Results: From a total of 301 statements shown to the expert panel, 172 were endorsed as helping statements to be including in the re-developed guidelines.

Conclusions: Aboriginal and Torres Strait Islander suicide prevention experts were able to reach consensus on appropriate strategies for providing mental health first aid to an Aboriginal or Torres Strait Islander person experiencing suicidal thoughts or behaviour. The re-development of the guidelines has resulted in more comprehensive guidance than the earlier version, for which the panel had rated 166 helping statements and had endorsed 52. These re-developed guidelines can be used to inform Indigenous suicide gatekeeper training courses.

Keywords: Suicide, Indigenous, Aboriginal and Torres Strait islander people, Mental health first aid, Prevention, Helping behaviour, Assistance

* Correspondence: g.armstrong@unimelb.edu.au
[1]Nossal Institute for Global Health, Melbourne School of Population and Global Health, University of Melbourne, 333 Exhibition St, Melbourne, VIC 3000, Australia
Full list of author information is available at the end of the article

Background

Suicide is a leading cause of mortality for Aboriginal and Torres Strait Islander peoples in Australia, ranking in as the fifth leading cause of death in 2014 [1]. The suicide death rate for Aboriginal and Torres Strait Islander peoples is estimated to be 23.0 per 100,000, which is twice the rate for non-Indigenous Australians [1]. The issue is particularly pronounced among Aboriginal and Torres Strait Islander youth, with a suicide death rate of 52.5 per 100,000 among those aged 15–24, which is approximately four times the rate of their non-Indigenous counterparts [1].

The high rate of Indigenous suicide is a distressing phenomenon that is similarly plaguing several other postcolonial countries, including Canada, the United States and New Zealand [2]. Suicide among Indigenous peoples is a complex socio-cultural, political, biological and psychological phenomenon that needs to be understood in the context of colonisation, loss of land and culture, trans-generational trauma, grief and loss, and racism and discrimination [3–5]. Additionally, the higher levels of social disadvantage experienced by Indigenous peoples increases their exposure to mental disorders, substance abuse and a suite of stressful life events, for example, unemployment, homelessness, incarceration and family breakdown, all of which are well-documented suicide risk factors [6–11].

Despite the high level of need, there is a lack of documented and rigorously evaluated Indigenous suicide prevention programs, and it is evident that there is no one solution [12, 13]. One evidence-based suicide prevention tool is known as 'gatekeeper training' [14]. The underlying premise of gatekeeper training is that family, friends and frontline workers (for example, teachers, youth workers) are often best positioned to identify and provide initial assistance to individuals experiencing suicidal thoughts or displaying suicidal behaviour. Gatekeeper training teaches groups of people in the community how to identify and support individuals who are at high risk of suicide and to refer them to appropriate community supports, including mental health services. [15] A systematic review of suicide interventions targeting Indigenous populations in Australia, Canada, New Zealand and the United States found that gatekeeper-training demonstrated encouraging results, with significant short-term increases in participant knowledge, skills, intentions to assist, and confidence in identifying and assisting individuals at risk of suicide [13]. However, there is still limited evidence regarding the maintenance of these changes and there remains a need for future research to examine longer-term outcome measures, for example, referral and treatment patterns and the impact on rates of suicide attempts and deaths. There is also a need for further research to inform the pedagogical approach to developing and delivering Indigenous suicide gatekeeper training programs and how best to harness existing local community knowledge.

'Mental health first aid' is defined as the help provided to a person developing a mental health problem, experiencing the worsening of an existing mental health problem or in a mental health crisis, until appropriate professional treatment is received or until the crisis resolves [16]. In 2001, a Mental Health First Aid training program was established in Australia in response to the need for public education about mental illness and its treatment [17]. Later, an Aboriginal and Torres Strait Islander Mental Health First Aid (AMHFA) program was established [18]. The first edition of the AMHFA course was based around a cultural adaptation of the Standard Mental Health First Aid course guided by an Indigenous working group. Subsequently, a second edition was produced based on a series of guideline documents that were developed using Delphi expert consensus studies with Aboriginal or Torres Strait Islander mental health professionals as expert panellists [19]. Based on this series of guideline documents, the AMHFA program sought to provide recommendations as to how to provide initial assistance to an Aboriginal or Torres Strait Islander person with a mental health problem or in a mental health crisis, including depression, psychosis, substance use, or experiencing a traumatic event, a panic attack, suicidal thoughts or engaging in non-suicidal self-injury. AMHFA guidelines were also developed around 'Cultural Considerations and Communication Techniques' and, later in 2014, around 'Communicating with an Aboriginal or Torres Strait Islander Adolescent' [19, 20].

The AMHFA program is run through Mental Health First Aid Australia (MHFAA) who use a train-the-instructor style model, whereby they train their pool of accredited AMHFA Instructors, who are Aboriginal or Torres Strait Islander people, in how to deliver the course material to Indigenous community members and non-Indigenous frontline workers in their respective communities, where they are already embedded and have local support. An initial evaluation of the AMHFA program based on roll-out data and qualitative data obtained from focus group discussions found the program to be both culturally appropriate and acceptable to Aboriginal and Torres Strait Islander people [18].

As part of the process outlined above, AMHFA guidelines for assisting an Aboriginal or Torres Strait Islander person experiencing suicidal thoughts or suicidal behaviour were developed in 2009 [19]. The aim of this current study was to use the Delphi methodology to re-develop these guidelines in order to ensure that they reflect current evidence and best practice in suicide prevention, and contain the most current recommended helping actions that can be shared with Indigenous community members and non-Indigenous frontline workers. Further, this study aimed to expand upon the previous guidelines and provide more comprehensive guidance as to how members of the public can provide mental health first aid to an Aboriginal or Torres Strait Islander person experiencing suicidal thoughts or suicidal behaviour. The re-development of these guidelines will help to ensure they are well placed to inform the development of Indigenous suicide prevention gatekeeper training programs developed by MHFAA and others.

Methods

The Delphi consensus method has been used extensively in health and social research as a method for decision-making processes, including mental health research [21]. The Delphi method provides a platform for obtaining expert consensus on what constitutes best practice in scenarios that cannot be feasibly or ethically subject to a randomised controlled trial. The process involves a series of questionnaires being sent to a group of experts, who do not have to attend group meetings and can respond anonymously. Traditionally, the Delphi method has involved a number of iterations before consensus is achieved. Feedback is given at each stage in order to help experts assess their opinions against those of the group.

We used the Delphi consensus method to elicit consensus on potential helping statements to be included in the guidelines. The development of the guidelines using the Delphi method involved four steps: 1) formation of the expert panel, 2) questionnaire development, 3) data collection and analysis, and 4) guideline development. The same Delphi process was also used to redevelop the mental health first aid guidelines for supporting an Aboriginal or Torres Strait Islander person who is engaging in non-suicidal self-injury, which was also published in this journal [22].

Panel formation

A panel was recruited, comprising of 27 Aboriginal and Torres Strait Islander people who had expertise in Indigenous suicide prevention through their professional experience. A recruitment advertisement was sent out via the Aboriginal Mental Health First Aid Instructor email list, the Onemda VicHealth Koori Health Unit (University of Melbourne) email list, and the Lowitja Institute email list. The advertisement encouraged people to distribute the flyer across their broader networks. Potential candidates were asked to contact the research coordinator with information on their expertise in Indigenous suicide prevention and were sent a Plain Language Statement prior to participation. The research was approved by the Human Research Ethics Sub-Committee at the University of Melbourne (HREC No.1443056.1). Expert

panel members were reimbursed AUD$250 for completing all three survey rounds.

Questionnaire development

The questionnaire contained statements describing helping actions that Indigenous community members and non-Indigenous frontline workers can take, and information they should have, to help an Aboriginal or Torres Strait Islander person who is experiencing suicidal thoughts or behaviour. Statements were considered acceptable for inclusion in the questionnaire if the working group (comprising the authors) agreed that they described how someone can help a person who is suicidal with clear and non-ambiguous actions.

The statements were sourced from two previous Delphi questionnaires; the first questionnaire was designed to develop the original Aboriginal mental health first aid guidelines for suicidal thoughts and behaviour in 2009 and the second questionnaire was designed to re-develop the mainstream mental health first aid guidelines for suicidal thoughts and behaviour in 2014 [19, 23]. These previous questionnaires were formed through systematic searches of peer-reviewed literature, grey literature, books, websites and online materials, and existing suicide intervention courses, and these literature searches are described in detail elsewhere [19, 23]. The statements in the questionnaire were divided into ten sections based on common themes. The statements derived from the literature were kept as intact as possible to remain faithful to the original wording of the information. Statements were only modified to ensure consistency of format, or where there was concern about the comprehensibility or cultural appropriateness of the information.

Data collection and analysis

Once panel members had been recruited, they were sent an electronic link to an online questionnaire hosted by SurveyMonkey. Participants responded by rating how important the first aid action statements were to the development of a set of guidelines on providing mental health first aid to an Aboriginal or Torres Strait Islander person who is experiencing suicidal thoughts or displaying suicidal behaviour. Each statement was rated using a five-point scale with the following options: *Essential, Important, Don't know/It depends, Unimportant, Should not be included.*

Pre-determined criteria were used to assess the outcome for each statement. Statements were immediately included in the guidelines if they were endorsed by ≥90% of panellists as either essential or important. Statements were re-rated in the Round 2 questionnaire if they were rated as essential or important by 80–89.9% of the panel. Statements were immediately excluded from the guidelines if they were rated as essential or important by less than 80.0% of both panel members.

In Round 1, panel members were also invited to make comments on any ambiguity or wording of the statements presented, and to suggest new statements that had not yet been considered, through a feedback textbox at the end of each section of the questionnaire. The working group reviewed all of these comments. Suggestions that contained novel ideas were used to create new helping statements to be included in the subsequent Round 2 questionnaire. Statements that received comments suggesting ambiguity in the interpretation of its meaning were re-phrased to make them clearer and were also included in the Round 2 questionnaire.

The Round 3 questionnaire comprised new statements that were developed from Round 1 feedback and had been presented for the first time in Round 2, but required re-rating in a further round. Statements that still did not achieve consensus after being re-rated were rejected from inclusion in the guidelines.

Following each round of the three rounds, each panellist was sent a report containing a summary of the results from the previous round, with the report personalised to include the individual panellist's rating for each statement, as well as a table summary of the overall panel's rating for the statement. This allowed the panellists to compare their rating with the level of endorsement given by the group as a whole and to inform their future ratings for those statements that needed to be re-rated.

Guideline development

All statements endorsed as either Essential or Important by ≥90% of the panel members were written into a guideline document. One author (NI) drafted the guidelines by writing the list of endorsed statements into sections of prose based on common themes. Where possible, statements were combined and repetition deleted to reduce length. The draft was then presented to the working group, who edited the document to create a set of guidelines that were written in plain English and were easy to follow. A number of drafting iterations were completed before the group agreed upon the final document, a copy of which was sent to each panel member for review. While panellists could not suggest new content at this stage, they were able to provide feedback on the wording and layout of the document to improve clarity and reduce ambiguity.

Results
Expert panel members

We recruited 27 expert panel members (19 female, 8 male, age range 28 to 58 years) who completed the Round 1 questionnaire. Of the 27, 92.6% ($n = 25$) were retained in the study, completing the Round 2 and 3 questionnaires. Approximately one-third (37.0%, $n = 10$) of the panel heard about the study through the Onemda VicHealth Koori Health Unit email list, 11.1% ($n = 3$) through the Aboriginal Mental Health First Aid Instructor list, 7.4% ($n = 2$) through a colleague, 3.2% ($n = 1$) through the Lowitja Institute email list, and 40.7% ($n = 11$) were recruited through other pathways, which is unsurprising given that the advertisement encouraged people to distribute the flyer across their broader networks. The panel members came from a range of health and community services roles: 6 panel members were social workers, 6 were Aboriginal Mental Health Workers, 3 were nurses, 2 were GPs, 2 were academics, 2 were Aboriginal Health Workers, 2 were Aboriginal Mental Health Policy Advisors, 1 was an Aboriginal Community Support Worker, 1 was an Indigenous Public Health Officer and 2 were other types of health workers. Many members of the panel also held multiple other community roles (for example, participation in Indigenous suicide prevention evaluations), indicating a high level of community engagement.

Further socio-demographic information on the panel members is provided in Table 1. In summary, the majority of panel members identified as being Aboriginal, with one identifying as Torres Strait Islander and one identifying as both Aboriginal and Torres Strait Islander. There was a broad representation of States and Territories across Australia, with panel members from Victoria, Queensland, Western Australia, New South Wales, Northern Territory, South Australia, Australian Capital Territory and Tasmania. On average, panel members had 11.6 years (range: 1–27 years) of experience in Indigenous suicide prevention. It is important to note that while we recruited a panel of people with professional expertise in suicide prevention, all panel members reported also having had personal experience (outside of their professional role) with suicidal thoughts and behaviour in either themselves, their families, their friends, or in their broader community network. This indicates that panel members were able to draw on both professional and personal experiences when rating the statements in the questionnaires, adding an important richness to their expertise.

Ratings of the statements

An overview of the three rounds of the Delphi study is provided in Fig. 1 and a breakdown of the number of endorsed and rejected statements for each section of the Delphi questionnaire is provided in Table 2. We started with a total of 283 statements in the Round 1 questionnaire, and included an additional 18 new

Table 1 Characteristics of panel members ($n = 27$)

	% (n)
Age group (range:28–58, mean:45.0 years)	
25–40 years	22.2% (6)
41–50 years	44.4% (12)
51–60 years	33.3% (9)
Gender	
Female	70.4% (19)
Male	29.6 (8)
Indigenous identification	
Aboriginal	92.6% (25)
Torres Strait Islander	3.7% (1)
Both Aboriginal and Torres Strait Islander	3.7% (1)
Years of experience in suicide prevention (mean = 11.6)	
1–4 years	7.4% (2)
5–9 years	37.0% (10)
10+ years	55.6% (15)
State where currently working	
Victoria	25.9% (7)
Queensland	14.8% (4)
Western Australia	11.1% (3)
New South Wales	11.1% (3)
Northern Territory	7.4% (2)
South Australia	7.4% (2)
Australian Capital Territory	7.4% (2)
Tasmania	3.7% (1)
Australia wide	11.1% (3)
Personal (i.e. not professional) experience with suicidal thoughts or behaviour ($n = 25$)	
In myself	48.0% (12)
In my family	76.0% (12)
In my friends	80.0% (20)
In my broader community network	84.0% (21)
No personal experience	0.0% (0)
I'd rather not say	0.0% (0)

statements based on feedback from the panel, resulting in a total of 301 different statements being rated by the panel across the three rounds. Of these 301 statements, 172 (57%) were endorsed as being either *Important* or *Essential* for the guidelines by ≥90% of panellists; 136 statements were endorsed in Round 1, 35 in Round 2 and 1 in Round 3. A total of 129 (43%) statements were not endorsed for the guidelines; 69 statements were rejected in Round 1, 55 in Round 2 and 5 in Round 3 (see Additional file 1 for a list of all the statements and their respective levels of endorsement).

Comparison with the original aboriginal mental health first aid guidelines for suicidal thoughts and behaviour

The re-development of the guidelines has resulted in more comprehensive guidance than the earlier version; for the development of the original version, panellists had rated 166 helping statements and had endorsed 52 statements [19]. The re-developed guidelines contain some familiar features while also incorporating some important new guidance for first aiders.

Culturally appropriate mental health first aid

The re-developed guidelines reaffirmed some important cultural elements of the original guidelines that are important for people to know when assisting an Aboriginal or Torres Strait Islander person who is having suicidal thoughts. The importance of cultural context and cultural competence was again prominent in the re-developed guidelines, with the endorsement of statements such as the first aider needs *"to be aware that Aboriginal people understand mental health within a wider context of health and well-being, which includes concepts of social and emotional functioning"* and the first aider needs *"to learn about the behaviours that are considered warning signs for suicide in the person's community, and in doing so take into consideration the spiritual and/or cultural context of the person's behaviour"*. Cultural safety was also again prominent, for example, with the need for first aiders to be aware of the *"cultural concept of 'shame' within the person's community, and that shame may be triggered by discussing behaviours that may be considered unusual or embarrassing"*; that *"the term 'help' may carry negative connotations for some Aboriginal people"*; and that the person has the *"right to make decisions about seeking culturally-based care"*. However, the idea of culturally appropriate first aid was qualified by endorsement of the following statements: *"it is more important to make the person feel comfortable, respected and cared for, than to do all the 'right things' and follow all the 'rules' when communicating with an Aboriginal person"* and *"it is more important to genuinely want to help than to be of the same age, gender or cultural background"*. The importance of family and community was also prominent, again with a qualification: *"family and friends are a very big part of Aboriginal culture and you should expect involvement by the family and friends in caring for the person. However, you should not assume that all Aboriginal people will want their family involved and respect that the person has the right to choose who they want involved"*. Several statements also noted the need for first aiders to consider that there may be a broad range of potential community supports that may be preferred as sources of support by Aboriginal and Torres Strait Islander people, for example, respected Elders, family and friends, Aboriginal health

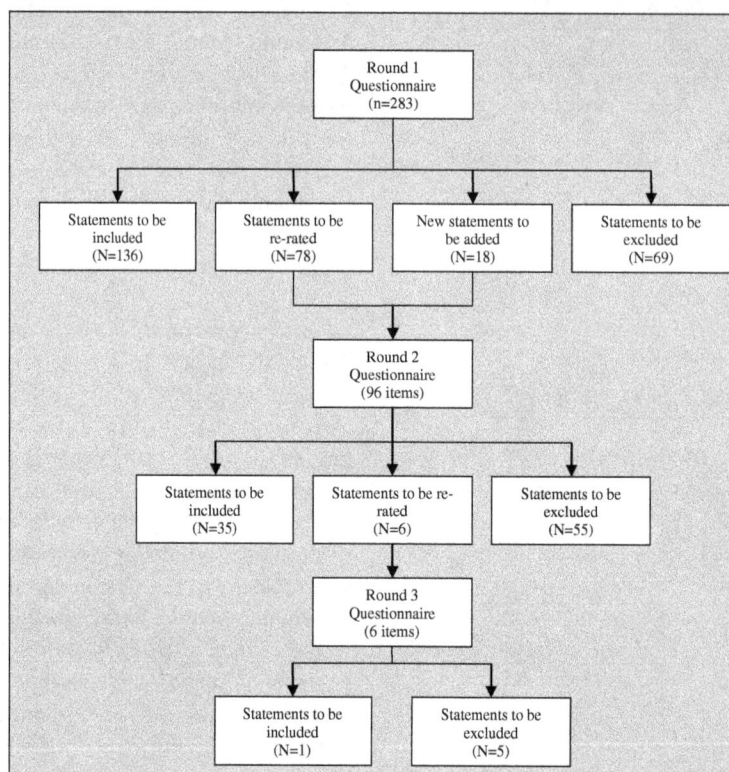

Fig. 1 Overview of the three rounds of the Delphi method

workers, community liaison officers, youth workers, sports coaches and teachers.

Extended guidance in basic communication skills around talking with a suicidal person

An important addition to the re-developed guidelines is the inclusion of extended guidance around the use of basic communication skills in relation to talking with a suicidal person and asking about thoughts of suicide. The re-developed guidelines give more detailed advice around avoiding stigmatising language when asking the

suicidal person about suicidal thoughts and specifically addresses an important myth that can stop people from asking about suicidal thoughts: *"If a person is not suicidal, asking them about suicide cannot put the idea in their head. If a person is suicidal, asking them about suicidal thoughts will not increase the risk that they will act on these thoughts, rather, it will allow them the chance to talk about their problems and will show them that somebody cares".*

Furthermore, while both the original and the re-develop guidelines discuss sourcing professional help,

Table 2 Sections in the Delphi questionnaire, and the number of statements endorsed and rejected

Section	Topic	Number of statements endorsed	Number of statements rejected	Total
1	What the first aider should know	27	10	37
2	Identification of suicide risk	29	20	49
3	Assessing seriousness of risk	19	11	30
4	Initial assistance	20	24	44
5	Talking with the suicidal person	39	27	66
6	Safety plan	13	8	21
7	Ensuring safety	1	5	6
8	Passing time during the crisis	1	4	5
9	Confidentiality	8	1	9
10	Adolescent specific	15	19	34
	TOTAL	172	129	301

the re-developed guidelines provides additional guidance in basic counselling skills that the first aider can themselves implement when talking with the suicidal person, for example: "*do something to help comfort the person, such as sitting with them, making them a cup of tea, offering them time, friendship and encouragement*"; "*allow the suicidal person to do most of the talking*"; and, "*encourage the person to discuss their reasons for dying and their reasons for living, validate that they are considering both options and emphasise that living is an option for them*". The re-developed guidelines also emphasise new basic communication tips related to 'listening' and 'what not to do', for example: "*show that you are listening by summarising what the person is saying*"; "*be conscious of your body language, ensuring that it doesn't communicate a lack of interest or negative attitude*"; "*don't use guilt or threats to prevent suicide, e.g. do not tell the person they will go to hell or ruin other people's lives if they die by suicide*"; and, "*don't give glib reassurance such as 'don't worry', 'cheer up', 'you have everything going for you' or 'everything will be alright'*".

Additional considerations when assisting an adolescent who is suicidal

The original guidelines offered no specific guidance for supporting Aboriginal and Torres Strait Islander adolescents. Our recent panel reviewed and endorsed a range of statements that allow the re-developed guidelines to provide additional guidance for when the first aider is supporting an adolescent who is feeling suicidal. These statements appear to be underscored by a major concern about the potential for impulsiveness in youth suicides and the need to closely monitor a suicidal adolescent, while balancing this against the need to involve them in making decisions about the next steps. For example: "*do not leave an adolescent who is feeling suicidal on their own*"; "*make sure someone stays close by them (in the same room, in visual contact) and engage whatever outside resources are available, e.g. family, friend, emergency mental health care or, if necessary, the police*"; "*if the adolescent is reluctant to seek help, you should talk to a helpline or health professional for advice and make sure that someone who is close to the adolescent is aware of the situation*"; and, "*treat the suicidal adolescent with respect and involve them in decisions about who else knows about the suicidal crisis*".

Other areas of difference

Aside from the abovementioned themes, there were a number of other areas where new guidance has emerged in the re-developed guidelines. These include: detail on the use of safety plans; a discussion around times when the first aider may need to breach the confidentiality of the suicidal person; and, a small section on the need for first aiders to look after themselves.

Comparison with the mainstream (i.E. non-indigenous specific) mental health first aid guidelines for suicidal thoughts and behaviour

There were 217 statements that appeared in both the first round of the current Delphi study and a 2014 Delphi study designed to develop the mainstream (i.e. not specific to Aboriginal and Torres Strait Islander people) mental health first guidelines for suicidal thoughts and behaviour. The 2014 Delphi study had two panels, a consumer panel and a professional panel, whereas the current study only had a professional panel (all of whom also had personal exposure to suicide). The ratings given by our panel of Aboriginal and Torres Strait Islander suicide prevention experts were, on average, statistically significantly higher than those ratings given by the mainstream Delphi panel in 2014. On average, 85.4% of our panel rated each statement as either important or essential for the AMHFA suicide guidelines, compared to an average of 78.1% (t (432) = 4.7, $p < 0.001$) of professionals and 81.1% (t (432) = 3.2, $p = 0.017$) of consumers in the 2014 mainstream Delphi study.

Among those statements rated in both studies, the endorsement ratings given by our Aboriginal and Torres Strait Islander suicide expert panel were strongly correlated across items with both the consumer panel r (221) = 0.79, $p < 0.05$ and the professional panel r (221) = 0.77, $p < 0.05$ from the 2014 mainstream Delphi study. In terms of comparing whether statements were endorsed or not between the two Delphi studies for each of the 223 statements, there was a strong level of inter-rater agreement with a kappa co-efficient of 0.74. In practical terms, the two Delphi studies came to the same conclusion about endorsing or not-endorsing an item on 87.6% of occasions; 92.1% of statements endorsed in the 2014 mainstream Delphi were also endorsed in the current study and 81.3% of statements rejected in the 2014 mainstream Delphi study were also rejected in the current study. The strongly correlated ratings across the two Delphi studies suggest a high degree of overlap in terms of suicide prevention knowledge.

Nevertheless, there were some differences in the ratings among those statements rated in both studies. There were 10 statements endorsed in the 2014 mainstream Delphi that were rejected in the current study and 17 statements that were rejected in the 2014 mainstream Delphi that were endorsed in the current study. Of these 27 statements, there were 16 statements for which our Aboriginal and Torres Strait Islander expert panel had given a markedly different (i.e. ±10%) rating than that given by either the professional or consumer panels in the 2014 mainstream study; 9 statements where there was a marked difference with both the professional and consumer panels, 4 statements where there was a marked difference with the professional panel only, and 3 statements where there was a marked difference with the consumer panel only.

There appeared to be some themes that emerged where there were marked differences with the professional and consumer panels in the 2014 mainstream Delphi study. Firstly, our Aboriginal and Torres Strait Islander panel endorsed items that may reflect the sense of emergency around the issue of suicide in some Aboriginal and Torres Strait Islander communities. For example, our Aboriginal and Torres Strait Islander panel endorsed the following items that were not endorsed in the 2014 mainstream Delphi study: 'the first aider should be aware of how commonly suicide occurs'; 'the first aider should not let the person convince them that it is not serious or that they can handle it on their own'; and, 'if the suicidal person won't make a safety plan, it is not safe to leave them alone for any period of time'. Secondly, our Aboriginal and Torres Strait Islander panel endorsed statements that may reflect some important cultural communications issues that need to be appreciated by the first aider, with particular emphasis on using a narrative or 'yarning' approach so as to avoid asking too many direct questions and taking charge of the situation at the expense of respecting the suicidal person. For example, our Aboriginal and Torres Strait Islander panel endorsed the following items that were not endorsed in the 2014 mainstream Delphi study: 'the first aider should begin the conversation by asking the person about how they are feeling'; 'the first aider should keep in mind that asking too many questions can provoke anxiety in the suicidal person'; and, 'the first aider should respect the suicidal person and not try to take charge of the situation'.

Additionally, there were 33 statements (11.0% of the 301 statements) that were presented to our Aboriginal and Torres Strait Islander expert panel that had not been presented to the earlier 2014 mainstream Delphi panel. These were statements specifically related to cultural competence and cultural safety and new statements that had been derived from the Aboriginal and Torres Strait Islander panel throughout the Delphi study, as well as statements that were similar but had been significantly re-worded to refer to culturally appropriate examples of community supports (for example, respected Elders, Aboriginal Health Workers and community liaison officers) when encouraging the suicidal person to choose someone they would like and would trust to support them. There were another 45 statements (14.6% of the 301 statements) that had been either derived from panellists' suggestions in the 2014 mainstream Delphi study (and thus had not been rated in the first round of

that study) or had been re-worded to the extent that they no longer had exactly the same meaning.

Discussion

The aim of this study was to re-develop the Aboriginal mental health first aid guidelines for members of the public in providing assistance to an Aboriginal or Torres Strait Islander person experiencing suicidal thoughts or displaying suicidal behaviour. This was achieved by engaging Aboriginal and Torres Strait Islander people who have expertise in the field of Indigenous suicide prevention. Despite being from diverse backgrounds and geographical locations across Australia, the expert panel was able to reach a high level of consensus on a range of mental health first aid techniques, and 172 statements endorsed by ≥90% of panellists were included in the re-developed guidelines.

The re-development of the guidelines has resulted in more comprehensive guidance than the earlier version; our panellists rated 301 statements and endorsed 172, while the previous panel rated 166 helping statements and had endorsed 52 statements [19]. The increase in the number of statements rated by panellists and included in the guidelines is a reflection of the growth of suicide prevention expertise and advice available in the published literature, grey literature, on websites, and other sources. This highlights the importance of conducting revisions of guideline documents, as the advice provided by the literature and expert opinion can change across the span of a few years.

The re-developed guidelines contain some familiar features, while also incorporating some important new guidance for first aiders. They reaffirmed some important cultural elements, under the broad themes of cultural context, cultural competence and cultural safety, as well as reaffirming the importance of family and community when supporting an Aboriginal and Torres Strait Islander person who is experiencing suicidal thoughts. Meanwhile, there were a number of areas where new guidance has emerged in the re-developed guidelines. An important new contribution has been the inclusion of a section on additional considerations when assisting an adolescent who is suicidal. The inclusion of adolescent-specific statements provides recognition that suicidal adolescents may need tailored support, and the statements endorsed by our panel appeared to be underscored by a major concern about the potential impulsiveness of youth suicide [24]. This section carries additional weight given the major concerns around the high rates of suicide among Aboriginal and Torres Strait Islander youth [25], and future re-developments of these guidelines should place greater emphasis on this section as the literature grows in terms of specific advice around Indigenous youth suicide.

The re-developed guidelines also offer extended guidance in basic communication skills around talking with a suicidal person, including communication tips related to 'listening' and 'what not to do'. This guidance is broadly underpinned by the use of a narrative or 'yarning approach' that allows the person to do most of the talking and avoids asking too many questions. As Adams, Drew & Walker [26] highlight, when talking about mental health and wellbeing with an Aboriginal or Torres Strait Islander person it is often best to use a narrative or 'yarning' approach. Asking too many direct questions or trying to take charge of their situation may make the individual feel 'shame', and can result in responses that provide inaccurate information and a sense of disempowerment [26, 27]. Additionally, new guidance has emerged in a section on the use of safety plans, a discussion around times when the first aider may need to breach the confidentiality of the suicidal person, and a small section on the need for first aiders to look after themselves. All of this additional guidance may be especially useful for situations where the first aider is required to be engaged as the primary support for longer periods of time. This is particularly relevant in remote areas where access to immediate 'professional' help is not always available or culturally appropriate for Aboriginal and Torres Strait Islander people [28], and situations where the suicidal person is reluctant to talk with others about their suicidal feelings. The extended emphasis on communication tips gives first aiders a greater suite of skills to use when talking to a suicidal person, without detracting from the need to work with the person to identify sources of appropriate help from relevant professionals, family or community leaders.

We observed a high degree of agreement in terms of suicide prevention knowledge between our panel of professional Aboriginal and Torres Strait Islander experts and the non-Indigenous consumer and professional panels who helped construct the mainstream MHFA suicide guidelines [23], in relation to the sub-set of 217 statements that were presented to both the current and former panels. The high proportion of these statements that were endorsed by both panels indicates a moderate degree of transferability of action statements between the mainstream guidelines and the Aboriginal mental health first aid suicide guidelines. We also observed that our panel of professional Aboriginal and Torres Strait Islander experts gave, on average, higher ratings of endorsement for the items compared to the non-Indigenous consumer and professional panels who helped construct the mainstream MHFA suicide guidelines. Future research with Delphi panels comprising Aboriginal and Torres Strait Islander professionals could examine if this is a consistent pattern.

Important considerations when using the guidelines to support the development of indigenous suicide gatekeeper training programs

The guidelines developed through this study are unique in having been developed using a Delphi methodology to harness the expertise of Indigenous suicide prevention experts from across Australia. The specific purpose of the guidelines is to inform the actions undertaken by mental health first aiders, and the guidelines will be used by MHFAA to revise the curriculum of the AMHFA course to a third edition and to develop a new Indigenous suicide prevention gatekeeper training course to be rolled out by their AMHFA Instructors.

Nonetheless, the guidelines may be useful to others working in Indigenous suicide prevention, particularly those developing or implementing other Indigenous suicide gatekeeper training programs. For example, community members and frontline workers may be hesitant to ask someone directly if they are thinking of suicide for fear that it may put the idea in their head [29]. These guidelines can offer a level of confidence that a panel of Indigenous suicide prevention experts have agreed that it is okay to ask an Aboriginal or Torres Strait Islander person directly if they are having thoughts of suicide. The guidelines make many other important and useful recommendations, for example: taking people seriously when they tell you they are thinking of suicide; providing space to talk about both the person's reasons for living and their reasons for dying; and not taking charge of the situation for the person but rather encouraging them to make decisions regarding how and by whom they would like to be supported during a crisis, including tapping into important community-based resources like family, friends, Aboriginal health workers, respected Elders and mental health services.

However, it is important to consider some of the following issues before using these guidelines to inform Indigenous suicide gatekeeper training programs. Firstly, the guidelines should not be used in isolation. There are other Aboriginal Mental Health First Aid Guidelines that could also be referred to, most notably the guidelines on 'Cultural Considerations and Communication Techniques' and 'Communicating with an Aboriginal or Torres Strait Islander Adolescent' [19, 20]. Those implementing the recommendations as first aiders will also need other local knowledge relevant to their respective communities. Aboriginal and Torres Strait Islander communities are not homogenous and, as such, reading these generalised guidelines in isolation is unlikely to be sufficient.

Secondly, while the guidelines do offer recommendations about how an Indigenous community member or non-Indigenous frontline health worker may support someone having suicidal thoughts, and what they may need to know to be able to do this, they don't specify how Indigenous suicide gatekeeper training programs should be developed, packaged and integrated within broader community-based programs. In developing training programs based on these guidelines, it is important to consider the findings of two recent reviews of Indigenous suicide prevention programs that both strongly indicated how important it is that programs have a commitment to Indigenous leadership, community consultation, and the use of culturally appropriate frameworks for talking holistically about mental health and suicide (for example, the concept of social and emotional wellbeing) [12, 30]. The Aboriginal and Torres Strait Islander Suicide Prevention Evaluation Project led by the University of Western Australia found that Indigenous suicide prevention programs that were culturally appropriate and had a strong basis in community engagement and ownership from the outset were more likely to be effective [30]. A review of the literature on Aboriginal suicide prevention programs conducted by the Black Dog Institute in Sydney found that while there was a dearth of rigorous program evaluations, the results that were available indicated the importance of employing a 'whole of community' approach and focusing on connectedness, belongingness and cultural heritage [12]. They found that program longevity appeared to be linked to community ownership, with those programs still in operation after several years being those that started small, were wholly owned and run by the communities in which they were originated, and were connected to a broader suite of community developments. Additionally, they recognised that those Indigenous suicide programs that were wholly or partly Indigenous owned tended to employ creative methods of delivery, including art classes, dancing events, theatrical showcases, cultural camps and community activities, which may all be highly effective ways for some Indigenous communities to engage with the recommendations in these guidelines.

Thirdly, one common strategy of suicide gatekeeper-training programs, including those that would evolve from these guidelines, is to support people 'at risk' to link with mental health services. We must acknowledge that referring Aboriginal or Torres Strait Islander people to mental health services is neither unproblematic nor apolitical. There are important barriers that prevent formal mental health services from being an ideal source of care for Indigenous people. These have been documented in Australia, Canada the United States and elsewhere, for example: 1) the stigma and shame Indigenous people may experience when accessing formal mental health services; 2) experiences of discrimination and racism within the broader health system, which can in turn worsen psychological distress; 3) the provision of individualised care, rather than community- or family-based interventions, that diminishes the value that many Indigenous people place on interconnectedness; 4) a heavy reliance on individualised treatment options (predominantly pharmacological and psychological) that can be seen to de-contextualise experiences of suicidality in connection to structural issues like intergenerational trauma, racism, discrimination and disempowerment; 5) concerns that formal mental health services may not be provided in a way that is compatible with the holistic and strengths-based nature of the social and emotional wellbeing framing of Indigenous mental health; and 6) a lack of engagement with cultural and/or spiritual approaches to nurturing social and emotional wellbeing (for example, community gatherings, intergenerational transmission of knowledge and stories, dancing, healing ceremonies, and nature-based activities), which are largely distanced as being outside the bounds of evidence-based mental health care [12, 31–40]. Formal mental health services are a critical resource for Aboriginal and Torres Strait Islander people experiencing suicidal thoughts, however, the challenges are many for them to become culturally safe and appropriate sources of care. Indigenous suicide gatekeeper programs can acknowledge these shortcomings and work with communities to discuss and establish acceptable ways of accessing support and care from different sources, while advocating with mental health services around the need to develop holistic, flexible and culturally appropriate approaches.

Limitations and future research

These guidelines have utilised the expertise of Indigenous suicide experts to offer recommendations as to how to support an Aboriginal or Torres Strait Islander who is experiencing suicidal thoughts or displaying suicidal behaviour. An important next step will be to conduct a trial to evaluate the outcomes of training programs that are based on these guidelines, in terms of their effect on participant knowledge, skills, intentions to assist and confidence in identifying and assisting individuals at risk of suicide. It will also be important to examine longer-term outcome measures, for example, assessing actual experiences of providing support against the guidelines and monitoring patterns of referrals to community supports and health services. Additionally, it is important to assess the perceived cultural appropriateness of these training programs for the participants.

Our panel was formed entirely of Aboriginal and Torres Strait Islander people with professional experience in Indigenous suicide prevention. Future research could consider also having a panel of people who identify as consumers of suicide prevention services or carers of people who are or have been suicidal, as such people would bring a different type of equally important expertise that would add great value to the re-development of these guidelines. However, given the high rate of suicide deaths in Aboriginal and Torres Strait Islander communities, it is not surprising that all of our professional panel members had personal exposure to suicidal thoughts and behaviour in either themselves, their families, their friends, or in their broader community network.

It must be kept in mind that the helping actions endorsed in the guidelines are based on expert opinion; these are the recommendations of experts in the absence of evidence from experimental studies about how best to provide mental health first aid to an Aboriginal or Torres Strait Islander person experiencing suicidal thoughts. Additionally, the use of these guidelines is recommended for use by mental health first aiders only. While the actions endorsed in these guidelines may be useful in different aspects of the Indigenous suicide prevention continuum, from preventing the onset of suicidal ideation itself to supporting the suicidal person in a professional setting, these are specific to the recommended support that can be provided by first aiders. These guidelines take into consideration the limitations in the first aiders' support role, and guide the first aider on how to act within these. Nonetheless, these guidelines may be useful to those working on Indigenous suicide prevention outside the scope of the mental health first aid paradigm. Indeed, qualitative research should be undertaken to examine the perceived utility of these guidelines for those developing or implementing Indigenous suicide prevention programs, including suicide gatekeeper training courses, across Australia.

The majority of the suicide prevention literature is based on studies and reports that are not specific to Aboriginal and Torres Strait Islander peoples, or other Indigenous communities in other countries. Thus, the majority of the statements presented to our Aboriginal and Torres Strait Islander panel, for endorsement or otherwise, were generated from the mainstream suicide prevention literature, which does not necessarily embody the holistic and Indigenous-preferred concept of social and emotional well-being. This put a great onus on our expert panel to either suggest new culturally appropriate helping statements or to suggest re-wording of existing actions so that they were more culturally appropriate. This was a difficult task for panel members given they were already faced with reviewing a large number of helping statements.

Finally, only two panel members identified as Torres Strait Islander, which may affect the generalisability of the findings for Torres Strait Islander peoples.

Conclusions

Through the Delphi process, the Aboriginal mental health first aid guidelines for supporting an Aboriginal or Torres Strait Islander person experiencing suicidal thoughts or displaying suicidal behaviour have been updated to ensure they are current and include the most recent and appropriate helping actions. This re-development has added depth to the previous version of the guidelines. These guidelines will now be made freely available for download on the MHFAA website, and will also be used to form the basis of an AMHFA Indigenous suicide prevention gatekeeper training course aimed at educating members of the public in providing first aid to an Aboriginal or Torres Strait Islander person who is experiencing suicidal thoughts.

Abbreviations
AMHFA: Aboriginal Mental Health First Aid; MHFAA: Mental Health First Aid Australia

Acknowledgements
The authors gratefully acknowledge the time and effort of the panel members, without whom this study would not have been possible. We would also like to acknowledge the support for the study provided by Professor Margaret Kelaher at The University of Melbourne and Ms. Betty Kitchener, CEO of Mental Health First Aid Australia. Funding was provided by the National Health and Medical Research Council in Australia.

Authors' contributions
AFJ developed the study methodology. GA implemented the study, including recruiting panel members, administering the Delphi questionnaires, analyzing the data and coordinating the working group. NI supported the data analysis and coordinated the drafting of the final guidelines document. All authors contributed to the development of the Delphi questionnaires and participated in the working group that reviewed the responses of the expert panel. GA and NI wrote the first draft of this manuscript with all authors suggesting improvements before approving the final manuscript. Three authors (NI, KA, KD) identify as Aboriginal or Torres Strait Islanders and provided critical cultural direction at working group meetings and throughout the development of this paper. All authors read and approved the final manuscript.

Consent for publication
This manuscript does not contain data relating to any particular individual participants. The plain language statement confirmed to participants that only aggregate data would be presented in publications.

Competing interests
The authors declare that they have no competing interests.

Author details
[1]Nossal Institute for Global Health, Melbourne School of Population and Global Health, University of Melbourne, 333 Exhibition St, Melbourne, VIC 3000, Australia. [2]Centre for Mental Health, Melbourne School of Population and Global Health, The University of Melbourne, 207 Bouverie St, Carlton, VIC 3010, Australia. [3]Mental Health First Aid Australia, Level 6, 369 Royal Parade, Parkville, VIC 3053, Australia. [4]Indigenous Health Equity Unit, Melbourne School of Population and Global Health, University of Melbourne, 207 Bouverie St, Carlton, VIC 3010, Australia.

References
1. Causes of Death, Australia, 2014 [http://www.abs.gov.au/AUSSTATS/abs@.nsf/DetailsPage/3303.02014?OpenDocument].
2. McLoughlin AB, Gould MS, Malone KM. Global trends in teenage suicide: 2003-2014. QJM. 2015;108(10):765–80.

3.   Hunter E, Harvey D. Indigenous suicide in Australia, New Zealand, Canada, and the United States. Emerg Med (Fremantle). 2002;14(1):14–23.
4.   Elias B, Mignone J, Hall M, Hong SP, Hart L, Sareen J. Trauma and suicide behaviour histories among a Canadian indigenous population: an empirical exploration of the potential role of Canada's residential school system. Soc Sci Med. 2012;74(10):1560–9.
5.   Coupe NM. Maori suicide prevention in New Zealand. Pac Health Dialog. 2000;7(1):25–8.
6.   Hawton K, van Heeringen K. Suicide. Lancet. 2009;373(9672):1372–81.
7.   Gracey M, King M. Indigenous health part 1: determinants and disease patterns. Lancet. 2009;374(9683):65–75.
8.   King M, Smith A, Gracey M. Indigenous health part 2: the underlying causes of the health gap. Lancet. 2009;374(9683):76–85.
9.   Elliott-Farrelly T. Australian aboriginal suicide: the need for an aboriginal suicidology? Advances in Mental Health. 2004;3(3):1–8.
10. Cwik M, Barlow A, Tingey L, Goklish N, Larzelere-Hinton F, Craig M, Walkup JT. Exploring risk and protective factors with a community sample of American Indian adolescents who attempted suicide. Arch Suicide Res. 2015;19(2):172–89.
11. Barlow A, Tingey L, Cwik M, Goklish N, Larzelere-Hinton F, Lee A, Suttle R, Mullany B, Walkup JT. Understanding the relationship between substance use and self-injury in American Indian youth. Am J Drug Alcohol Abuse. 2012;38(5):403–8.
12. Ridani R, Shand FL, Christensen H, McKay K, Tighe J, Burns J, Hunter E. Suicide prevention in Australian aboriginal communities: a review of past and present programs. Suicide Life Threat Behav. 2015;45(1):111–40.
13. Clifford AC, Doran CM, Tsey K. A systematic review of suicide prevention interventions targeting indigenous peoples in Australia, United States, Canada and New Zealand. BMC Public Health. 2013;13:463.
14. Mann JJ, Apter A, Bertolote J, Beautrais A, Currier D, Haas A, Hegerl U, Lonnqvist J, Malone K, Marusic A, et al. Suicide prevention strategies: a systematic review. JAMA. 2005;294(16):2064–74.
15. Isaac M, Elias B, Katz LY, Belik SL, Deane FP, Enns MW, Sareen J, Swampy Cree Suicide Prevention T. Gatekeeper training as a preventative intervention for suicide: a systematic review. Can J Psychiatr. 2009;54(4):260–8.
16. Kitchener BA, Jorm AF, Kelly CM. Mental Health First Aid International Manual. Melbourne: Mental Health First Aid International; 2015.
17. Jorm AF, Korten AE, Jacomb PA, Christensen H, Rodgers B, Pollitt P. "Mental health literacy": a survey of the public's ability to recognise mental disorders and their beliefs about the effectiveness of treatment. Med J Aust. 1997; 166(4):182–6.
18. Kanowski LG, Jorm AF, Hart LM. A mental health first aid training program for Australian aboriginal and Torres Strait islander peoples: description and initial evaluation. Int J Ment Health Syst. 2009;3(1):10.
19. Hart LM, Jorm AF, Kanowski LG, Kelly CM, Langlands RL. Mental health first aid for indigenous Australians: using Delphi consensus studies to develop guidelines for culturally appropriate responses to mental health problems. BMC Psychiatry. 2009;9:47.
20. Chalmers KJ, Bond KS, Jorm AF, Kelly CM, Kitchener BA, Williams-Tchen A. Providing culturally appropriate mental health first aid to an aboriginal or Torres Strait islander adolescent: development of expert consensus guidelines. Int J Ment Health Syst. 2014;8(1):6.
21. Jorm AF. Using the Delphi expert consensus method in mental health research. Aust N Z J Psychiatry. 2015;49(10):887–97.
22. Armstrong G, Ironfield N, Kelly CM, Dart K, Arabena K, Bond K, Jorm AF. Re-development of mental health first aid guidelines for supporting aboriginal and Torres Strait islanders who are engaging in non-suicidal self-injury. BMC Psychiatry. 2017;17(1):300.
23. Ross AM, Kelly CM, Jorm AF. Re-development of mental health first aid guidelines for suicidal ideation and behaviour: a Delphi study. BMC Psychiatry. 2014;14:241.
24. Bridge JA, Goldstein TR, Brent DA. Adolescent suicide and suicidal behavior. J Child Psychol Psychiatry. 2006;47(3–4):372–94.
25. Armstrong G, Pirkis J, Arabena K, Currier D, Spittal MJ, Jorm AF. Suicidal behaviour in indigenous compared to non- indigenous males in urban and regional Australia: prevalence data suggest disparities increase across age groups. Aust N Z J Psychiatry. 2017;51(12):1240–8. Published online first April 2017
26. Adams Y, Drew N, Walker R. Principles of practice in mental health assessment with Aboriginal Australians. In: Dudgeon P, Milroy H, Barton WR, editors. Working together: Aboriginal and Torres Strait Islander mental health and wellbeing principles and practice edn. A.C.T: Commonwealth of Australia; 2014. p. 271–87.
27. Westerman TG. Engagement of Indigenous clients in mental health services: what role do cultural differences play? Australian e-Journal for the Advancement of Mental Health (AeJAMH). 2004;3(3):1–8.
28. Reeve C, Humphreys J, Wakerman J, Carroll V, Carter M, O'Brien T, Erlank C, Mansour R, Smith B. Community participation in health service reform: the development of an innovative remote aboriginal primary health-care service. Aust J Prim Health. 2015;21(4):409–16.
29. World Health Organization. Preventing suicide: A global imperative. Geneva: World Health Organization; 2014.
30. Aboriginal and Torres Strait Islander Suicide Prevention Evaluation Project. Solutions that work: What the evidence and our people tell us. Western Australia: University of Western Australia; 2016.
31. Farrelly T. The aboriginal suicide and self-harm help-seeking quandary. Aboriginal & Islander Health Worker Journal. 2008;32(1):11–5.
32. Kelaher MA, Ferdinand AS, Paradies Y. Experiencing racism in health care: the mental health impacts for Victorian aboriginal communities. Med J Aust. 2014;201(1):44–7.
33. Wexler LM, Gone JP. Culturally responsive suicide prevention in indigenous communities: unexamined assumptions and new possibilities. Am J Public Health. 2012;102(5):800–6.
34. Wexler L, White J, Trainor B. Why an alternative to suicide prevention gatekeeper training is needed for rural indigenous communities: presenting an empowering community storytelling approach. Critical Public Health. 2016;25(2):205–17.
35. Battiste K. Indigenous Knowledge and Pedagogy in First Nations Education. In: A literature review with recommendations. Ottawa: Prepared for the National Working Group on Education and the Minister of Indian Affairs; 2002. Retrieved from http://www.afn.ca/uploads/files/education/24._2002_oct_marie_battiste_indigenousknowledgeandpedagogy_lit_review_for_min_working_group.pdf.
36. Isaacs AN, Pyett P, Oakley-Browne MA, Gruis H, Waples-Crowe P. Barriers and facilitators to the utilization of adult mental health services by Australia's indigenous people: seeking a way forward. Int J Ment Health Nurs. 2010;19(2):75–82.
37. Fielke K, Cord-Udy N, Buckskin J, Lattanzio A. The development of an 'Indigenous team' in a mainstream mental health service in South Australia. Australas Psychiatry. 2009;17(Suppl 1):S75–8.
38. Hepworth J, Askew D, Foley W, Duthie D, Shuter P, Combo M, Clements LA. How an urban aboriginal and Torres Strait islander primary health care service improved access to mental health care. Int J Equity Health. 2015;14:51.
39. Kirmayer LJ. Cultural competence and evidence-based practice in mental health: epistemic communities and the politics of pluralism. Soc Sci Med. 2012;75(2):249–56.
40. McKenna B, Fernbacher S, Furness T, Hannon M. "cultural brokerage" and beyond: piloting the role of an urban aboriginal mental health liaison officer. BMC Public Health. 2015;15:881.

20

Using photo-elicitation to understand reasons for repeated self-harm

Amanda J. Edmondson[1*], Cathy Brennan[2] and Allan O. House[2]

Abstract

Background: Reasons for self-harm are not well understood. One of the reasons for this is that first-hand accounts are usually elicited using traditional interview and questionnaire methods. This study aims to explore the acceptability of using an approach (photo-elicitation) that does not rely on solely verbal or written techniques, and to make a preliminary assessment of whether people can usefully employ images to support a discussion about the reasons why they self-harm.

Method: Interviews with eight participants using photo elicitation, a method in which photographs produced by the participant are used as a stimulus and guide within the interview.

Results: Participants responded positively to using images to support a discussion about their self-harm and readily incorporated images in the interview. Four main themes were identified representing negative and positive or adaptive purposes of self-harm: self-harm as a response to distress, self-harm to achieve mastery, self-harm as protective and self-harm as a language or form of communication.

Conclusions: Employing this novel approach was useful in broadening our understanding of self-harm.

Keywords: Self-harm, Self-injury, Photo elicitation, Visual methods, Motive, Reason, Function, Qualitative research, Experience

Background

Self-harm is a major public health concern which incurs large costs to healthcare systems [1]. One of its most intractable features is the high prevalence of repeated self-harm, especially in younger people - 15-25% present to the same hospital following a repeat episode within a year [2]. There is also an increased risk of eventual suicide for people who repeatedly self-harm [3].

Most explanations for repeated self-harm focus on deficits such as disordered affect regulation or interpersonal relationship problems (for reviews see Suyemoto [4] Klonsky [5], Edmondson et al. [6]). Current therapeutic approaches typically treat self-harm as a symptom of such underlying pathology and have faced criticism from service users as tending to primarily problematize

rather than understand [7]. Focussing on solutions to the problem, mainly through development of interventions with problem solving elements, is a research priority [8]. Yet the evidence so far that such interventions are effective in reducing repetition has not been overwhelming. [9–11]. For example, a Cochrane review of interventions for self-harm in children and adolescents concluded that there is a lack of evidence of effective interventions. Of the relatively few trials of interventions ($n = 11$), most were of low quality [12]. Similar findings were also reported in a Cochrane review of psychosocial interventions for self-harm in adults [13]. Although the number of trials of interventions was greater ($n = 55$) the evidence was reported as "inconclusive" due to the moderate to low quality of the trials, and of those interventions that showed some effectiveness in reducing repetition of self-harm (e.g. cognitive behavioural - based psychotherapy and dialectical behaviour therapy), further trials were needed. It is conceivable therefore that to develop effective

* Correspondence: A.Edmondson@hud.ac.uk
[1]Centre for Applied Research in Health, School of Human and Health Sciences, University of Huddersfield, Queensgate, Huddersfield HD1 3DH, UK
Full list of author information is available at the end of the article

interventions which are likely to meet the needs of people who self-harm, a better understanding of why individuals repeatedly self-harm is still required.

A challenge for research in this area is the difficulty experienced by people in verbalising reasons for their self-harm [14–18]. For example, when asked why they have self-harmed people often report feeling unable to put it into words [17]. The act itself has been described as their 'primary language' [19].

Despite suggestions that affect can be indescribable and sometimes unknown to the person experiencing it [20], and evidence which shows an association between the trait Alexythymia 'lacking words for emotion' and self-harm [21], there is still an assumption that we can articulate our distress effectively [14]. This may explain why first person (verbal) accounts of self-harm often focus on precipitating events ("I had an argument") rather than a more nuanced exploration of its function in the context of these events [22, 23], consequently restricting our understanding.

It has been suggested therefore that future research in self-harm may benefit from an approach that does not rely on purely verbal or written accounts [17]. The value of adopting a visual approach with people who find it difficult to express themselves verbally has been well documented [24–29]. Using participant generated photographs during an interview for example is said to promote expression and communication [30–32]. The visual information evokes a deeper level of consciousness which elicits more of an emotional response than verbal questioning alone, and highlight issues of significance [33]. The benefits of adopting a visual approach when researching sensitive subject areas are also well documented [29, 31–33]. For example, photographs are helpful in introducing difficult subject matter [34]. The photograph(s) can create a sense of distance between the participant and their experience [35] enabling them to opt in/out of direct personal association and talk about an issue more broadly [33].

In this study we therefore undertook an initial exploration using photo elicitation, a method in which photographs or pictures are used as a stimulus or guide in interviews [36]. We aimed to explore the acceptability of using an approach (photo-elicitation) that does not rely on solely verbal or written techniques, and to make a preliminary assessment of whether people can usefully employ images to support a discussion about the reasons why they self-harm.

Method

Participants

Working age adults (18 – 65 yrs) admitted to the clinical decision unit or the medical assessment unit of an acute general hospital following a self-harm injury were informed of the research following their self-harm assessment, using information sheets handed out by self-harm team. Service users from a community organisation supporting people who self-harm were also invited to participate through distribution of an information sheet featuring details of the study and contact details of the researcher. Given only a small proportion of people who self-harm attend hospital [37] it was anticipated that capturing experiences from both groups would offer a broader discussion. After initial approaches by staff working in those organisations, those who gave consent to be contacted/expressed an interest were followed up to establish consent and arrange participation. Those people clearly expressing suicidal intent requiring immediate clinical care, requiring translation, or lacking mental capacity were not approached. This was assessed by the self-harm team, where possible.

Data collection

Participants were asked to take photographs over a two week period of anything that would help them describe their experience of self-harm. Due to ethical concerns and principles of consent, participants were asked to avoid taking pictures of others. All participants were offered the use of a digital camera, although some chose to use their own equipment.

Once the participants had taken their photographs, arrangements were made to meet and discuss the images. Some participants chose to print their images prior to this meeting and brought them along, others selected which images they wanted printing and images were printed by the researcher immediately before the interview. All images were viewed and discussed in A4 colour printed format.

At interview the technique of auto-driving was employed. In this approach a prior topic guide is not used by the researcher but the participant leads or 'drives' the interview by choosing which pictures to discuss, in what order and how they talk about the pictures: the researcher adopts the role of 'active listener' [38]. Prompts were used to explore thoughts and feelings about presented images and how they represented the participants' experiences. An ad hoc topic guide was used with one participant who presented without images; this included a discussion around images they might have considered and possible difficulties they encountered. At the end of the interview each participant was informed that the researcher may invite them for a second interview to discuss their experiences further. This was to enable further exploration of any themes following preliminary analyses. Additional consent was obtained from all participants. However, although no further interviews were requested by the researcher, three participants expressed a wish for a further interview. Two of the participants had additional images and issues they wished to discuss, including homosexuality. One participant expressed how after the first interview she had "figured it out"; the uniqueness of the research task appeared to create some initial anxiety. By the end of the first interview she seem reassured and expressed a wish to take more photographs and discuss her experience further. Further interviews were arranged with all three participants two weeks following the first interview though due to varying circumstances (cancellations, intoxication) some interviews took up to six weeks to complete. Interviews were audio-recorded and transcribed verbatim and a copy of the pictures was retained, with the consent of the participants, to be used in the analysis.

To assess the acceptability of using images, the interviewer kept field notes about the tone and conduct of sessions and the use to which images were put during discussions, and reviewed audio recordings for what they said about the use of images as well as what was said about self-harm. Each participant was also asked how they felt about using the method at the end of each interview.

Analysis

There is currently little guidance on how to analyse combined visual and textual data [39, 40]. Instead, studies reporting visual methods typically employ methods of analysis designed to manage textual data only [30, 41]. In this study however, the aim of the analysis was to capture both the verbal and the visual data. A polytextual thematic analysis developed by Gleeson [39] was therefore undertaken. This method allows the exploration of more than one type of data set whilst working with the assumption that these data sets are linked; meaning is explored by moving back and forward between the data sets rather than seeing them as separate.

Each participant's transcript and set of images was scrutinised for themes in an iterative process that involved moving back and forward from text to images. Initially, textual excerpts and individual images were scrutinised and extracts of text that were felt to say something were highlighted and qualities within the pictures were noted. The next stage was the creation of explanatory codes (a basic unit of meaning) that could be applied to the textual excerpts and individual images that conveyed the interpreted meaning. Following this stage the data were managed as one source (a list of codes with their associated images and text from an individual); separating the analysis by method of collection was avoided [42]. All coded textual data and images were then reviewed for fittingness by reviewing the text and visual data associated with each code to ensure all the data shared the same meaning. If different extracts of data or images differed in meaning then codes were

expanded (or collapsed if different codes had a shared meaning). Deleting codes was avoided in case they became pertinent further down the process of analysis. Codes with similar properties were grouped into tentative themes which were then refined and their boundaries demarcated by further scrutiny of the images and text that had informed the themes. Finally, each theme was defined and named.

This process was repeated for each participant individually and then the themes across the whole data corpus were explored. A framework of tentative master themes was generated from the individual analysis. Tentative master themes were also assessed for fittingness; data were re-examined to explore the ways in which the data were divergent or convergent across individual participants. Where necessary, themes were collapsed or expanded. NVivo, a qualitative data analysis computer software package was used throughout the analysis [43].

Initial analysis was undertaken by the first author and then codes and themes were refined through discussion by all three authors. Using this integrated method of analysis enabled a rigorous and systematic analysis of the textual and visual data from individual experiential accounts of self-harm in the first instance, before concentrating on themes which were common across cases.

As part of the interview, the participants were asked about their experience of photo-elicitation. During analysis, the authors held extensive discussions on the nature of the images presented and on the types of images that were not present. Notes from these discussions and from the participants' responses were used to make an assessment of the role of images in the interviewing process, as reported elsewhere [44, 45] .

Results

Consent to be contacted by a researcher was obtained from 28 people; however contact could only be established with 20 people. Of these, thirteen consented to participate in the research; two declined due to housing difficulties; two declined due to low mood; and three people declined due to feeling unable to discuss their self-harm at the time of the research.

Of these thirteen, eight people provided data; three withdrew consent (reasons included further inpatient treatment and issues with probation) and two did not respond to attempts to contact them.

The participants

Eight adults, two males and six females, aged between 21 and 65 participated in the study. A total of eleven interviews lasting between 40 min and two hours were carried out and 143 photographs were collected (mean number 18 images; range 0–66). One participant, presented without images and an ad hoc topic guide was used.

Five of the participants reported a long history of self-harm using varied methods. Of those, one participant also reported a long history of an eating disorder and addiction to alcohol. Three participants, reported self-poisoning only during a particularly difficult period of their life.

Participants also reported having suffered varied mental health problems. Self-reported diagnoses included schizophrenia, drug induced psychosis, depression, alcoholism, bulimia, and dissociative identity disorder.

Observations about the use of images
Number and variety of images
In addition to the number of images presented by participants we noted their variety. For example, familial and intimate relationships as well as close friendships were represented through images, as were interior and outdoor spaces. The range and number of images facilitated detailed discussions about self-harm in terms of specific triggers, methods of harm and functions; they also elicited discussions of the significance of people and place.

We were struck by the absence of some images that are frequently present on internet sites and accessible via social media. We were shown no pictures at all of actual injuries. This might reflect a difference in the personal uses to which people will put images, from those which lead others to place images in the public domain. Since the purpose of the study was to explore the reasons why people self-harm, participants may have chosen images that would enable a discussion of the purpose it served for them, rather than the end result. Alternatively our proscription of pictures of identifiable individuals may have been interpreted as an implicit instruction that only certain more impersonal images were acceptable.

Use of images in interviews
The images were readily incorporated into the interviews and there were many occasions where seemingly mundane images, such as a road works sign, unveiled complex narratives relating to self-harm; the interaction between image and narrative was important in understanding what was being communicated.

Both males in this study, participants 3 and 8, talked about their experiences in a very visual way. Participant 3 in particular presented pictures to represent the contents of his flashbacks; four out of five images represented traumatic experience which he found difficult to verbalise. One of the images captured two birds, see Fig. 1. He discussed how he wanted to capture an image of a heron; he described a fear of herons and how the sight of one would trigger an act of self-harm. He

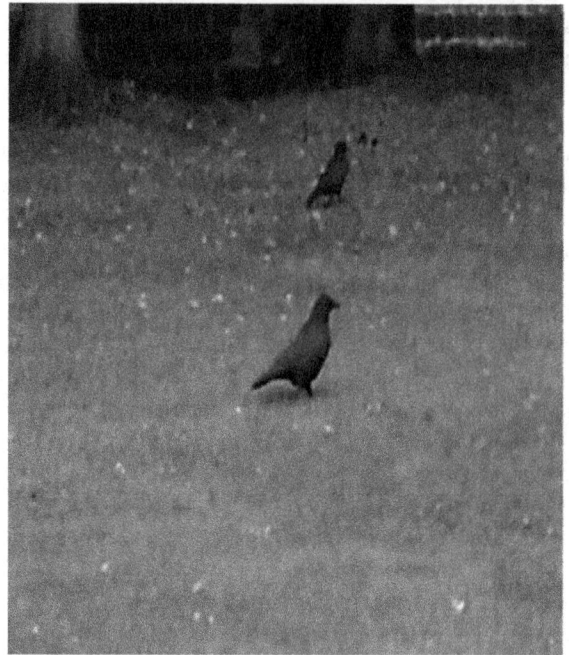

Fig. 1 The birds

went onto describe how the image (of a replacement bird) represented a very abusive relationship with his mother. His other images also featured images to represent different abusers and places of abuse.

Engagement with use of imagery
Some participants seemed energised by the task of producing images; participant 2 had arranged some of her images into a collage for the interview. Participant 6 described how the use of visuals had allowed her to express her experiences in a way others could understand:

> "You could translate into something that somebody else could understand like, like the volcano, how would you explain that? Whereas you show them the volcano it's more obvious than words. I suppose people will understand volcanos." (Participant 6, p.14 line 614)

We noted that some people seemed more familiar with, or receptive to, the idea of taking photographs than others. Only one participant (participant 5) produced no pictures despite consenting. Some respondents seemed more innately "visual" in their thinking. Participant 1 for instance noted how a change in her emotional status also saw a change in her physical appearance:

> "every time I've done it [overdosed], I've dyed my hair...it's a bit weird that like every time I've done it I've kind of tried to change my appearance as well" (Participant 1, p.12 line 483 interview 1)

A positive experience

Participants reported having enjoyed using photographs to describe their experience of self-harm. They described it as "helpful", "a good thing" and "interesting". Participant 1 described how the photograph served as a tool which helped her begin and continue talking about her experience:

> "it's quite a good thing because if you were just to say come in and talk about it I wouldn't know where to start and its good like, it's a talking point, like the picture you can say I've taken this because and then it leads, like the picture of my dog, it's a picture of a dog but it causes this and that you know what I mean" (Participant 1, p.11 line 511, interview 1)

Participants reported feeling able to capture images which represented their personal experience of self-harm. Each participant led their interview and for the most part they seemed at ease throughout. Having prepared for the interview by taking and choosing images in advance, (and perhaps considering what they wished to discuss in relation to each image prior to the interview), served to facilitate the interview.

A challenging experience

Almost certainly, capturing images to represent experience of self-harm was more of a challenge for some than others. For some the biggest challenge seemed to be getting started and thinking about what they wanted to capture, and then finding the image (e.g. a heron). Most of the participants described the process as something which gathered momentum. Finding images to express emotional states was described as difficult by participant 1 but then she came up with her own solution:

> "I don't understand how I can take a picture of anger, like I guess I could take a picture of something that causes the anger which I did" (Participant 1, p.12, line 526, interview 1)

Some participants apologised for their images and seemed to lack confidence when showing them. Some seemed embarrassed and perhaps felt under pressure to produce images of great interest, which in turn might have inhibited their ability to express their experience of self-harm.

Explanations for self-harm
A response to distress

The analysis identified a number of themes that support commonly recognised explanations for self-harm such as: self-harm as punishment, self-harm as a relief from pain (affect regulation) and self-harm as a counter to loneliness.

Loneliness was a common theme across all participants with discussion often centred on the scarcity of human contact. Many of the images presented seemed to depict loneliness with a predominance of bare rooms sometimes with single cups on a table.

Self-harm as a form of punishment was also a common theme. Participant 4 presented a number of images of barbed wire and one of a rusty medieval looking arrow tip. She described how her self-harm was an act of punishment for bad thoughts and deeds as well as things not done:

> "...it was punishment but it was kind of good punishment because it hurt but I got a satisfaction out of it as well, and it served a purpose so it was, it's always been a very contradictory thing of pain only being soothed by more pain." (Participant 4, p.12 line 656)

There was much discussion of self-harm as a way to manage emotions when things got too much. For example, one of the images presented by participant 6 was of a closed door and she described her self-harm as a way to take a pause on her life, not in the sense of contemplating suicide, but temporarily taking a respite when things got too difficult.

> "Yeah just sick of dealing with all the shit cos it's one thing after another after another sometimes you think just let me step off for a bit and I can't deal with anymore shit thrown my way" (Participant 6, p.11 line 461)

Participant 1 described how self-harm was a way to help her sleep and reach a sense of calm when things became overwhelming and she presented a picture of her lying in front of a car seemingly "at rest" see Fig. 2.

It was an interesting choice of picture in that it could be interpreted as quite the opposite, for example it might suggest vulnerability, risk and disorder. This interaction between the image and narrative was important to really understand what was being communicated. Showing images which depicted the opposite of what was said, and how they preferred to be perceived was particularly notable in the narratives of participants 1 and 3. They both discussed a need to present a hardy persona. Participant 1 described how she preferred her friends think that she is fine, rather than "a mental bitch". Participant 4 similarly presented a number of images which depicted a desire to appear strong, yet on the inside she felt completely broken. The discussion of images helped reveal both their internal and external

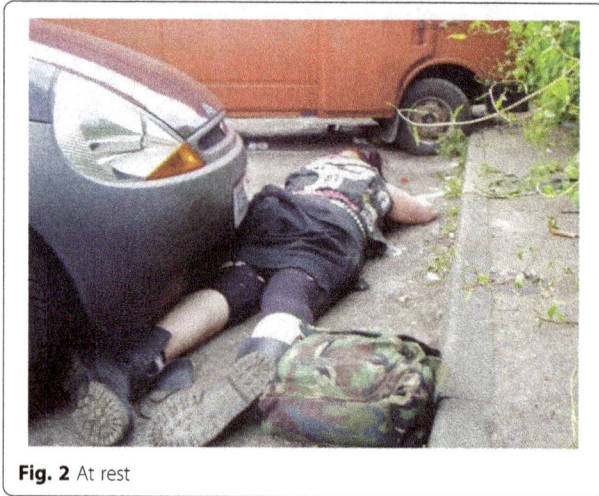

Fig. 2 At rest

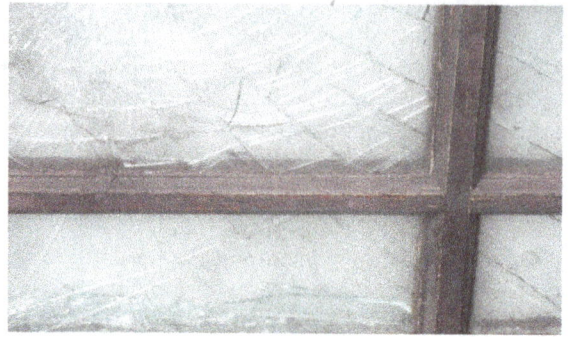

Fig. 3 Broken glass

selves and describe how self-harm can be protective in that it allows the internal self to remain hidden, whilst offering a sense of mastery (being in control of the perception of others).

Self-harm as protective:

Many of the participants reported experiencing adverse events throughout their lives, such as sexual abuse, death of significant others and bullying. When discussing these experiences a common thread throughout the narratives was the apparent lack of protective factors within their life. This was usually expressed through feelings of vulnerability, loneliness and a perceived lack of care from others.

A sense of vulnerability was visually represented by participant 4 through images of glass sheets that had been shattered but had not yet fallen apart. Her narrative picked up this theme by describing how she always felt she was shattered on the inside but never actually broken. Whilst reflecting on the images, she described how her experiences had left her internally damaged but that she felt she needed to project an external sense of herself as someone who would never break; they depicted something brutally damaged but still intact, see Fig. 3. Participant 4 also presented an image of a brick wall which could both depict external strength but also act as a barrier to conceal her inner turmoil:

"Stay upright, stay together and not cross those boundaries so people would find out what was going on because that was something that I couldn't do so I had to internalise it." (Participant 4, p.4 line 136)

A sense of mastery

The theme of self-harm as a sense of mastery captures how feelings of control (or a lack thereof) were

experienced in different and complex ways as both an antecedent to and a function of self-harm. Fundamentally control was something participants felt they lacked. It was described in terms of a generalised feeling of lack of agency and also as a result of being controlled by another or others. Participant 4, a young woman who had a long history of self-harm, discussed a dislike of her life of 'chaos' and disorder and central to her account was the value of being able to reduce her sense of 'chaos' through the act of self-harm. For example, to represent her chaotic life she chose images of winding paths and dark stairwells which for her captured a sense of uncertainty. To counter this she presented an image of a road sign to indicate roadworks ahead. She described the roadworks sign, which for her represented the act of self-harm, as an indication that she could now sense what was happening ahead and that there was the possibility of repairs to the chaos, see Fig. 4.

Some participants reported feeling as though their lives were heavily controlled and manipulated; their sense of control was lacking as they felt controlled by someone or something else. Participant 4 described an 'evil' inside her and self-harm was a way to exert some control over this, see Fig. 5

"I had so many times where I was like, I need to cut because I need to, I can't stop the evil, I can't stop it taking over and putting all these pictures in my head and I thought ultimately it was going completely take over my personality and I was going do all these horrible pictures that I was seeing in my head to other people. So I needed to slow it down so it was very logical of ok how do I slow down something that's in my blood would be to cut cos I'm releasing the blood therefore I can slow down the evil" (Participant 4, p.15 line 671)

This sense of control the participants gained through self-harm was also evident when participant 4 talked about being her own master of hurt; self-harm gave her

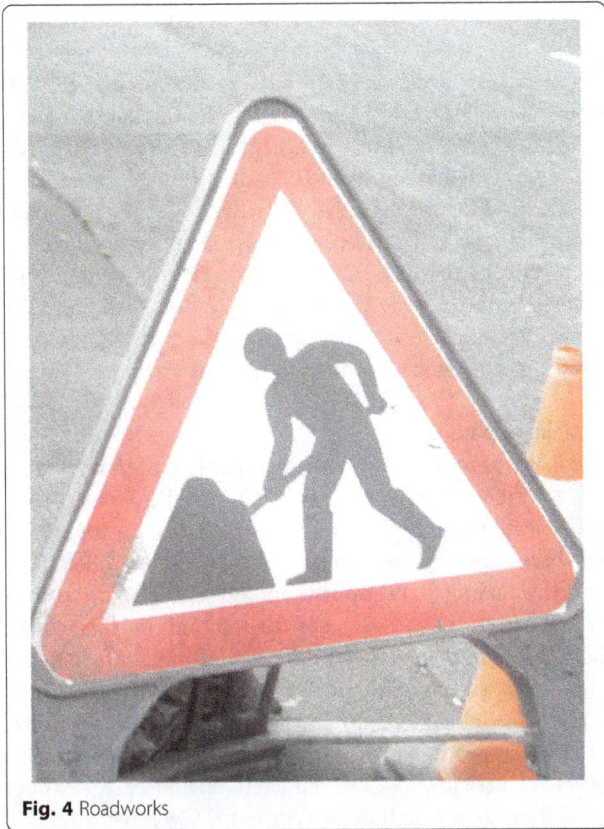

Fig. 4 Roadworks

control and although she was able to reflect that this might seem irrational, she gained positive benefits from this thought.

Self-harm and communication

Across participants' accounts of self-harm the theme of communication was very apparent. Many of the participants discussed images representative of communication difficulties.

For example, participant 6 presented an image of a women's mouth crossed shut with black strips, see Fig. 6. She discussed how she had tried to talk to people about her self-harm in the past but she felt that they "just didn't get it".

Being unable to communicate satisfactorily was expressed in several ways. First, the use of words was sometimes described as inappropriate and ineffective, some difficult and sensitive experiences were felt to be 'beyond words'. Some participants expressed an inability and reluctance to express themselves through words because of negative experiences or a lack of experience in using words to communicate issues of a sensitive nature.

*"Actions speak louder than words don't they"
(Participant 7, p.3 line 112)*

"I don't use my words, so the pressure builds then I, I cut and that's how I deal with that" (Participant 4, p.9 line 415)

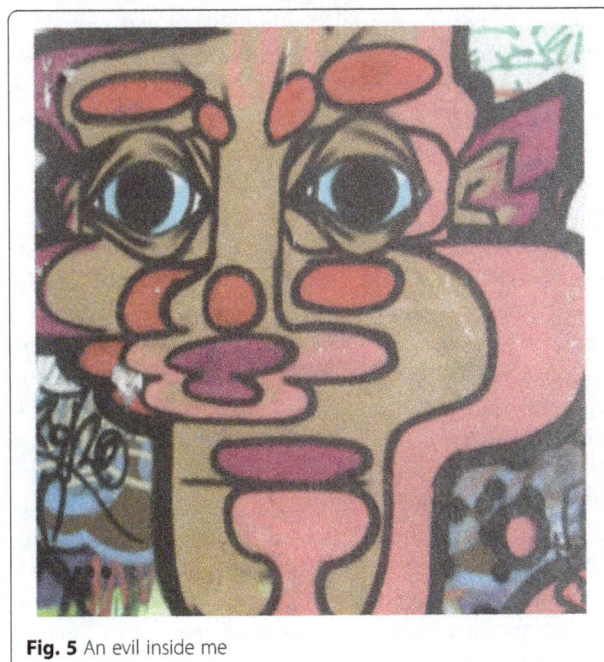

Fig. 5 An evil inside me

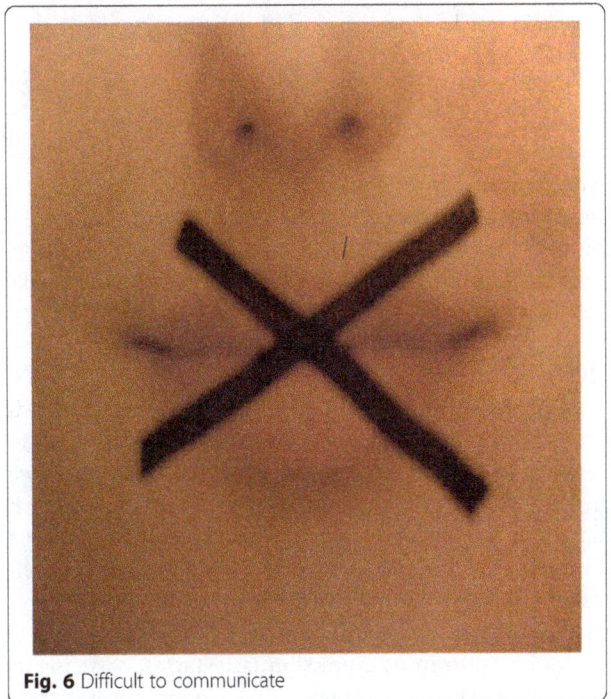

Fig. 6 Difficult to communicate

Some participants did describe their self-harm as a form of communication to others of inner turmoil or pain that they either could not find the words for or did not think the words were understood.

However, in this theme self-harm was more nuanced than simply social communication, seeking attention or help. The act or injury was often seen as a signifier to the self that things were different, or might be different going forward.

For example, participant 3 used a grammar metaphor to describe his self-harm. In this sense, the communication was not with others but as a message to himself:

> *"Self-harm is like a full stop, like punctuation, it's punctuation, it's a sort of punctuation to moods or emotions or to a series of memories" (Participant 3, p. 8 line 359)*

There was a recognition from some of the participants that using self-harm as communication could be problematic; participant 7 described how she had been criticised by others and at this point in the interview she presented an image of her notebook which symbolised a shift in the way she now expresses herself.

> *"my notebook and erm since like the erm self-harming happened and stuff I've started like writing like my negative thoughts and feelings down it's like, its more about how I'm dealing with it now...I find it really helpful to just write things down that I'd want to say to him like angry feelings and how he made me feel so that I won't say them to him or to anybody else or I'll like get back in that bad place" (Participant 7, p.12 line 601)*

Discussion

The aim of this article was to explore whether using a novel method to elicit reasons for self-harm would help participants talk about their experiences and therefore provide a more nuanced understanding of why people self-harm.

Utility of the method

One of the main purposes of adopting a visual methods study with people who self-harm was to enable them to feel as though they were in control of the research process and offer them a different form of expression. It has been interesting to see how those key features were discussed by the participants as their functions of self-harm. Perhaps through enabling a different form of expression (from conventional methods), yet similar to their chosen form of expression (self-harm), participants felt more able to express and communicate their

experience of self-harm. For example, others have suggested that people draw upon visual images during times of psychological distress [46–48] . Holmes et al. [47] and Hales et al. [46] both reported how participants experienced detailed mental imagery about future suicide attempts, which they termed 'flash forwards'. They suggested 'flashforward' imagery warrants further investigation for formal universal clinical assessment procedures.

Moreover, the use of metaphorical and figurative speech featured widely throughout most of the participants' accounts which would suggest a propensity to describe experiences of distress through imagery.

Explaining self-harm

Self-harm as a response to distress and to punish oneself

As described in reviews by Suyemoto [4], Klonsky [49] and more recently Edmondson et al. [6], evidence of self-harm serving to regulate affect (to get relief from negative feelings) and punish oneself (show anger toward oneself to self-soothe) were also found in this study. Both functions are particularly well documented in the literature; a systematic review of self-reported reasons for non-suicidal self-injury, which included accounts of 29,350 participants, found the majority of studies (49/152 articles, 98%) reported evidence of affect regulation as a function of self-harm. Over half (92/152, 60%) reported punishment as a function of self-harm [6].

Self-harm and sense of mastery

Self-harm was described as a behaviour through which feelings of control, empowerment and ownership could be sought. The subject of control has been well documented and the evidence suggests that self-harm offers a feeling of control through feeling able to rid oneself of or reduce unpleasant affective states, commonly referred to as affect regulation [4, 5, 18, 50–53]. The findings from this study and others however have shown how control can be gained through the behaviour in and of itself, for example through controlling the level of pain, depth of cut and the amount of blood [18, 49, 51–55]. Moreover, our participants and others described a sense of ownership over their behaviour, remarks such as *"it's mine"*, *"there are certain things they can't have and that's [self-harm] one of them"*. Such statements suggest there are positive experiences to be gained through self-harm. These sorts of experiences resonated with those participant responses in Shearer's [55], Demming's [51] and Brooke and Horn's [53] studies who all studied women's reflections of their self-harm. One participant in Demming's [51] study described her self-harm as something that belonged to her, that she controlled and only she could stop it. Shearer [55] on the other hand included the statement *"to do something I have control over and no one else can control"* within a questionnaire and the item was ranked one of the top three functions by 22% of participants.

Self-harm as protective

Experiences of sexual abuse, death of significant others and mental health problems were common in our participants as they are among most populations where repeated self-harm is found. In response to such experiences self-harm seemed to function as a protection. Usually protective factors - "predictors of positive outcomes among people at risk for developing problems as a result of adverse life events or experiences" [56] - are thought of as a supportive network of family or friends [57]. How can self-harm act as a substitute?

The protective properties of self-harm were expressed in different ways, again, some of which resonated with functions such as affect regulation [4, 5] and anti-suicide (where a person self-harms to avoid suicide) [4, 5].

The experiences captured in this study however, again, seemed encompassing of something more than affect regulation and anti-suicide. For example, self-harm was described as a behaviour through which feelings of protection and preservation could be sought. Similar descriptors have been reported in other studies and articles, for example, metaphorical statements such as "it's my life raft...a sort of safety shield," [58].

Collectively these findings support the idea that self-harm serves to regulate feelings of distress, but they also suggest that self-harm can be adaptive and can offer something positive beyond the elimination of distress. For a more detailed discussion about positive and adaptive functions of self-harm see [6].

Self-harm and communication

The theme of communication was very apparent throughout the personal accounts of self-harm. Klonsky [5] and Suyemoto [4] both described how people use self-harm as a way of interacting with their environment. Klonsky [5] refers to the 'interpersonal influence' model to describe how people use self-harm to influence or manipulate people in their environment. Suyemoto [4] refers to the environmental model to describe how self-harm creates environmental responses that are reinforcing.

The four function model [59, 60] proposes that people use self-harm as a language to serve a social function that relates to items such as "to get other people to act differently or change", "to try and get a reaction from someone, even if it's negative", and "to make others angry". Nock [61] also compared self-harm as a language to somatoform behaviours, whereby physical symptoms are presented as an alternative means to communicating psychological distress.

Although the environmental model does include how self-harm can be used to express the inexpressible, which might seem related to the idea of using self-harm as a language, these models do not satisfactorily explain how people used self-harm as a language in this study.

Messages were 'written on the body' in the same way Adshead [14] described, through the act of self-harm and this was used to do the talking that participants felt unable to for the reasons discussed – not just to seek help or for an immediate social function but in a more personal way – described in other research as a form of remembrance, like creating physical reminders of important events [49].

Strengths and limitations

To the best of our knowledge this is the first study to use photo elicitation to explore reasons for self-harm and to an extent, this method encouraged participants' to use images in the same way they use their body, as a way of expression. This visual way of expression allowed the researcher to 'see' what was often hidden and private but in a controlled way. All of the images were generated by the participant which facilitated a safer, more controlled disclosure. For some, it was reported as the first time they had ever spoken in such an honest and detailed way about their self-harm. The study yielded rich, distinct, visual and verbal data (over ten hours of interview, featuring 143 images). However, given the small sample size ($n = 8$) we cannot be confident of saturation or transferability to the population as a whole. Similarly, although some participants were interviewed on more than one occasion, further interviews with all participants following a preliminary analysis would have allowed further exploration of some of the more novel themes (i.e. protection and mastery), and a more detailed discussion of all the images in cases where excessive numbers of images were generated. More emphasis on the process of taking images could also have been discussed in subsequent interviews to enable a more comprehensive critique of the method. Future research into self-harm should consider the strengths and limitations of certain research approaches to ensure a more complete understanding of the reasons why people self-harm, to help develop interventions which are likely to meet the needs of people who self-harm.

Conclusions

Taking pictures is familiar; personal lives now seem perpetually pictorially documented through social media. However, on reflection taking pictures to represent difficult experiences is not as familiar and requires more thought. Using pictures to represent experiences of self-harm required effort, abstract thinking and reflexivity [30] which some people struggled with more than others. For some this approach was possibly perceived as a measure of their ability – observations made in a different context by Mannay [62], Packard [63] and Frith and Harcourt [36].

These characteristics of photo-elicitation – the degree to which it requires concerted and unfamiliar effort from the informant, and yet offers control over the content of what is discussed – are differences from traditional language-based methods and arise directly from its use of images. We found that most participants responded positively, produced multiple appropriate images and discussed them actively – revealing aspects of their reasons for self-harm that are less well documented. These observations suggest that photo-elicitation has potential as a method for clinical or research use in self-harm work and further evaluation is justified.

Acknowledgements
We would like to thank all the service users who participated in the research, including those involved in the design of the study. We are also grateful to the self-harm team based at Leeds and York Partnership Foundation Trust (LYPFT) who helped with the research design and recruitment.

Funding
This study was funded by a studentship from the Economic and Social Research Council (ESRC). The funders had no role in study design, data collection and analysis, decision to publish, or preparation of the manuscript.

Authors' contributions
Conception & design of the work (AE, CB AH); Data collection (AE); Data analysis and interpretation (AE, CB, AH); Drafting the article (AE, CB, AH); Critical revision of the article (AE, CB, AH); Final approval of the manuscript for publication (all authors).

Consent for publication
Consent for publication (i.e. copies of all images) in journal publications was obtained in written form from all participants.

Competing interests
The authors declare that they have no competing interests.

Author details
[1]Centre for Applied Research in Health, School of Human and Health Sciences, University of Huddersfield, Queensgate, Huddersfield HD1 3DH, UK. [2]Institute of Health Sciences, School of Medicine, University of Leeds, 101 Clarendon Rd, Leeds LS2 9LJ, UK.

References
1. Tsiachristas A, McDaid D, Casey D, Brand F, Leal J, Park AL, Geulayov G, Hawton K: General hospital costs in England of medical and psychiatric care for patients who self-harm: a retrospective analysis. The Lancet Psychiatry. 2017;4(10):759-67.
2. Hawton K, Harriss L. Deliberate self-harm by under-15-year-olds: characteristics, trends and outcome. J Child Psychol Psychiatry. 2008;49(4):441-8.
3. Hawton K, Bergen H, Kapur N, Cooper J, Steeg S, Ness J, Waters K. Repetition of self-harm and suicide following self-harm in children and adolescents: findings from the multicentre study of self-harm in England. J Child Psychol Psychiatry. 2012;53(12):1212-9.
4. Suyemoto K. The functions of self mutilation. Clin Psychol Rev. 1998;18(5):531-54.
5. Klonsky ED. The functions of deliberate self-injury: a review of the evidence. Clin Psychol Rev. 2007;27(2):226-39.
6. Edmondson AJ, Brennan CA, House AO. Non-suicidal reasons for self-harm: a systematic review of self-reported accounts. J Affect Disord. 2016;191:109-17.
7. Hunter C, Chantler K, Kapur N, Cooper J. Service user perspectives on psychosocial assessment following self-harm and its impact on further help-seeking: a qualitative study. J Affect Disord. 2013;145(3):315-23.
8. Self-harm in over 8s: long-term management : Clinical guideline [CG133] [https://www.nice.org.uk/guidance/cg133/chapter/2-Research-recommendations].
9. Hawton K, Arensman E, Townsend E, Bremner S, Feldman E, Goldney R, Gunnell D, Hazell P, Kv H, House A, et al. Deliberate self harm: systematic review of efficacy of psychosocial and pharmacological treatments in preventing repetition. BMJ. 1998;317(7156):441-7.
10. Owens C. Interventions for self-harm: are we measuring outcomes in the most appropriate way? Br J Psychiatry. 2010;197(6):502-3.
11. Kapur N, Cooper J, Bennewith O, Gunnell D, Hawton K. Postcards, green cards and telephone calls: therapeutic contact with individuals following self-harm. Br J Psychiatry. 2010;197(1):5-7.
12. Hawton K, Witt KG, Taylor Salisbury TL, Arensman E, Gunnell D, Townsend E, van Heeringen K, Hazell P. Interventions for self-harm in children and adolescents. Cochrane Database Syst Rev. 2015;(Issue 12). Art. No.: CD012013. https://doi.org/10.1002/14651858.CD012013.
13. Hawton K, Witt KG, Taylor Salisbury TL, Arensman E, Gunnell D, Hazell P, Townsend E, van Heeringen K. Psychosocial interventions for self-harm in adults. Cochrane Database Syst Rev. 2016;Issue 5. Art. No.: CD012189. https://doi.org/10.1002/14651858.CD012189.
14. Adshead G. Written on the body: deliberate self-harm as communication. Psychoanal Psychother. 2010;24(2):69-80.
15. Horrocks J, Hughes J, Martin C, House A, Owens D. Patients experience of hospital care following self-harm, a qualitatvie study. In: University of Leeds. 2002. https://www.researchgate.net/publication/228359199_Patient_Experiences_of_Hospital_Care_Following_Self-Harm-A_Qualitative_Study
16. Pembroke L (ed.): Self-Harm : Perspectives from personal experience; 1994.
17. Spandler H. Who's hurting who? : Young people, self-harm and suicide. Handsell: Gloucester; 2001.
18. Sutton J. Healing the hurt within. Understand self injury and self-harm, and heal the emotional wounds. In: 3 edn: how to books ltd.; 2007.
19. Reece J. The language of cutting: initial reflections on a study of the experiences of self-injury in a group of women and nurses. Issues in mental health nursing. 2005;26(6):561-74.
20. Cromby J. Feeling the way: qualitative clinical research and the affective turn. Qual Res Psychol. 2012;9(1):88-98.
21. Norman H, Borrill J. The relationship between self-harm and alexithymia. Scand J Psychol. 2015;56(4):405-19.
22. Michel K, Valach L, Waeber V. Understanding deliberate self-harm: the patients' views. Crisis: The J of Crisis Intervent and Suicide Prev. 1994;15(4):172-8.
23. Rodham K, Hawton K, Evans E. Reasons for deliberate self-harm: comparison of self-poisoners and self-cutters in a community sample of adolescents. J Am Acad Child Adolesc Psychiatry. 2004;43(1):80-7.
24. Pink S. More visualising, more methodologies: on video, reflexivity and qualitative research. Sociol Rev. 2001;49(4):586-99.
25. Sweetman P. Revealing habitus, illuminating practice: Bourdieu, photography and visual methods. Sociol Rev. 2009;57(3):491-511.
26. Bagnoli A. Beyond the standard interview: the use of graphic elicitation and arts-based methods. Qualitative Res. 2009;9(5):547-70.
27. White A, Bushin N, Carpena-Méndez F, Ní Laoire C. Using visual methodologies to explore contemporary Irish childhoods. Qual Res. 2010;10(2):143-58.
28. Erdner A. Photography as a method of data collection: helping people with long-term mental illness convey their life world. Perspectives in Psychiatric Care. 2010;47:145-50.
29. Whitehurst T. Liberating silent voices - perspectives of children with a profound and complex learning needs on inclusion. Br J Learn Disabil. 2006;35:55-61.
30. Drew S, Duncan R, Sawyer S. Visual storytelling: a beneficial but challenging method for health research with young people. Qual Health Res. 2010;21(12):1677-88.
31. Pain H. A literature review to evaluate the choice and use of visual methods. Int J Qual Methods. 2012;11(4):303-19.
32. Pyle A: Engaging young children in research through photo elicitation. Early Child Development and Care 2013(ahead-of-print):1-15.
33. Harrison B. Seeing health and illness worlds – using visual methodologies in a sociology of health and illness: a methodological review. Sociology of Health & Illness. 2002;24(6):856-72.

34. Lachal J, Speranza M, Taïeb O, Falissard B, Lefèvre H, Moro MR, Revah-Levy A. Qualitative research using photo-elicitation to explore the role of food in family relationships among obese adolescents. Appetite. 2012;58(3):1099–105.

35. Balmer C, Griffiths F, Dunn J. A review of the issues and challenges involved in using participant-produced photographs in nursing research. J Adv Nurs. 2015;71(7):1726–37.

36. Frith H, Harcourt D. Using photographs to capture Women's experiences of chemotherapy: reflecting on the method. Qual Health Res. 2007;17(10): 1340–50.

37. Hawton K, Saunders KEA, O'Connor RC. Self-harm and suicide in adolescents. Lancet. 2012;379(9834):2373–82.

38. Heisley D, Levy S. Autodriving : a photo elicitation approach. J Consum Res. 1991;18:257–72.

39. Gleeson K. Polytextual thematic analysis for visual data. In: Visual methods in psychology. Reavey P: Psychology Press; 2011.

40. Frith H, Riley S, Archer L, Gleeson K. Editorial. Qual Res Psychol. 2005;2:187–98.

41. Frith H, Harcourt D, Fussell A. Anticipating an altered appearance: women undergoing chemotherapy treatment for breast cancer. Eur J Oncol Nurs. 2007;11(5):385–91.

42. Bazeley P. Analysing qualitative data: more than Identyfying themes. Malaysian Journal of Qualitative Research. 2009;2:6–22.

43. NVIVO: Software for Qualitative Data Analysis [http://www.qsrinternational. com/product].

44. Edmondson A. Listening with your eyes: using pictures and words to explore self-harm: University of Leeds; 2013.

45. Edmondson A, Brennan C, House A. A research encounter with self-harm. In: edn E w s-h, editor. Baker C, Shaw,C. Biley, F: PCCS Books; 2013.

46. Hales S, Deeprose C, Goodwin G, Holmes E. Cognitions in bipolar affective disorder and unipolar depression: imagining suicide. Bipolar Disord. 2011;13:651–61.

47. Holmes E, Crane C, Fennell M, Williams M. Imagery about suicide in depression : flashforwards. J Behav Ther Exp Psychiatry. 2007;38:423–34.

48. Holmes E, Grey N, Young KA. Intrusive images and hotspots of trauma memories in PTSD: an exploratory investigation of emotions and cognitive themes. J Behav Ther Exp Psychiatry. 2005;35:3–17.

49. Klonsky ED. The functions of self-injury in young adults who cut themselves: clarifying the evidence for affect-regulation. Psychiatry Res. 2009;166(2–3):260–8.

50. Bancroft J, Hawton K, Simkin S, Kingston B, Cumming C, Whitwell D. Reasons people give for taking overdoses - further enquiry. Br J Med Psychol. 1979;52(DEC):353–65.

51. Demming V. Women's reflection on their adolescent self injury in relation to grief and los. In: Faculty of Saybrook Graduate School and Research Center. PhD in Psychology; 2008.

52. Haas B, Popp F. Why do people injure themselves? Psychopathology. 2006;39(1):10–8.

53. Brooke S, Horn N. The meaning of self-injury and overdosing amongst women fulfilling the diagnostic criteria for 'borderline personality disorder. Psychol Psychother-Theory Res and Prac. 2010;83(2):113–28.

54. Osuch EA, Noll JG, Putnam FW. The motivations for self-injury in psychiatric inpatients. Psychiatry-Interpers and Biological Processes. 1999;62(4):334–46.

55. Shearer S. Phenomenology of self injury amongst inpatient women with BPD. J Nerv Ment Dis. 1994;182:524–6.

56. Lopez S. The encyclopedia of positive psychology. In: Blackwell Reference Online; 2009.

57. McDougall T, Armstrong M, Trainor G. Helping children and young people who self-harm. In: An introduction to self-harming and suicidal behaviours for health professionals. London and New York: Routledge; 2010.

58. Collins D. Attacks on the body: how can we understand self-harm. Psychodyn Pract. 1996;2(4):463–75.

59. Nock MK, Prinstein MJ. A functional approach to the assessment of self-mutilative behavior. J Consult Clin Psychol. 2004;72(5):885–90.

60. Nock MK, Prinstein MJ. Contextual features and behavioral functions of self-mutilation among adolescents. J Abnorm Psychol. 2005;114(1):140–6.

61. Nock M. Actions speak louder than words: an elaborated theoretical model of the social functions of self injury and other harmful behaviours. Appl Prev Psychol. 2008;12:159–68.

62. Mannay D. Making the familiar strange: can visual research methods render the familiar setting more perceptible. Qual Res. 2010;10(1):91–111.

63. Packard J. I'm gonna show you what it's really like out here: the power and limitation of participatory visual methods. Vis Stud. 2008;23(1):63–77.

21

Attempted suicide of ethnic minority girls with a Caribbean and Cape Verdean background: rates and risk factors

Diana D. van Bergen[1*], Merijn Eikelenboom[2] and Petra P. van de Looij-Jansen[3]

Abstract

Background: WHO data shows that female immigrants in Europe attempt suicide at higher rates than 'native' women and 'native' and immigrant men. Empirical studies addressing attempted suicide of female immigrants of Caribbean (Antillean-Dutch and Creole-Surinamese-Dutch) as well as Cape Verdean descent in Europe are however scarce. We aim to increase knowledge about rates and risk factors of girls of Caribbean and Cape Verdean descent living in the Netherlands.

Methods: We conducted logistic regression on a dataset that consisted of self-reported health and well-being surveys filled out by 5611 female students, age 14–16, in Rotterdam, the Netherlands (Antillean Dutch $N = 357$, Creole-Surinamese-Dutch $N = 130$, and Cape Verdean-Dutch $N = 402$, and Dutch 'natives' $N = 4691$). We studied if girls of these minority groups had elevated risk for attempted suicide. Risk indicators that were suspected to play a role were investigated i.e. household composition, socio-economic class, externalizing problems, emotional problems and sexual abuse.

Results: We found that rates of attempted suicide among Antillean (14%), Creole-Surinamese young women (15.4%) were higher than of 'native' Dutch girls (9.1%), while rates of Cape-Verdean girls (8.3%) were rather similar to those of 'native' girls. Not living with two biological parents was a risk factor for 'native' girls, but not for girls of Caribbean and Cape Verdean descent. Emotional problems and sexual abuse seems to be a risk indicator for suicidality across all ethnicities. Aggressive behaviour was a risk factor for Antillean Dutch and 'native' girls.

Conclusions: Our findings underscore the need for developing suicide prevention programs for minority girls in multicultural cities in western Europe, in particular those of Caribbean descent. Results suggest the importance of addressing socio-economic class and educational background for suicide prevention, which bear particular relevance for Caribbean populations. Referral in the case of sexual trauma and low psychological wellbeing seems critical for reducing suicidal behaviour in girls, regardless of ethnicity.

Background

Attempted suicide in young women and the relationship with ethnicity

Attempted suicide in adolescence is an important concern for public health [1]. Knowledge about attempted suicide of youth in Europe is mostly guided by studies among its majority ('white') populations. However demographic trends show that the number of ethnic minorities in Europe is increasing. Specific immigrant and ethnic minority groups in Europe [2] are at increased risk for attempting suicide, a finding also observed for the USA [3].

Attempted suicide is more often found among females than males [4]. Especially the period of mid adolescence (14–16 years), shows a peak in the risk for attempted suicide for females health [1]. Considering an increased risk for attempting suicide exists for (some) ethnic minority groups on the one hand, and among young females on the other hand, a heightened risk of suicidal behavior could be expected for minority females. Underpinning this assumption, females from Turkish descent in Germany, Switzerland and the Netherlands and

* Correspondence: d.d.van.bergen@rug.nl
[1]Research Unit for Youth Studies, Department of Education, University of Groningen, Groningen, The Netherlands
Full list of author information is available at the end of the article

females of South Asian descent in the United Kingdom and The Netherlands attempt suicide at higher rates than 'native' women and 'native' and immigrant men [2]. Additionally, girls with a Hispanic background in the USA demonstrate disproportionate suicide risk [3]. Thus, young females of certain ethnic minority groups seem to be a vulnerable group with regard to suicidal behavior in Europe and in the USA. However, there is an incomplete picture on rates of and risk factors for attempted suicide in immigrant female populations in Europe at present.

There are indicators that young women of African and Caribbean descent in the west are at risk for suicidal behavior. Young Caribbean and 'Black' British women aged 16 to 34 had the highest rates of suicide attempts of all ethnicities in the United Kingdom [5]. In the Netherlands, Creole-Surinamese women were shown to have increased suicide rates [6]. In the US, 'black' young females have an increased risk of attempting suicide resulting in medical treatment, compared to white young US women [3]. Therefore, the present study aims to investigate the rates and risks for suicidal behavior of young women of Caribbean and (mixed) African descent in the Netherlands, that is, Caribbean Dutch (Antillean and Creole-Surinamese) girls and Cape-Verdan Dutch girls.

Migration history of Caribbean and Cape-Verdean immigrants in the Netherlands

Caribbean-Dutch constitute the second largest immigrant group in the Netherlands (500.000 people). The first wave of Antillean and Surinamese migrants to the Netherlands consisted of people who came for educational purposes in the 1950's and 1960's. During the eighties and nineties, Antillean migration to the Netherlands rapidly increased, especially by economically deprived individuals. Among the Surinamese, a second large migration wave occurred in the late seventies, just after the country gained its independence from the Netherlands [7]. While Cape Verdean immigrants are a relatively small immigrant group in the Netherlands (20.000 persons), the city of Rotterdam (The Netherlands) is however host to the second largest community of Cape Verdeans in Europe. The harbor of Rotterdam had a central function for the sea trade in the 1970's where many immigrant Cape Verdeans sought and found jobs, started families, and continued to reside in The Netherlands.

Risk factors for attempted suicide among girls of Caribbean and Cape-Verdean descent

Attempted suicide in adolescence is best understood as an interplay between socio-economic dimensions, family, individual and socio-cultural factors [8]. An immigrant status often coincides with a low socio-economic position, which influences the wellbeing of immigrant children, including the risk of attempting suicide [8]. Many Creole-Surinamese, Antillean and Cape Verdean families in the Netherlands have been found to have minimal financial resources compared to majority Dutch families.

Next, risks for attempting suicide may also exist in relation to the family structure. In Caribbean as well as Cape Verdean cultures, the family is traditionally shaped within a matrifocal system, in which the upbringing of children is *a joint venture* among female (extended) family members and the (biological) father's role is considered to be marginal [9]. Many researchers argue that the matrifocal system is a non-problematic future of Caribbean and African societies [9]. However, upon migration, this may change, since the support system that used to surround the mother has often eroded. Thus, Caribbean and African family households may then start resembling single-parent families 'western style', for which there is evidence for risks of suicidal behavior amongst children [10].

On the individual level, both internalizing (emotional) and externalizing problems [11]. independently seem to enhance the propensity to attempt suicide. Emotional problems often coincide with feelings of hopelessness and depressed mood that precedes suicidal behaviour. In Europe, 'Black' British female adolescents [12] as well as Antillean Dutch girls [13] were found to have higher scores of emotional disorders compared to 'native' girls. Surinamese Dutch girls did not differ much from majority females [13] (no information available on Cape Verdan girls). Furthermore, externalizing problems were reported among black female adolescent European populations at a higher rate than 'natives', including 'Black' British girls [14] as well as Antillean and Creole-Surinamese Dutch girls [13]. (No information available on Cape Verdean Dutch).

Research of Western majority samples show that sexual abuse has a strong association to suicidality [4], and that this relationship also exists among immigrant young female populations in the Netherlands [8]. As Caribbean-Dutch girls on average report their first sexual intercourse at a much younger age than 'native' girls [13], this may convey a risk for negative sexual experiences, potentially including sexual abuse.

On the basis of the aforementioned literature, in the present study we expect and explore whether socio-economic factors, household structure, sexual trauma, and emotional and externalizing problems are risk factors for attempted suicide among Dutch girls of Caribbean and Cape Verdean descent.

Methods
Study design and procedure
Data were obtained from the YMR, a child and adolescent health surveillance monitor carried out by the

Municipal Public Health Service. All YMR data were obtained within routine health examinations which had been ethically approved by the local government previously.

For the present study we used data of 14 to 16 year old students. About 85% of all secondary schools in Rotterdam participated in the YMR. The survey was filled out in the classroom on a voluntary basis between September 2003 and July 2006. Parents received written information on the YMR and could withdraw their child's participation. The response rate was about 90%.

Ethnicity

The ethnicity of the youngsters was established by using the country of birth of the father and mother. However, three exceptions existed: Girls with a mixed ethnic background, third generation immigrant girls, and Creole-Surinamese girls (since the Surinamese population consists of a number of ethnic subgroups) could only be identified through ethnic self-identification in the dataset. This was done through the item "Which group do you identify mostly with?" 1.Dutch 2. Surinamese 3. Surinamese/Creole 4. Surinamese/South Asian 5. Antillean or Aruban 6. Moroccan 7. Turkish 8. Cape Verdean 9. Other. Thus, respondents considered to be part of the aforementioned exceptional three cases were categorized as minorities only when youngsters self-identified mostly with the specific minority culture. Third generation immigrant youth concerned 6 Antillean Dutch youth and one Cape Verdean Dutch youth.

Dependent variable

Life time prevalence of attempted suicide was measured through the following item 'Have you ever made an attempt to end your life?'[three point scale: never, once or more than once]. In the analyses we dichotomized the answers (Never = no. Once/more than once = yes).

Independent variables
Household structure

Respondents filled out whether they lived with two biological parents in one household, or if they lived in a different household composition. For the analyses, we dichotomized this variable into: Lives not with two biological parents (no versus yes).

Emotional problems

Emotional problems were examined with 9 items of a shortened version of the Child Health Questionnaire [15]. The items relate to the presence of certain feelings in the past 4 weeks (e.g. loneliness, pleasure, depressed mood, self-image, anxiety and worrying). Each item is scored on a 5-point likert scale ranging from very often to never. A total sumscore is calculated, which varies between 0 and 100 (a higher score means fewer emotional problems). Chronbach's alpha of the scale was 0.86.

Externalizing problems

Four items about aggression in the past 4 weeks were used [16] (e.g. "have you physically attacked someone?"). Answers were on a 5-point scale ranging from never (0) to very often (4) and showed and alpha of .74. In the analyses the answers were put into three categories 1) never 2) sometimes and 3) frequently.

Sexual abuse

Lifetime prevalence of sexual abuse was investigated through asking 'Have you ever been sexually abused (for instance forced against your will into sexual activities, harassed, raped)'. Never = no. Once/more than once = yes.

Socio-economic status and educational track

The postal code of respondents was used as a proxy for socioeconomic class, since no other information was available from the survey regarding this element. Factor scores that link the postal code to socioeconomic class were available from the National Statistics Office. These factor scores are based on a scale of items, e.g., income, hours of work, and educational level. Next, several types of education exist in Dutch secondary school: a 'vocational track' (=1) which takes 4 years and where students focus particularly on acquiring vocational skills. The university track (=3) is a 6 year long theoretical program which prepares students for a study at university. The general continued education program ('middle track' = 2) prepares students for continued education for professional degrees at college level, and takes 5 years. Students enrolled in vocational tracks often have parents belonging to lower socio-economic strata.

Statistical analyses

Sample characteristics were obtained using descriptive statistics. Rates of attempted suicide in the minority groups were reported, and their difference with the 'native' Dutch group were tested using logistic regression. To examine whether demographics, sexual abuse, emotional and externalizing problems contributed to suicidality in each ethnic group; bivariate (chi-square tests and t-tests) and multivariate analyses (multivariate logistic regression) were conducted. Finally, to examine if differences in rates of attempted suicide between ethnicities remained significant, we controlled for the independent variables step by step. All statistical analyses were performed using the Statistical Package for Social Sciences (SPSS), version 20.0 and two-tailed tests were used with $\alpha = 0.05$.

Results

Sample description

Minority girls were overrepresented in vocational educational tracks and among the lower socio-economic strata, and they disproportionately lived in families that are not composed of two biological parents. Rates of emotional problems and sexual abuse were quite comparable across ethnicities, while aggressive behavior was twice as common among minorities compared to 'native's (see Table 1).

Rates of attempted suicide

Nine percent of Dutch girls reports having survived at least one suicide attempt. The rates of Creole-Surinamese and Antillean Dutch girls were about 1.5 times higher (15.4% and 14.0% respectively). Cape Verdean Dutch girls reported less suicidal behavior (8.2%) than 'native' girls, albeit not significantly (see Table 2).

Associations between risk indicators and attempted suicide within the Caribbean groups, Cape Verdean Dutch group and majority Dutch group

Table 3 shows bivariate associations between socio-economic class, educational track, household structure, sexual abuse, emotional- and aggression problems to suicide attempts in four ethnic groups. For Dutch 'native' girls, all these aforementioned factors constituted a significant risk to suicidal behavior. Sexual abuse and emotional problems emerged as a significant risk for attempting suicide in both Caribbean groups and Cape Verdeans. Frequent aggression was more often found among suicide attempters in all minority groups, however only among Antillean Dutch girls this indicator reached significance.

Table 4 shows the multivariate analyses of the aforementioned risk indicators of attempted suicide in four

Table 2 Non-fatal suicidal behavior by ethnicity of female students aged 14–16 in Rotterdam, The Netherlands 2003–2006

	Dutch		Creole-Surinamese		Antillean		Cape-Verdean	
	N = 4691		N = 130		N = 357		N = 433	
	N	(%)	N	(%)	N	(%)	N	(%)
Attempted Suicide								
No	4264	(90.9)	110	(84.6)	307	(86.0)	397	(91.7)
Yes	427	(9.1)	20	(15.4)[a]	50	(14.0)[b]	36	(8.3)

[a]Significant difference with Dutch females (the reference group) at level ≤ 0.05
[b]Significant difference with Dutch females (the reference group) at level ≤ 0.01

Table 1 Sample characteristics by ethnicity of female students (N = 5611), aged 14–16 in Rotterdam, The Netherlands 2003–2006

	Dutch	Creole-Surinamese	Antillean	Cape- Verdean
	N = 4691	N = 130	N = 357	N = 433
	%, mean (sd)[a]	%, mean (sd)[a]	%, mean (sd)[a]	%, mean (sd)[a]
Socio-demographic factors				
Age				
14	56.6%	48.5%	36.4%	37.9%
15	38.4%	36.2%	48.5%	51.3%
16	4.9%	15.4%	15.1%	10.9%
Level of Education				
Vocational Track	43.0%	76.0%	89.5%	82.0%
Middle Track	25.7%	14.7%	6.8%	9.2%
University Track	31.3%	9.3%	3.7%	8.8%
SES score (−2.7–3.8)[b]	0.16 (1.13)	1.59 (1.35)	1.71 (1.12)	2.13 (1.09)
Does not live with 2 biological parents (yes)	22.9%	71.1%	75.2%	55.0%
Trauma				
Sexual abuse (yes)	8.0%	9.2%	11.0%	8.9%
Problems				
Emotional problems (0–100)	73.9 (15.1)	70.7 (18.3)	72.2 (18.2)	73.9 (17.2)
Aggressive behavior				
Never	75.4%	42.3%	40.8%	46.2%
Occasional	21.5%	42.3%	46.2%	42.5%
Frequent	3.1%	15.4%	13.0%	11.4%

Note: *SES* Socio-Economic Status
[a]Based on descriptive statistics
[b]Highest socioeconomic status = −2.7

Table 3 The bivariate association between socio-demographic characteristics, household structure, sexual abuse, wellbeing and externalizing problems to suicide attempts among female students in four ethnic groups ($N = 5611$), aged 14–16 in Rotterdam, The Netherlands 2003–2006

	Dutch ($N = 4691$)			Creole-Surinamese ($N = 130$)			Antillean ($N = 357$)			Cape Verdean ($N = 433$)		
	No SA ($N = 4264$)	SA ($N = 427$)	P	No SA ($N = 110$)	SA ($N = 20$)	P	No SA ($N = 307$)	SA ($N = 50$)	P	No SA ($N = 397$)	SA ($N = 36$)	P
Level of Educational, %												
Low	40.6	67.1	<.001	75.2	80.0	.77	89.8	87.8	.61	81.6	86.1	.75
Middle	26.3	19.7		14.7	15.0		6.9	6.1		9.3	8.3	
High	33.1	13.1		10.1	5.0		3.3	6.1		9.1	5.6	
SES score, mean (SD)	.15 (1.12)	.32 (1.23)	.003	1.54 (1.40)	1.84 (1.06)	.37	1.68 (1.13)	1.97 (0.98)	.12	2.12 (1.11)	2.22 (0.81)	.62
Not living with 2 biological parents, %	21.5	36.5	<.001	68.5	85.5	.14	75.7	72.0	.57	53.9	66.7	.14
Sexual abuse, %	6.2	26.5	<.001	5.5	30.0	<.001	7.9	30.0	<.001	6.9	30.6	<.001
Emotional problems, mean (SD)	75.3 (14.1)	60.0 (18.0)	<.001	74.3 (14.8)	51.3 (23.1)	<.001	74.9 (16.5)	55.8 (19.4)	<.001	75.4 (16.2)	58.3 (20.3)	<.001
Aggressive behavior, %												
Never	78.0	48.6	<.001	43.6	35.0	.72	42.8	28.6	<.001	47.5	31.4	.19
Occasional	19.6	40.6		41.8	45.0		47.4	38.8		41.4	54.3	
Frequent	2.3	10.8		14.5	20.0		9.8	32.7		11.1	14.3	

Note: *SA* Attempted Suicide, *SES* Socio-Economic Status

ethnic groups. In the majority Dutch group all risk indicators except socio-economic status, demonstrated a significant risk to attempting suicide. Socio-economic status was not a risk indicator for suicidality in minorities. Sexual abuse was a significant risk indicator among Antillean Dutch and Cape Verdean Dutch girls. Fewer emotional problems were significantly related to less suicidal behavior in all three minority groups. Frequent aggression increased the odds for attempting suicide in Antillean Dutch girls.

Table 4 Multivariate analyses of risk indicators of suicidal behavior in four different ethnic groups of female students, aged 14–16 in Rotterdam, The Netherlands 2003–2006. (Four separate models)

	Dutch ($N = 4691$)	Creole-Surinamese ($N = 130$)	Antillean ($N = 357$)	Cape Verdean ($N = 433$)
	OR (95% CI)	OR (95% CI)	OR (95% CI)	OR (95% CI)
Level of education				
Vocational track	REF	REF	REF	REF
Middle track	0.56 (0.42–0.74)**	0.38 (0.04–3.75)	0.16 (0.02–1.52)	0.68 (0.17–2.67)
University track	0.35 (0.25–0.49)**	0.10 (0.00–2.73)	2.18 (0.45–10.48)	0.60 (0.13–2.79)
SES	0.99 (0.90–1.09)	1.39 (0.85–2.29)	1.38 (0.95–2.10)	1.24 (0.83–1.84)
Not living with 2 biological parents	1.44 (1.13–1.84)**	0.92 (0.19–4.37)	0.63 (0.26–1.52)	1.21 (0.54–2.70)
Sexual abuse	2.52 (1.87–3.40)**	4.00 (0.63–25.65)	4.21 (1.56–11.35)**	4.39 (1.79–10.78)**
Emotional problems	0.86 (0.85–0.88)**	0.80 (0.71–0.91)**	0.86 (0.81–0.91)**	0.88 (0.83–0.93)**
Aggressive behavior				
Never	REF	REF	REF	REF
Sometimes	2.09 (1.63–2.68)**	0.63 (0.16–2.47)	1.06 (0.43–2.60)	2.07 (0.88–4.84)
Frequent	4.40 (2.81–6.88)**	0.58 (0.08–4.11)	4.88 (1.71–13.94)**	1.12 (0.29–4.27)
R square of the model (Nagelkerke)	0.26	0.41	0.34	0.22

Note: *SES* Socio-Economic Status
**Significant at level ≤ 0.01

Testing a model of risk indicators of suicidal behavior across majority Dutch, Caribbean and Cape Verdean ethnicity

Table 5 demonstrates differences in suicidality associated with a Caribbean or Cape Verdean ethnicity compared to Dutch ethnicity, when controlling through separate steps for; socioeconomic variables, household structure, sexual abuse, emotional problems and aggression. Creole-Surinamese and Antillean ethnicity showed a significant positive association with suicidal behavior (model 1). However, when controlling for socio-demographics, sexual abuse, emotional problems and externalizing behavior this significant positive association disappears (model 6). Moreover, in model 6 Antillean ethnicity and Cape Verdean ethnicity showed a negative association with suicidal behavior. The change from a risk factor to a protective factor was caused by

socio-demographic factors (model 2) and aggression (model 5). Furthermore, when comparing only those girls from all four ethnic groups who were enrolled in vocational educational tracks, levels of attempted suicide were not significantly elevated anymore in the ethnic minority groups compared to the Dutch 'native' group (Dutch, 14.2%, Creole-Surinamese 16.3%, Antillean 13.6%, Cape Verdean 8.7%) (not presented in table).

Discussion

To our knowledge, this study is the first to investigate suicide attempts of girls of Caribbean and Cape Verdean descent in mainland Europe (i.e. the Netherlands). The increased rates of attempted suicide of Antillean Dutch girls underpin results of a Dutch report by the

Table 5 The association between ethnicity and suicidal behavior controlling for socio-demographics, abuse, internalizing problems and externalizing behavior in female students, aged 14–16 in Rotterdam, The Netherlands 2003–2006

	Suicidal behavior (Model 1)[a] OR (95% CI) P	Suicidal behavior (Model 2)[a] OR (95% CI) P	Suicidal behavior (Model 3)[a] OR (95% CI) P	Suicidal behavior (Model 4)[a] OR (95% CI) P	Suicidal behavior (Model 5)[a] OR (95% CI) P	Suicidal behavior (Model 6)[a] OR (95% CI) P
Ethnicity						
Dutch	REF	REF	REF	REF	REF	REF
Creole-Surinamese Dutch	1.82 (1.12–2.95) .02	1.11 (0.67–1.86) .68	1.83 (1.11–3.03) 02	1.51 (0.89–2.58) .13	1.12 (0.68–1.87) .65	0.80 (0.45–1.44) .47
Antillean Dutch	1.63 (1.19–2.23) .002	0.73 (0.50–1.06) .10	1.57 (1.14–2.18) .007	1.39 (0.98–1.98) .06	1.00 (0.72–1.39) .99	0.59 (0.39–0.89) .01
Cape Verdean Dutch	0.91 (0.64–1.29) .58	0.53 (0.36–0.80) .002	0.90 (0.62–1.29) .56	0.82 (0.56–1.20) .82	0.57 (0.40–0.83) .003	0.41 (0.27–0.64) < .001
Socio-demographic factors						
Level of education						
Vocational track		REF				REF
Middle track		0.52 (0.40–0.66) < .001				0.55 (0.42–0.72) < .001
University track		0.30 (0.22–0.40) < .001				0.38 (0.27–0.51) < .001
Socioeconomic status		1.03 (0.95–1.12) .49				1.04 (0.95–1.14) .37
Not living with 2 biological parents		1.75 (1.43–2.15) < .001				1.37 (1.09–1.71) .006
Trauma						
Sexual abuse			5.54 (4.43–6.92) < .001			2.72 (2.09–3.54) < .001
Internalizing Problems						
Emotional problems				0.85 (0.84–0.87) < .001		0.86 (0.85–0.88) < .001
Externalizing behavior						
Aggressive behavior						
Never					REF	REF
Occasional					2.95 (2.42–3.60) < .001	1.94 (1.55–2.43) < .001
Frequent					6.19 (4.51–8.47) < .001	3.72 (2.56–5.39) < .001

[a]Model 1 only ethnicity; Model 2 ethnicity and socio-demographics; Model 3 ethnicity and trauma; Model 4 ethnicity and internalizing problems; Model 5 ethnicity and externalizing problems; Model 6 all independent variables

Amsterdam Municipal Public Health Services showing a higher 12- months incidence of suicidal ideation (27.8 versus 17.7%) and attempts (5.3 versus 1.8%) among Antillean-Dutch girls in Amsterdam (The Netherlands) compared to 'native' girls [17]. This suggests that the vulnerability of Antillean-Dutch girls is not limited to living in Rotterdam. Our results are also in line with a study that showed increased rates of attempted suicide of 'Black' young females in the UK [5], and may thus point at a vulnerability to suicidality among young female Caribbean populations across Western Europe. Rates of attempted suicide of Cape-Verdean Dutch girls were much lower than Caribbean as well as 'native' Dutch, and self-reported rates of Cape-Verdean immigrant girls residing elsewhere in Europe were unavailable (to the best of our knowledge).

We were unable to retrieve self-reported rates of attempted suicide of Cape Verdean girls living on Cape Verde, and of Antillean and Creole-Surinamese girls living in the Dutch Caribbean. However, self-reported life time rates of suicide attempts (13%) of girls 13 to 18 years old living in other countries in the Caribbean region (e.g. Bahamas and Jamaica) are in quite similar to those of Caribbean immigrant girls in our study (14/ 15.4%, see [18]. This may suggest that the role of migration to suicidality is modest, yet this would need to be further examined.

Next, important risk indicators such as emotional problems and sexual abuse were associated with an elevated level of attempted suicide in both 'native' and Caribbean groups. (although among Creole-Surinamese Dutch this was only visible in the bivariate test). Furthermore, the propensity for aggression increased the risk for attempting suicide of Antillean- and 'native' females. Next, girls living in Caribbean- or Cape-Verdean Dutch families not composed of a biological father and mother (highly common for these ethnic groups) were not at heightened risk for suicidal behaviour, while 'native' girls in households without two biological parents were more at risk for suicidality. Possibly, the long standing tradition of matrifocalism [9] in Caribbean and African cultures can explain this result.

Once the demographics, sexual abuse, psychological wellbeing and aggression were controlled for, Antillean Ducth had a lower instead of higher risk of suicidal behavior, and the heightened risk in the Creole-Surinamese Dutch group to attempt suicide was no longer observed. This underpins the relevance of socio-economic class to the epidemiology of suicidal behavior, as pointed out by suicide researchers of the WHO multicenter study in Europe [19]. Suggestions for future research include a larger sample size for Creole Surinamese girls, as well as a longitudinal rather than cross sectional design.

Conclusion

The present study indicates that the apparently increased propensity to suicidal behavior of Caribbean Dutch girls compared to Dutch 'native' girls can be explained by their differences in socio-economic status, education, household structure and increased level of aggressive behavior. Hence, our study underpins the idea that immigrants and their children share certain risk factors with mainstream populations in Europe to the manifestation of suicidal behavior (e.g. sexual abuse and emotional problems as well as they seem to have unique features regarding suicide risk (e.g. no detrimental impact of growing up without biological father in Caribbean immigrant households). Considering the very large proportion of our Caribbean sample that lives in deprived socio-economic circumstances compared to majority Dutch girls, and given that the disproportionate rates of attempted suicide ceased to exist when controlling for these socio-economic aspects, our study sheds a light on the high mental health burden on girls who grow up in poverty and who lack access to higher education. Therefore, our study underpins the need for suicide prevention programs that would target socio-economic and educational disparities in both Caribbean and 'native' groups.

Abbreviation
YMR: Youth Health Monitor, conducted in Rotterdam, The Netherlands

Acknowledgements
Authors want to acknowledge all secondary schools in Rotterdam for their involvement in the YMR study.

Funding
Authors did not receive funding for the present study. The YMR is funded by municipality of Rotterdam, The Netherlands.

Authors' contributions
DDVB designed the study, commented on the analyses, and did the writing and interpretation. ME oversaw the project design, conducted analyses, and commented on drafts and the interpretation of data. PMVdeLJ designed the questionnaire, coordinated participant recruitment, and commented on drafts and the interpretation of data. All authors read and approved the final manuscript.

Ethics approval and consent to participate
Data were obtained from the Youth Health Monitor Rotterdam (YMR), a longitudinal youth health surveillance system carried out by the the the Rotterdam-Rijnmond Public Health Services (GGD, Gemeentelijke gezondheidsdienst) in Rotterdam, The Netherlands. Activities of the preventive youth health care system of Rotterdam, of which the RYM is part, have been approved by the Dutch government (Ministery of Health). The data of the RYM are protected by the Municipal Health Service of Rotterdam, which follows the Code of Conduct Health Research of the Netherlands. Adolescents received verbal information about the questionnaires each time they were applied, and their parents received written information regarding every assessment. Adolescents and their parents were free to decline participation. The questionnaires were completed on a voluntary basis, and confidentiality of responses was guaranteed. Observational research (ie, not experimental) with confidential data gathered in routine health care does not fall

Attempted suicide of ethnic minority girls with a Caribbean and Cape Verdean background: rates...

193

within the ambit of Dutch Medical Research Involving Human Subjects Act (WMO), and therefore does not require the approval of an ethics review board; separate informed consent was therefore not required. [20] Data were de-identified before the analyses.

Consent for publication

Not applicable

Competing interests

The authors declare that they have no competing interests.

Author details

[1]Research Unit for Youth Studies, Department of Education, University of Groningen, Groningen, The Netherlands. [2]Department of Psychiatry and the Amsterdam Public Health research institute, VU University Medical Center Amsterdam / GGZ inGeest, Amsterdam, The Netherlands. [3]Department of Research and Business Intelligence, Municipality of Rotterdam, PO BOX 1130, 3000 BC Rotterdam, The Netherlands.

References

1. Boeninger DK, Masyn KE, Feldman BJ, Conger RD. Sex differences in developmental trends of suicide ideation, plans, and attempts among European American adolescents. Suicide Life Threat Behav. 2010;40(5):451–64. doi: https://doi.org/10.1521/suli.2010.40.5.451.

2. Heredia-Montesinos A, Heinz A, Schouler-Ocak M, Aichberger MC. Precipitating and risk factors for suicidal behaviour among immigrant and ethnic minority women in Europe: a systematic review. Suicidol Online. 2013;4:60–80.

3. Eaton DK, Kann L, Kinchen S, Shanklin S, Flint KH, Hawkins J, et al. Youth risk behavior surveillance - United States, 2011. MMWR Surveill Summ (Washington, DC: 2002). 2012;61(4):1–162.

4. Schrijvers DL, Bollen J, Sabbe BGC. The gender paradox in suicidal behavior and its impact on the suicidal process. J Affect Disord. 2012;138(1–2):19–26. doi: https://doi.org/10.1016/j.jad.2011.03.050.

5. Cooper J, Murphy E, Webb R, Hawton K, Bergen H, Waters K, Kapur N. Ethnic differences in self-harm, rates, characteristics and service provision: three-city cohort study. Br J Psychiatry. 2010;197:212–8. doi: https://doi.org/10.1192/bjp.bp.109.072637.

6. Garssen MJ, Hoogenboezem J, Kerkhof AJ. Zelfdoding onder Nederlandse Surinamers naar etniciteit. Tijdschr Psychiatr. 2007;49(6):373–81.

7. Vermeulen H, Penninx R. Immigrant integration: the Dutch case. Amsterdam: Het Spinhuis; 2000.

8. Van Bergen DD, Eikelenboom M, Smit JH, van de Looij-Jansen PM, Saharso S. Suicidal behavior and ethnicity of young females in Rotterdam, The Netherlands: rates and risk factors. Ethn Health. 2010;15(5):515–30. doi: https://doi.org/10.1080/13557858.2010.494719.

9. Roopnarine JL. Fathers in Caribbean cultural communities. Fathers Cult. Context; 2013. p. 203–27.

10. Weitoft GR, Hjern A, Haglund B, Rosén M. Mortality, severe morbidity, and injury in children living with single parents in Sweden: a population-based study. Lancet. 2003;361(9354):289–95.

11. Kerr DC, Reinke WM, Eddy JM. Trajectories of depressive symptoms and externalizing behaviors across adolescence: associations with histories of suicide attempt and ideation in early adulthood. Suicide Life Threat Behav. 2013;43(1):50–66. doi: https://doi.org/10.1111/j.1943-278X.2012.00127.x.

12. Green, H., McGinnity, A., Meltzer, H., Ford T. & Goodman, R. (2004). Mental health of children and young people in great Britain. The Office for National Statistics on behalf of the Department of Health and the Scottish Executive.

13. Van de Broek A, Kleijnen E, Keuzenkamp S. Verschillen in gebruik van hulp bij opvoeding, onderwijs en gezondheid tussen autochtonen en migranten. Den Haag: The Netherlands Institute for Social Research; 2010. [Ethnic differences in health care use]

14. Maynard MJ., Harding S., Minnis H. (2007). Psychological well-being in black Caribbean, Black African, and White adolescents in the UK. Medical Research Council.

15. Landgraf J, Abetz L. Functional status and well-being of children representing three cultural groups: initial self-reports using the cHQ-CF87. Psychol Health. 1997;12(6):839–54.

16. Junger-Tas J, Van der Laan PH, Kruisink M. Ontwikkeling van de jeugdcriminaliteit en de justitiële jeugdbescherming: periode 1980–1990. Arnhem: Gouda Quint; 1992. [Trend in Youth Crime in the Netherlands, 1980-1990]

17. Van Vuuren, L., Stegeman, H., Van Dieren, L., Verhagen, C., Van der Wal M. (2012). Report on the health and wellbeing of youth in Amsterdam. Amsterdam Municipal Public Health Services [Report in Dutch].

18. Halcon L, Blum RW, Beuhring T, Pate E, Campbell-Forrester S, Venema A. Adolescent health in the Caribbean: a regional portrait. Cajanus. 2005;38(4):214–29.

19. Schmidtke A, Bille-Brahe U, De Leo D, Kerkhof A, Lohr C, Weinacker B, et al. Sociodemographic characteristics of suicide attempters in Europe: combined results of the monitoring part of the WHO/EURO multicentre study on suicidal behaviour. In: Unni Bille-Brahe AS, De Leo D, Kerkhof A, editors. Suicide behaviour in Europe: results from the WHO/EURO multicentre study on suicidal behaviour. Gottingen: Hogrefe & Huber Publishers; 2004. p. 29–43.

20. Nogueira Avelar e Silva R, Wijtzes A, van de Bongardt D, van de Looij-Jansen P, Bannink R, Raat H. Early Sexual Intercourse: Prospective Associations with Adolescents Physical Activity and Screen Time. PLoS ONE. 2016;11(8):e0158648. doi:https://doi.org/10.1371/journal.p one.0158648.

Permissions

All chapters in this book were first published in PSYCHIATRY, by BioMed Central; hereby published with permission under the Creative Commons Attribution License or equivalent. Every chapter published in this book has been scrutinized by our experts. Their significance has been extensively debated. The topics covered herein carry significant findings which will fuel the growth of the discipline. They may even be implemented as practical applications or may be referred to as a beginning point for another development.

The contributors of this book come from diverse backgrounds, making this book a truly international effort. This book will bring forth new frontiers with its revolutionizing research information and detailed analysis of the nascent developments around the world.

We would like to thank all the contributing authors for lending their expertise to make the book truly unique. They have played a crucial role in the development of this book. Without their invaluable contributions this book wouldn't have been possible. They have made vital efforts to compile up to date information on the varied aspects of this subject to make this book a valuable addition to the collection of many professionals and students.

This book was conceptualized with the vision of imparting up-to-date information and advanced data in this field. To ensure the same, a matchless editorial board was set up. Every individual on the board went through rigorous rounds of assessment to prove their worth. After which they invested a large part of their time researching and compiling the most relevant data for our readers.

The editorial board has been involved in producing this book since its inception. They have spent rigorous hours researching and exploring the diverse topics which have resulted in the successful publishing of this book. They have passed on their knowledge of decades through this book. To expedite this challenging task, the publisher supported the team at every step. A small team of assistant editors was also appointed to further simplify the editing procedure and attain best results for the readers.

Apart from the editorial board, the designing team has also invested a significant amount of their time in understanding the subject and creating the most relevant covers. They scrutinized every image to scout for the most suitable representation of the subject and create an appropriate cover for the book.

The publishing team has been an ardent support to the editorial, designing and production team. Their endless efforts to recruit the best for this project, has resulted in the accomplishment of this book. They are a veteran in the field of academics and their pool of knowledge is as vast as their experience in printing. Their expertise and guidance has proved useful at every step. Their uncompromising quality standards have made this book an exceptional effort. Their encouragement from time to time has been an inspiration for everyone.

The publisher and the editorial board hope that this book will prove to be a valuable piece of knowledge for researchers, students, practitioners and scholars across the globe.

List of Contributors

Maria Giuseppina Petruzzelli, Mariella Margari, Antonia Peschechera, Concetta de Giambattista, Andrea De Giacomo and Emilia Matera
Child Neuropsychiatry Unit, Department of Basic Medical Sciences, Neuroscience and Sense Organs, University of Bari "Aldo Moro", Azienda Ospedaliero-Universitaria Policlinico di Bari, Piazza Giulio Cesare 11, 70124 Bari, Italy

Francesco Margari
Psychiatry Unit, Department of Basic Medical Sciences, Neuroscience and Sense Organ, University of Bari "Aldo Moro", Azienda Ospedaliero-Universitaria Policlinico di Bari, Piazza Giulio Cesare 11, 70124 Bari, Italy

Amanda J. Edmondson
Centre for Applied Research in Health, School of Human and Health Sciences, University of Huddersfield, Queensgate, Huddersfield HD1 3DH, UK

Cathy Brennan and Allan O. House
Institute of Health Sciences, School of Medicine, University of Leeds, 101 Clarendon Rd, Leeds LS2 9LJ, UK

Sarah Steeg, Leah Quinlivan, Rebecca Nowland, Caroline Clements and Jayne Cooper
Centre for Mental Health and Safety, Manchester Academic Health Science Centre, University of Manchester, Manchester, England

Nav Kapur
Centre for Mental Health and Safety, Manchester Academic Health Science Centre, University of Manchester, Manchester, England
Greater Manchester Mental Health NHS Foundation Trust, Manchester, England

Deborah Casey and Keith Hawton
Centre for Suicide Research, University of Oxford Department of Psychiatry, Warneford Hospital, Oxford, England

Jennifer Ness
Centre for Self-harm and Suicide Prevention Research, Derbyshire Healthcare NHS Foundation Trust, Derby, England

Robert Carroll, Duleeka Knipe and David Gunnell
Population Health Sciences, Bristol Medical School, University of Bristol, Bristol, England

Linda Davies
Institute of Population Health, University of Manchester, Manchester, England

Rory C. O'Connor
Suicidal Behaviour Research Laboratory, Institute of Health and Wellbeing, University of Glasgow, Glasgow, Scotland

Vivian Isaac
Flinders Rural Health South Australia, Flinders University, Renmark, Australia

Chia-Yi Wu
School of Nursing, National Taiwan University College of Medicine, Taipei, Taiwan
Taiwan Suicide Prevention Center, Taipei, Taiwan

Ming-Been Lee
Taiwan Suicide Prevention Center, Taipei, Taiwan
Departments of Psychiatry, National Taiwan University College of Medicine & National Taiwan University Hospital, Taipei, Taiwan
Department of Psychiatry, Shin Kong Wu Ho-Su Memorial Hospital, Taipei, Taiwan

Craig S. McLachlan
Rural Clinical School, University of New South Wales, Sydney, Australia

Anthony F. Jorm, Angela Nicholas, Jane Pirkis, Alyssia Rossetto and Nicola J. Reavley
Centre for Mental Health, Melbourne School of Population and Global Health, The University of Melbourne, 207 Bouverie St, Carlton, VIC 3010, Australia

Ruth Wilson
Community Eating Disorder Service, East London NHS Foundation Trust, London, UK

Tim Weaver
Department of Mental Health, Social Work and Integrative Medicine, Middlesex University, London, UK

Daniel Michelson
Department of Population Health, Centre for Global Mental Health, London School of Hygiene & Tropical Medicine, London, UK

Crispin Day
CAMHS Research Unit, IOPPN, King's College London, Michael Rutter Centre, De Crespigny Park, Camberwell, London SE5 8AZ, UK

Masahiro Takeshima, Takashi Kanbayashi and Tetsuo Shimizu
Department of Neuropsychiatry, Akita University Graduate School of Medicine, 1-1-1,Hondo, Akita City, Akita 010-8543, Japan

Hiroyasu Ishikawa
Department of Neuropsychiatry, Akita University Graduate School of Medicine, 1-1-1,Hondo, Akita City, Akita 010-8543, Japan
Department of Neuropsychiatry, Nakadori Rehabilitation Hospital, 6-1-58, Nakadori, Akita City, Akita 010-0001, Japan

Akihiro Kitadate
Division of Hematology/Oncology, Department of Medicine, Kameda General Hospital, 929 Higashi-chou, Kamogawa City, Chiba 296-8602, Japan

Ryo Sasaki
Department of Neuropsychiatry, Akita City Hospital, 4-30, Matsuoka-machi, Kawamoto, Akita City, Akita 010-0933, Japan

Takahiro Kobayashi
Department of Hematology, Nephrology and Rheumatology, Akita University Graduate School of Medicine, 1-1-1, Hondo, Akita City, Akita 010-8543, Japan

Hiroshi Nanjyo
Division of Clinical Pathology, Akita University Graduate School of Medicine, 1-1-1, Hondo, Akita City, Akita 010-8543, Japan

Rebecca C. Brown, Stefanie Heines, Andreas Witt, Joerg M. Fegert, Daniela Harsch and Paul L. Plener
Department of Child and Adolescent Psychiatry/Psychotherapy, University of Ulm, Steinhoevelstr, 5, 89075 Ulm, Germany

Department of Child and Adolescent Psychiatry, Medical University of Vienna, Waehringerguertel 18-20, 1090 Vienna, Austria

Elmar Braehler
Department of Psychosomatic Medicine and Psychotherapy, University Medical Center of the Johannes Gutenberg University of Mainz, Langenbeckstraße 1, 55131 Mainz, Germany
Department of Medical Psychology and Medical Sociology, University of Leipzig, Leipzig, Germany

Angelique Lowrie
School of Psychology, University of Birmingham, Edgbaston, Birmingham, UK

Kareen Heinze
School of Psychology, University of Birmingham, Edgbaston, Birmingham, UK
Institute for Mental Health, University of Birmingham, Edgbaston, Birmingham, UK

Stephen J. Wood
School of Psychology, University of Birmingham, Edgbaston, Birmingham, UK
Institute for Mental Health, University of Birmingham, Edgbaston, Birmingham, UK
Orygen, the National Centre of Excellence in Youth Mental Health, Melbourne, Australia
Centre for Youth Mental Health, University of Melbourne, Melbourne, Australia

Rachel Upthegrove
School of Psychology, University of Birmingham, Edgbaston, Birmingham, UK
Institute for Mental Health, University of Birmingham, Edgbaston, Birmingham, UK
Institute of Clinical Sciences, University of Birmingham, Edgbaston, Birmingham, UK

Renate L. E. P. Reniers
Institute for Mental Health, University of Birmingham, Edgbaston, Birmingham, UK
Institute of Clinical Sciences, University of Birmingham, Edgbaston, Birmingham, UK

Ashleigh Lin
Telethon Kids Institute, Perth, Australia

Bo-Jian Wu
Department of Psychiatry, Ministry of Health and Welfare, Yuli Hospital, 448 Chung-Hua Road, Yuli Township, Hualien County 981, Taiwan, Republic of China

Barnaby Nelson
Orygen, the National Centre of Excellence in Youth Mental Health, Melbourne, Australia
Centre for Youth Mental Health, University of Melbourne, Melbourne, Australia

Latoya Clarke
Warwick Medical School, University of Warwick, Coventry, UK

Ayesha Roche
Department of Psychology, University of Sheffield, Sheffield, UK

Ping Qin, Anne Seljenes Bøe and Lars Mehlum
National Centre for Suicide Research and Prevention, Institute of Clinical medicine, University of Oslo, Sognsvannsveien 21, N-0372 Oslo, Norway

Barbara Stanley
National Centre for Suicide Research and Prevention, Institute of Clinical medicine, University of Oslo, Sognsvannsveien 21, N-0372 Oslo, Norway
Department of Psychiatry, Columbia University College of Physicians and Surgeons, New York, NY, USA

Shihua Sun
Department of Epidemiology, Shandong University School of Public Health and Shandong University Center for Suicide Prevention Research, Jinan, China

Gregory Armstrong
Nossal Institute for Global Health, Melbourne School of Population and Global Health, University of Melbourne, 333 Exhibition St, Melbourne, VIC 3000, Australia

Natalie Ironfield, Nicola Reavley and Anthony F. Jorm
Centre for Mental Health, Melbourne School of Population and Global Health, The University of Melbourne, 207 Bouverie St, Carlton, VIC 3010, Australia

Claire M. Kelly, Katrina Dart and Kathy Bond
Mental Health First Aid Australia, Level 6, 369 Royal Parade, Parkville, VIC 3053, Australia

Kerry Arabena
Indigenous Health Equity Unit, Melbourne School of Population and Global Health, University of Melbourne, 207 Bouverie St, Carlton, VIC 3010, Australia

M. S. Kim
Jeju Institute of Public Health and Health Policy, Jeju, Republic of Korea

J. Kim
Department of Nursing, Dongeui University, Busan, Republic of Korea

J. E. Lee
Department of Food and Nutrition, Seoul National University, Seoul, Republic of Korea

Birthe Loa Knizek and Heidi Hjelmeland
Department of Mental Health, Norwegian University of Science and Technology, NO-7491 Trondheim, Norway

Songli Mei, Gang Xu, Tingting Gao and Hui Ren
Department of Social Medicine and Health Management, School of Public Health, Jilin University, NO. 1163 Xinmin Street, Changchun, Jilin Province, China

Jingyang Li
Department of Mental Health, The First Hospital of Jilin University, NO. 71 Xinmin Street, Changchun, Jilin Province, China

María-Laura Parra-Fernández, María-Dolores Onieva-Zafra and Elia Fernández-Martinez
Faculty of Nursing, University of Castilla-La-Mancha, Ciudad Real, Spain

Teresa Rodríguez-Cano
Head of Mental Health, Castilla la Mancha Health Services, Ciudad Real, Spain

María José Perez-Haro
Biostatech Advice, Training and Innovation in Biostatistics, S.L Santiago de Compostela, A Coruña, Spain

Víctor Casero-Alonso
School of Industrial Engineers, University of Castilla-La Mancha, Ciudad Real, Spain

Blanca Notario-Pacheco
Faculty of Nursing, University of Castilla-La-Mancha, Cuenca, Spain

H. Jung
College of Nursing, Konyang University, Daejeon, Republic of Korea

Bertine de Vries
Department of clinical psychology and experimental psychopathology, faculty of behavioral and social sciences, University of Groningen, Grote Kruisstraat 2/1, 9712 TS Groningen, Netherlands

André Aleman
Department of clinical psychology and experimental psychopathology, faculty of behavioral and social sciences, University of Groningen, Grote Kruisstraat 2/1, 9712 TS Groningen, Netherlands
Department of Neuroscience, BCN Neuroimaging Center, University of Groningen, University Medical Center Groningen, Antonius Deusinglaan 2, 9713 AW Groningen, Netherlands

Gerdina H. M. Pijnenborg
Department of clinical psychology and experimental psychopathology, faculty of behavioral and social sciences, University of Groningen, Grote Kruisstraat 2/1, 9712 TS Groningen, Netherlands
Department of Psychotic Disorders, GGZ-Drenthe, Dennenweg 9, 9404 LA Assen, Netherlands

Elisabeth C. D. van der Stouwe
University of Groningen, University Medical Center Groningen, University Center of Psychiatry, Rob Giel Onderzoekcentrum, Hanzeplein 1, 9713 GZ Groningen, Netherlands
Department of Neuroscience, BCN Neuroimaging Center, University of Groningen, University Medical Center Groningen, Antonius Deusinglaan 2, 9713 AW Groningen, Netherlands

Jooske T. van Busschbach
University of Groningen, University Medical Center Groningen, University Center of Psychiatry, Rob Giel Onderzoekcentrum, Hanzeplein 1, 9713 GZ Groningen, Netherlands
Department of Human Movement and Education, Windesheim University of Applied Sciences, Campus 2-6, 8017 CA Zwolle, the Netherlands

Clement O. Waarheid, Stefan H. J. Poel and Johan Arends
Department of Psychotic Disorders, GGZ-Drenthe, Dennenweg 9, 9404 LA Assen, Netherlands

Erwin M. van der Helm
Helmsport, Vechtstraat 72B, 9725 CW Groningen, Netherlands

Su-Jung Liao
Department of Nursing, Ministry of Health and Welfare, Yuli Hospital, 448 Chung-Hua Road, Yuli Township, Hualien County 981, Taiwan, Republic of China
Department of Nursing, National Taipei University of Nursing Health Science, No.365, Mingde Rd., Beitou Dist., Taipei City 112, Taiwan, Republic of China

Jiin-Ru Rong
Department of Nursing, National Taipei University of Nursing Health Science, No.365, Mingde Rd., Beitou Dist., Taipei City 112, Taiwan, Republic of China

Tse-Tsung Liu
Department of Geriatrics, Mennonite Christian Hospital, 44, Minquan Rd., Hualien City, Hualien County 970, Taiwan, Republic of China

Chao-Ping Chou
Department of Psychiatry, Mennonite Christian Hospital, 44, Minquan Rd., Hualien City, Hualien County 970, Taiwan, Republic of China

Rose McCabe, Amy Backhouse and Penny Xanthopoulou
University of Exeter Medical School, Heavitree Road, Exeter EX1 2LU, UK

Ruth Garside
European Centre for Environment and Human Health, Knowledge Spa, Royal Cornwall Hospital, Truro TR1 3HD, UK

Hanna Y. Berhane and Yemane Berhane
Addis Continental Institute of Public Health, Addis Ababa, Ethiopia

Bethannie Jamerson-Dowlen, Lauren E. Friedman, Michelle A. Williams and Bizu Gelaye
Department of Epidemiology, Harvard T.H. Chan School of Public Health, Boston, MA, USA

O. Kim
Korean Nurses Association, Seoul, Republic of Korea
College of Nursing, Ewha Womans University, Seoul, Republic of Korea

Shuang Li, Zimri S. Yaseen, Hae-Joon Kim, Jessica Briggs, Molly Duffy, Anna Frechette-Hagan, Lisa J. Cohen and Igor I. Galynker
Department of Psychiatry, Beth Israel Medical Center NY, 1st Avenue and 15th Street, New York, NY 10003, USA

Diana D. van Bergen
Research Unit for Youth Studies, Department of Education, University of Groningen, Groningen, The Netherlands

Merijn Eikelenboom
Department of Psychiatry and the Amsterdam Public Health research institute, VU University Medical Center Amsterdam/GGZ inGeest, Amsterdam, The Netherlands

Petra P. van de Looij-Jansen
Department of Research and Business Intelligence, Municipality of Rotterdam, 3000 BC Rotterdam, The Netherlands

Index

www.ingramcontent.com/pod-product-compliance
Lightning Source LLC
Chambersburg PA
CBHW082018190326
41458CB00010B/3221